SBAQs for the FRCEM Primary

SBAQs for the FRCEM Primary

Edited by

Pawan Gupta MBBS, MS, FRCS, FRCEM, MSc (Medical Education)

Consultant in Emergency Medicine, Mid-Essex Hospital Services NHS Trust
Training Programme Director (CT3 & DRE-EM), Health Education,
East of England, UK

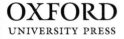

OXFORD
UNIVERSITY PRESS

Great Clarendon Street, Oxford, OX2 6DP,
United Kingdom

Oxford University Press is a department of the University of Oxford.
It furthers the University's objective of excellence in research, scholarship,
and education by publishing worldwide. Oxford is a registered trade mark of
Oxford University Press in the UK and in certain other countries

© Oxford University Press 2018

The moral rights of the author have been asserted

First Edition published in 2018
Impression: 1

Published in the United States of America by Oxford University Press
198 Madison Avenue, New York, NY 10016, United States of America

British Library Cataloguing in Publication Data
Data available

Library of Congress Control Number: 2017962706

ISBN 978-0-19-874863-2

Printed and bound by
CPI Group (UK) Ltd, Croydon, CR0 4YY

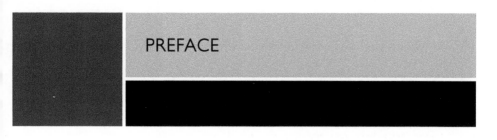

PREFACE

The assessment process in medicine has evolved from descriptive questions and answers to multiple true or false questions, to a more specific application of knowledge by way of single best answer (SBA) styles. The Royal College of Emergency Medicine has changed its specialty examination process at all steps; replacing the old MRCEM and FRCEM to new format of the FRCEM examinations. The FRCEM Primary examination, the Part A of the old MRCEM, constitutes multiple choice question paper of 180 single best answer questions (SBAQs) over three hours replacing the old true/false system following its Basic Sciences 2015 Curriculum. The first new Primary Examination took place in December 2016.

This book is unique as it includes questions very similar to that of the FRCEM Primary examination. The answer to each question is followed by a rationale of the correct choice and an explanation as to why the other options are incorrect/inappropriate. The explanations are extensive with appropriate references so that the reader's thoughts are stimulated and encouraged to read further. This allows the reader to explore and develop their knowledge of the relevant topic. Each question is based on a clinical scenario, most of which are taken from real-life experiences and correlated with the basic background sciences. The questions also cover the practical skills to improve understanding of the basics and their applicability in day-to-day life. It is also outside the scope of ability to include every topic in emergency medicine in this book. Therefore, the scenarios written in this book cover the regular clinical issues alongside the more serious ones with potentially catastrophic consequences.

This book is not only a simple question and answer book, but also provides additional descriptions to help readers prepare for the examination. Hence, the aim of this book is not to facilitate the cramming of questions and answers by the readers just for a successful exam result, but to provide a platform of stimulating, enjoyable, and thought-provoking experiences.

To enrich the learning of candidates, I would also highly recommend reading the book *Oxford Assess and Progress: Emergency Medicine*, which provides over 250 extra clinical questions (approximately) to ensure a solidification of emergency medicine knowledge. These consist of a mixture of SBAs and extended matching questions and answers based on real-life clinical scenarios.

Pawan Gupta

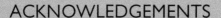

ACKNOWLEDGEMENTS

I would like to thank all of the contributors to this book providing invaluable materials in their own time. I am especially grateful to Dr Trisha Gupta, Dr David Thaxter, and Dr Daniel Walter for providing a significant number of questions within a short span of time, to whom this project owes its success. I am also grateful to Rachel Goldsworthy and Geraldine Jeffers for their support and guidance. I would like to thank the library staff of Broomfield Hospital (Essex) for their help with providing me with relevant literature and books for this project.

My thanks also go to the external medical reviewers whose comments have helped me in improving my original ideas.

Finally, this project would not have been completed without the support of my wife, Dr Ishita Gupta (PhD) and my daughter, Ms Celina Gupta, for providing constant support, encouragement, and patience in making this effort a success.

CONTENTS

Abbreviations   xi

Contributors   xv

Introduction: General advice on preparation for the examination   xvii

1   Anatomy

Questions   1

Answers   35

2   Physiology

Questions   79

Answers   116

3   Microbiology

Questions   165

Answers   174

4   Pharmacology

Questions   191

Answers   206

5   Evidence-based medicine

Questions   229

Answers   233

6 Pathology

Questions   241

Answers   249

7 Mock exam paper

Questions   261

Answers   289

Index   307

ABBREVIATIONS

ABG	arterial blood gas
ACE	angiotensin converting enzyme
ACL	anterior cruciate ligament
ACS	acute coronary syndrome
ACTH	adrenocorticotropic hormone
AD	Alzheimer's disease
ADH	antidiuretic hormone
AF	atrial fibrillation
AICA	anterior inferior cerebellar artery
AIDS	acquired immunodeficiency syndrome
AMI	acute myocardial infarction
AMTS	abbreviated mental test score
ANP	atrial natriuretic peptide
ARAS	ascending reticular activating system
ARR	absolute risk reduction
ASIS	anterior superior iliac spine
AV	atrioventricular
BNP	brain natriuretic peptide
BP	blood pressure
bpm	beats per minute
CCS	central cord syndrome
CI	confidence interval
CKD	chronic kidney disease
CNS	central nervous system
COPD	chronic obstructive pulmonary disease
COX	cyclooxygenase
CPK	creatinine phosphokinase
CPP	cerebral perfusion pressure
CPR	cardiopulmonary resuscitation

CRH	corticotropin-releasing hormone
CRP	C-reactive protein test
CRT	capillary refill time
CSF	cerebrospinal fluid
CT	computed tomography
CVA	cerebrovascular accident
CXR	chest X-ray
DI	diabetes insipidus
DKA	diabetic ketoacedosis
$DLCO_2$	diffusion capacity of the lungs for CO_2
DVT	deep vein thrombosis
EBM	evidence-based medicine
ECF	extracellular fluid
ECG	electrocardiogram
ED	emergency department
EHL	extensor hallucis longus
FAST	focused assessment sonography test
FCU	flexor carpi ulnaris
FDP	flexor digitorum profundus
FDS	flexor digitorum superficialis
FEV_1	forced expiratory volume in 1 second
FVC	forced vital capacity
GABA	gama amino butyric acid
GCS	Glasgow Coma Scale
GFR	glomerular filtration rate
GLUT	glucose transporter
GP	general practitioner
HBV	hepatitis B-virus
HIV	human immunodeficiency virus
HR	heart rate
HSV	human papilloma virus
IC	intercostal
ICP	intracranial pressure
IgE	immunoglobulin E
IgG	immunoglobulin G
IgM	immunoglobulin M

IGF	insulin growth factors
ILGF	insulin-like growth factor
IMA	internal mammary artery
INR	international normalized ratio
IP	interphalangeal joint
ISF	interstitial fluid
IV	intravenous
IVC	inferior vena cava
JVP	jugular venous pressure
LP	lumbar puncture
LV	left ventricle
MCA	middle cerebral artery
MCL	medial collateral ligament
MCV	mean corpuscular volume
MMR	measles, mumps, and rubella
MRSA	methicillin-resistant *Staphylococcus aureus*
MS	multiple sclerosis
MTP	metatarsophalangeal
NNH	number needed to harm
NNT	number needed to treat
NPV	negative predictive value
NSAIDs	non-steroidal anti-inflammatory drugs
PCL	posterior cruciate ligament
PCR	polymerase chain reaction
PD	Parkinson's disease
PE	pulmonary embolism
PEA	pulseless electrical activity
PEG	percutaneous endoscopic gastrostomy
PICA	posterior inferior cerebellar artery
PID	pelvic inflammatory disease
PNS	peripheral nervous system
PO	*Per os*, by mouth
PSA	procedural sedation and analgesia
PSNS	parasympathetic nervous system
PTH	parathyroid hormone
RASS	Richmond Agitation-Sedation Scale

RBC	red blood cell
RCT	randomized controlled trial
RIF	right iliac fossa
RR	respiratory rate
RSV	respiratory syncytial virus
RV	right ventricle
SaO_2	oxygen saturation
SC	subcutaneous
SCA	superior cerebellar artery
SLE	systemic lupus erythematosus
SMA	superior mesenteric artery
SNS	sympathetic nervous system
STEMI	ST-elevation myocardial infarction
T	temperature
T2DM	type 2 diabetes mellitus
TB	tuberculosis
TIA	transient ischaemic attack
TN	trigeminal neuralgia
UGI	upper gastrointestinal bleeding
UTI	urinary tract infection
VF	ventricular fibrillation
VP	venous pressure
V/Q	ventilation/perfusion (scan)
WBC	white blood cell

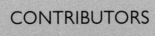

CONTRIBUTORS

In order of contribution:

David Thaxter
Department of Paediatrics
Kingston Hospital, Kingston Upon
Thames, UK

Trisha Gupta
Department of Emergency Medicine
Kingston Hospital NHS Foundation Trust
UK

Pawan Gupta
Consultant, Department of Emergency Medicine
Mid-Essex Hospital Services NHS Trust, UK

Daniel Walter
Bedford Hospital NHS Trust
Bedford Hospital
UK

Additional contributors:

Jennifer Currigan
Emergency Medicine Department Guys and St Thomas' NHS Trust
Evelina Hospital,
UK

Kaung Htet
Cardiology Department
Royal Free London NHS Foundation Trust
University College London
London, UK

INTRODUCTION

GENERAL ADVICE ON PREPARATION FOR THE EXAMINATION

There have been changes to the structure of the membership examination. From August 2016, the Part A of MRCEM examination will be replaced by FRCEM Primary examination. In the previously known format of the Part A examination, each question had four statements and the candidate had to answer all of them by marking the given statement as 'True' or 'False'. In the new system, it will consist of multiple choice question (MCQ) paper of single best answer questions (SBAQ). Each question has five choices and the candidate has to select the single best answer. The paper has 180 questions to be answered in three hours. The FRCEM Primary examination is mapped to the Emergency Medicine 2015 Curriculum, which is available on the RCEM website.

In order to prepare for the FRCEM Primary examination, it is imperative to acknowledge the extensive syllabus; it is easy to underestimate the time required to prepare and revise for it. It covers a vast array of topics, most of which may not have been revisited since your medical school days. Preparation time for this exam is recommended as six to nine months to achieve an appropriate standard.

Revising and spending substantial time on the topic that a candidate enjoys most is unfortunately not the most efficient method of reviewing information, as rewarding as it may seem. It would be advisable to start by revising the material that is disliked the most. This way, if you are running short on revision time, you will be left with topics that you already know a lot about. Hence, your revision should be easier and less stressful. With the busy unsocial shifts of the emergency department, one option may be to revise on the job. Whether you are working on the shop floor in the emergency department (ED) or rotating through acute medicine and anaesthetics, there are many opportunities for you to consolidate your knowledge. For example: talk yourself through local anaesthetic side effects while doing a hematoma block; calculate the A-a gradient on your COPD patients; or discuss hand anatomy when referring your metacarpal fractures, and so on. These are all practical and opportunistic methods of consolidating your knowledge.

Practice questions are a valuable resource during the revision period and are available in abundance. It is important that you are familiar with the format and structure of the questions that you will see in the exam and will therefore be able to discover the best ways to approach these questions. This can only be achieved carefully by reading the College guidelines, following them, and practising numerous questions. Inevitably, as with any exam, certain topics tend to be more popular with examiners than others and this is reflected in the practice questions that you will find. As such, there is a large section of questions dedicated to upper limb anatomy to reflect the proportion of questions in the FRCEM Primary exam. Do not limit yourself only to emergency medicine question banks. MRCS and MRCP exam questions are also excellent revision material. Additionally, the MRCS anatomy syllabus is very similar to that of the FRCEM Primary exam, as is the question typology. The same is also true in the microbiology and pharmacology sections of the MRCP examination.

Make sure that you practice under exam conditions. Time yourself doing mock exams so you are used to pacing yourself when it comes to the real situation. There is nothing worse than not answering the last five questions because you were short on time.

It is also worth noting that there is no negative marking in the FRCEM Primary exam, so make sure you attempt every question. If you guess the answers, you have a 20% chance of scoring a mark, but a blank question will always score 0.

Finally, read the question carefully. Marks are easily lost because you either misunderstood what was being asked or missed that all-important word in the question.

Good luck!

1. **A 75-year-old female has had paraesthesia on the inner surface of the right hand following a sprain to the neck after a fall. Which nerve root is the most likely to be affected?**
   A. C5
   B. C6
   C. C7
   D. C8
   E. T1

2. **A 26-year-old male has been stabbed with a knife in his left axilla during a fight. He is bleeding profusely. His blood pressure (BP) is 86/56 mmHg and heart rate (HR) is 116 bpm. Which statement is correct regarding the axilla?**
   A. Axillary artery becomes the brachial artery at the lower border of teres minor
   B. The axilla is irregular in shape and somewhat tilted rectangle
   C. The axillary artery is divided into three parts by pectoralis major
   D. The axillary artery commences at the medial border of the first rib as a continuation of subclavian artery
   E. The cervicoaxillary opening at the apex of axilla transmits subclavian artery and brachial plexus from the neck into the axilla

3. **A 30-year-old male, who is a martial art athlete, has had subcoracoid dislocation of his left shoulder joint. This has been successfully reduced in the emergency department. His shoulder has been immobilized in a poly sling. Which is the single best appropriate statement regarding the shoulder joint?**
   A. Abduction is initiated by deltoid muscle
   B. Movement around the shoulder girdle in a fused shoulder joint is very limited
   C. Movement of sternoclavicular joint is reciprocal to the scapular movement
   D. Movement of the shoulder joint itself can be divorced from those of the whole shoulder girdle
   E. Rotation of scapula begins when the abduction of the joint is near completion

4. **A 20-year-old male has a self-inflicted knife wound in his left antecubital fossa. He is bleeding profusely. Which is the correct statement regarding antecubital fossa?**

A. It is a diamond-shaped area in front of the elbow joint
B. The brachial artery bifurcates to radial and ulnar arteries at the level of the neck of radius
C. Brachial artery pulsation may not be visible on ultrasound examination
D. The median nerve lies lateral to the brachial artery in the antecubital fossa
E. The lateral margin is formed by bicipital tendon

5. **An 88-year-old lady has had fall on her outstretched right hand. She is unable to move her right thumb. Her wrist is swollen, bruised, and deformed. Injury to which single nerve supply may explain the patient's neurological sign?**

A. The abductor pollicis brevis is innervated by C6–7 component of the median nerve
B. The abductor pollicis brevis is innervated by the C8-T1 component of the median nerve
C. The adductor pollicis is innervated by C6-C7 componesnt of the ulnar nerve
D. The adductor pollicis is innervated by the C8-T1 component of median nerve
E. The opponens pollicis is innervated by the C7–8 component of the ulnar nerve

6. **A 28-year-old man has had a laceration on his palm with a Stanley knife while laying carpet. He is unable to flex his middle finger at the proximal interphalangeal (IP) joint. Which is the single most likely tendon might have been severed?**

A. Flexor digitorum profundus (FDP)
B. Flexor digitorum superficialis (FDS)
C. Lumbricals
D. Palmer interosseous
E. Palmaris longus

7. **A 25-year-old man has had his right index finger tip crushed when his seven-year-old son slammed the car door suddenly. Which is the single most likely statement correct regarding the nail bed?**

A. The germinal matrix is responsible for the growth of the nail bed
B. The nail bed is a thin layer of epithelial tissue
C. The skin edge at the distal nail is called eponychium
D. The skin that covers the proximal end of the nail is called hyponychium
E. The source of blood supply to the nail bed is median artery

8. **A 25-year-old man has had a motorbike accident. His right wrist is swollen and tender. Which is the single most likely statement correct regarding carpal bones?**
   A. Only the scaphoid articulates with distal radius
   B. The carpal bones are organized in proximal, middle, and distal rows
   C. The distal row of carpal bones is more mobile than the proximal row
   D. The lunate provides the main stability to the midcarpus
   E. The proximal row is made up of scaphoid, lunate, and triquetrum

9. **A 78-year-old lady has had a fall on her outstretched left hand. She has a comminuted fracture of the distal radius. Which single statement regarding the wrist joint is correct?**
   A. Carpal joint movements add to the range of extension of the wrist
   B. It is a condyloid joint
   C. It is a hinge joint
   D. Range of the abduction is more than the adduction
   E. The articular disc of the inferior radioulnar joint is attached to the radial styloid process

10. **A 40-year-old lady has had a fall on her outstretched left hand. She has a deformity of the left elbow joint and is unable to move. The X-ray confirms dislocation of the elbow joint. Which single statement regarding the elbow joint is correct?**
    A. The capsule of the joint is reinforced by ligaments on the anterior, posterior, medial, and lateral sides
    B. The lateral collateral ligament is attached distally to the radial neck
    C. The medial and lateral condyles are intracapsular
    D. The superior radioulnar joint is a part of the elbow joint
    E. The upper margin of the annular ligament is free to allow radial head movements

11. **A 28-year-old man has had a fall on his outstretched right hand. The radial side of his wrist is swollen and bruised. He has tenderness in the anatomical snuffbox. Which is the most likely correct statement about the anatomical snuffbox?**
    A. The abductor pollicis brevis forms the radial boundary
    B. The extensor pollicis brevis forms the ulnar boundary
    C. Radial artery can be palpated 5 mm away on the ulnar side of the 'snuffbox'
    D. The cephalic vein passes through the roof of the 'anatomical snuffbox'
    E. The floor is formed by the ulnar surface of the trapezium

12. **A 21-year-old football player was tackled from behind while running in a game of football. He lost his balance and landed on his head, resulting in a burst fracture dislocation of C6/7. He has neurological signs of injury in the upper limb. Which tendon reflex arc involves C6/7?**
    A. Biceps
    B. Brachioradialis
    C. Long finger flexors
    D. Supinator
    E. Triceps

13. **A 66-year-old woman has had paraesthesia on the axilla and medial surface of the upper arm after a radical axillary clearance because of breast cancer. Which nerve is affected?**
    A. Axillary
    B. Intercostobrachial
    C. Median
    D. Radial
    E. Ulnar

14. **A professional gymnast has injured her left shoulder during a contest. She found combing and dressing herself very painful. Rotator cuff muscle injury was suspected. Which muscle is not a part of the rotator cuff?**
    A. Infraspinatous
    B. Subscapularis
    C. Supraspinatous
    D. Teres major
    E. Teres minor

15. **A rugby player has injured his left shoulder during a match. He has subcoracoid dislocation of his shoulder joint and has anaesthesia on the 'regiment batch' area (skin on the lower part of the deltoid muscle). Which muscle is most likely to be affected in such nerve injury?**
    A. Infraspinatous
    B. Supraspinatous
    C. Serratus Anterior
    D. Teres major
    E. Teres minor

16. **A 26-year-old man has fallen off his motorbike and sustained an open fracture of the right clavicle. Brachial plexus injury is also suspected. Which statement is correct about the brachial plexus?**
    A. The cords pass under the clavicle
    B. The middle trunk is formed by the ventral rami of C8
    C. The roots pass in-between the middle and posterior scalene muscles
    D. The trunks are formed in the axilla
    E. There are three divisions—medial, lateral, and posterior

17. **A 79-year-old woman has right hip pain following a fall. She has deformity of the hip joint. The X-ray shows fracture neck of femur. To relieve pain, fascia iliaca block is performed. Which is the single most likely area of skin to be anaesthetized?**
    A. Anterior part of labia majora
    B. Lateral aspect of the lower leg
    C. Lateral aspect of the thigh
    D. Mid-inguinal point
    E. Web space between first and second toe

18. **A 40-year-old female attends the emergency department (ED) with groin pain and weakness with leg adduction on the left side. She recently underwent surgery for endometriosis. On examination, she has weak adduction of the hip joint and sensory loss over medial aspect of the thigh. Which nerve is most likely to be injured?**
    A. Genitofemoral
    B. Iliohypogastric
    C. Ilioinguinal
    D. Obturator
    E. Pudendal

19. **A 42-year-old man has tingling and burning sensation of his outer aspect of his left thigh. He has type 2 diabetes and is on metformin. His condition is diagnosed as meralgia paraesthetica. Which is the most likely nerve root affected?**
    A. L1–L2
    B. L2–L3
    C. L3–L4
    D. L4–L5
    E. L5–S1

20. **A 45-year-old female has had a fall on her buttocks. She is unable to stand on one leg. The Trendelenburg test is positive on the right. Which statement is correct regarding the muscles around the hip joint?**
   A. Gluteus maximus is an abductor
   B. Gluteus maximus is a lateral rotator
   C. Gemelli and quadratus femoris are medial rotators
   D. Gluteus medius and minimus are extensors of the joint
   E. Tensor fasciae latae are lateral rotatorss

21. **A 14-year-old boy has had a fall on his buttocks. He has pain in his right hip and unable to stand on the right leg. The Trendelenburg test is positive. Which muscle group is affected?**
   A. The left gluteus maximus and gluteus medius are affected
   B. The left gluteus medius and minimus are affected
   C. The right gluteus maximus and gluteus medius are affected
   D. The right gluteus medius and minimus are affected
   E. The tensor fasciae latae of the right is affected

22. **An 80-year-old female has had a fall and sustained an intracapsular fracture of the neck of left femur. Which of the following options may cause avascular necrosis of the head?**
   A. Branches from the obturator artery are interrupted to cause avascular necrosis
   B. Disruption of the cervical vessels and retinacular supply of the head are responsible for the necrosis
   C. Disruption to the cruciate anastomosis contributes mainly to the necrosis of the head
   D. The disruption of the branches from the superior gluteal artery is the chief contributor
   E. The ligament of the head of the femur (which carries the main blood supply to the femoral head) is disrupted

23. **A 29-year-old man has had pain and deformity to his left lower thigh/upper knee area after a road traffic collision. The X-ray is shown in Figure 1.1. Which statement is most likely correct?**
   A. Loss of the dorsalis pedis pulse is a likely clinical finding
   B. The distal fragment is angulated because of the pull from the adductor magnus
   C. The distal fragment is pulled up by hamstrings
   D. The great saphenous vein may be severed
   E. Tibial nerve is most likely to be injured

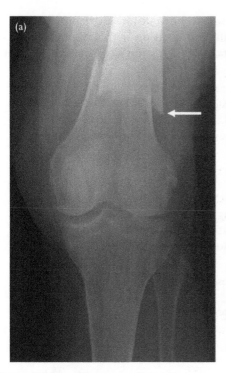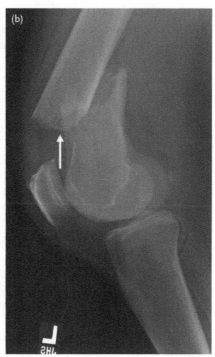

Figure 1.1 Knee X-rays.

Reproduced with permission from Hani Abujudeh (eds), *Emergency Radiology*, Figure 34.4. Copyright © 2016 with permission from Oxford University Press.

24. **A 23-year-old man has had a blunt injury to the back of his right thigh during a rough tackle while playing rugby. He is very tender on the middle third of his thigh posteriorly and finding it difficult to walk. Which is the most appropriate statement regarding muscles of the posterior compartment of the thigh?**

A. All hamstring muscles cause flexion of the hip and extension of the knee joints

B. Semimembranosus originates from the ischial tuberosity and is inserted to the lateral tibial condyle

C. Semimembranosus and semitendinosus muscles lie on the medial aspect

D. Semitendinosus at its insertion contribute to the formation of the ligaments and fascia around the joint

E. The biceps femoris is inserted into the medial collateral ligament of the knee joint

25. **A 15-year-old girl has had sudden pain in her left knee while playing netball. Her knee is fixed in a semiflexed position with deformity in the front of the knee. A lateral patellar dislocation is suspected. Which option is most likely correct?**
    A. Associated with disruption of the medial patellofemoral ligament and medial retinaculum
    B. Hyperextension of the knee with leg in extension may predispose this condition
    C. The displacing force on the patella is markedly increased during extension
    D. The forwards prominence of the lateral condyle of the femur contributes to lateral dislocation
    E. The pull by the quadriceps tendon on the patella is vertical

26. **A 65-year-old man has had pain in the left knee for few weeks, which has increased recently. He is finding difficult to walk. On examination, he has a cystic swelling in the popliteal fossa, which is suspected to be a popliteal cyst. Which is the most appropriate option regarding popliteal fossa?**
    A. The fat in the fossa may bulge in full extension of the knee, giving the appearance of a swelling
    B. The floor of the fossa is formed by the upper posterior surface of the tibia
    C. The fossa has semimembranosus tendon on the medial side and semitendinosus tendon on the upper lateral side
    D. The lower part of the fossa has the boundary of soleus on both sides
    E. The roof of the fossa is formed by the layer of biceps expansion covered with skin

27. **A 55-year-old man presented to ED with a large painful swelling in the popliteal fossa. There had been a puncture wound by a nail two days ago. On examination, there is a pulsatile mass in the popliteal fossa. Traumatic popliteal pesudoaneurysm is suspected. Which structure is not a content of the popliteal fossa?**
    A. The common peroneal nerve
    B. The deep peroneal nerve
    C. The posterior cutaneous nerve of thigh
    D. The superior genicular nerve
    E. The small saphenous vein

28. **A 25-year-old man has had right knee pain following an injury while playing football. He was going to kick a ball when the opposition player fell on his stance knee from the lateral side. He has a suspected medial collateral ligament sprain. Which option is correct?**
    A. In minimal medial ligament sprain, the extended knee may have an opening gap during abduction of the leg
    B. The collateral ligaments are liable to be injured when the knee is in flexion
    C. The lateral ligaments are torn more commonly than the medial
    D. The medial ligament may be torn when a violent abduction strain is applied
    E. The stability of the knee joint is mainly dependent on its ligaments

29. **A 22-year-old man has had an injury to the left knee pain during a rugby game. He has instantaneous swelling of the joint and in ability to weight bear. He has anterior drawer sign positive. The most probable diagnosis is anterior cruciate ligament (ACL) tear. Which option is correct regarding the cruciate ligaments?**

A. Distally, the ACL is attached to the posterior part of the tibial plateau

B. The ACL is attached to the posterolateral aspect of the medial femoral condyle

C. The ACL is shorter and stronger than the posterior cruciate ligament (PCL)

D. The ACL may be torn in violent hyperextension of the knee

E. The cruciate ligaments are intracapsular and intrasynovial

30. **A 58-year-old man with known type 2 diabetes has had a back-slab removed from his left leg last week. His leg was immobilized for a midshaft fibular fracture for about four weeks. He says he is finding it difficult to walk. He has to lift his leg high up while walking to avoid tripping over on his toes. He also has a pins and needles sensation in his foot. Which nerve is most likely affected?**

A. Common peroneal

B. Diabetic neuropathy

C. Femoral

D. Lateral femoral cutaneous

E. Posterior tibial

31. **A 28-year-old man, while running for bus, has sprained his right ankle joint which is now swollen and painful. He has bruising and tenderness on the lateral side of the joint. There is no tenderness on the medial side of the joint. Which ligament is injured in this case?**

A. Anterior talofibular ligament

B. Anterior tibiofibular ligament

C. Calcaneofibular ligament

D. Deltoid ligament complex

E. Transverse tibiofibular ligament

32. **An 80-year-old woman has had bleeding from a vein after she caught her leg on furniture. She has varicose veins for many years. Which statement is correct regarding the veins of the lower limb?**

A. The great saphenous vein drains the medial part of the dorsal foot

B. The great saphenous vein travel through popliteal fossa

C. The short saphenous vein commences behind the lateral malleolus

D. The position of the great saphenous vein is very variable

E. The sural nerve accompanies the great saphenous vein

33. **A 64-year-old man is bought in by ambulance with chest pain. A 12-lead electrocardiogram (ECG) is performed. This shows ST elevation in the 1, aVL, V3–V6 leads, and ST depression in the II, III, aVF. Which is the most likely artery to be occluded?**
    A. Left anterior descending artery
    B. Left circumflex artery
    C. Right coronary artery
    D. Right marginal branch
    E. Sinoatrial nodal artery

34. **Having been involved in a road traffic accident, a 25-year-old male arrives at the hospital complaining of chest pain that is worse on movement and breathing. He was the driver of a vehicle travelling at 60 mph and was wearing a seat belt. On examination he is very tender over his sternum. X-rays demonstrate a fracture of his sternum. Which statement is the most appropriate regarding the sternum?**
    A. It is made up of four parts
    B. The angle of Louis is at the level of T6
    C. The first rib does not articulate with the sternum
    D. The ribs attach to the sternum via its costal cartilage
    E. The xiphisternum has the false ribs attached to it

35. **A gentleman has had a red, itchy, and burning rash is like a band at the level of his right nipple around to his back. It does not cross the midline. He has shingles. Which is the most likely dermatome affected?**
    A. T3
    B. T4
    C. T5
    D. T6
    E. T8

36. **A 75-year-old man has fallen off a stepladder while cleaning his windows. He landed on his left side, hitting a small wall. He has pain on the left side of his chest, which is worse on breathing and movement. The X-rays show a fracture of his left sixth rib. Which statement is the most appropriate regarding ribs?**
    A. All ribs articulate with the thoracic vertebra above it, as well as its own
    B. The eleventh and twelfth ribs are sometimes called floating ribs
    C. The false ribs have no connection to the sternum
    D. There are 13 ribs positioned bilaterally in a man
    E. The ribs ossify anteriorly to posteriorly

37. **A 22-year-old male has had traumatic haemopneumothorax on the right side. An intercostal (IC) drain to be inserted through the fifth intercostal space in the midaxillary line. Which is the single most appropriate statement?**
    A. The blunt dissection for the drain insertion goes through the two layers of intercostal muscles
    B. The cutaneous nerve supply in the fifth IC space is usually through the sixth thoracic nerve
    C. The neurovascular bundle is organized as nerve, artery, and vein, from top to bottom
    D. The neurovascular bundle lies between the internal and innermost intercostal muscle layers
    E. The neurovascular bundle lies just above the sixth rib

38. **A 25-year-old male has had a penetrating injury to the left side of the neck. The chest X-ray shows significantly elevated left hemidiaphragm. A chest X-ray five years ago done for a different clinical reason was normal. He is suspected to have a phrenic nerve injury. Which is the single most appropriate statement?**
    A. The abnormality is an anatomical variant
    B. The phrenic nerve carries fibres from C5, C6, and C7 segments of the spinal cord
    C. The phrenic nerve is a purely motor nerve
    D. The sensation from the central diaphragm is carried by the phrenic nerve
    E. The sensory fibres from the peripheral part of the diaphragm runs through the phrenic nerve

39. **A 45-year-old male, who has a learning difficulty, has had a choking episode with a food bolus. He had a cough and cyanotic episode before settling down. A foreign body inhalation is suspected. Which is the most appropriate statement?**
    A. The foreign body has a tendency to go into left main bronchus
    B. The left main bronchus also gives off upper lobe branch like the right one before entering the lungs
    C. The left main bronchus enters the hilum of the lungs opposite T5
    D. The right main bronchus enters the root of the lungs at the level of T4
    E. The right main bronchus is shorter and wider than the left main bronchus

40. **A 40-year-old male has had cough with expectoration and fever for about four to five days. He is mildly short of breath. A provisional diagnosis of pneumonia is suspected. His chest X-rays are shown in Figure 1.2 Which is the single most likely site of consolidation on the right side?**
    A. The lower lobe
    B. The middle lobe
    C. The middle and lower lobes
    D. The subdiaphragmatic lesion
    E. The upper lobe

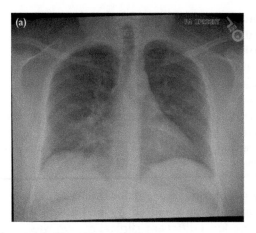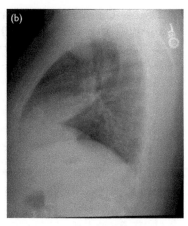

Figure 1.2 Chest X-rays (CXRs).

Reproduced with permission from Hani Abujudeh (eds), *Emergency Radiology*, Figure 11.2. Copyright © 2016 with permission from Oxford University Press.

41. **A 45-year-old woman has had shortness of breath and right-sided pleuritic chest pain for about a week. Her HR is 82 bpm, RR 24 breaths per minute, and BP124/78 mmHg. Pulmonary embolism (PE) is suspected. Which is the single most appropriate statement?**

    A. Hypoxaemia is purely caused by a reduction in blood supply to the lungs
    B. It is always due to blockage of the main pulmonary artery
    C. Left heart failure is the commonest cause of death
    D. Only 15% of patients with PE have signs of deep vein thrombosis (DVT)
    E. Pleuritic chest pain is caused by the sensation carried from the pulmonary arterial occlusion site

42. **A 75-year-old man has had sudden onset of central chest pain, which has radiated through to the back. He appears sweaty, clammy, and pale. His HR is 100 bpm, RR 28 breaths per minute, BP95/85 mmHg. The provisional diagnosis is thoracic aortic dissection. Which is the single most appropriate statement regarding aortic dissection?**

    A. Crack cocaine may be a high-risk condition for aortic dissection
    B. It most commonly presents in the descending thoracic aorta
    C. Pulse deficit is more common in ascending aortic dissection
    D. The mortality is lower in pulse deficit patients
    E. The primary event is an atheromatous plaque in the intimal layer of aorta

43. **A 25-year-old man, who is known to have asthma, has had shortness of breath and wheezes gradually developed over the last couple of days. His HR is 100 bpm, respiratory rate 32 breaths per minute, BP 122/75 mmHg, SaO$_2$ 88% on air. The provisional diagnosis is acute exacerbation of asthma. Which is the single most appropriate statement regarding acute asthma?**

    A. Airflow obstruction is contributed to by smooth muscle spasm, oedema, and mucus production

    B. Cartilaginous support in the intrapulmonary airways contributes to the airflow obstruction in this situation

    C. Mast cells are only evident in the bronchiolar walls after exposure to allergens

    D. The smooth muscles around the alveoli contribute to the air flow obstruction

    E. The alveoli have the same epithelia as that of the trachea

44. **An otherwise healthy 20-year-old man has had sudden onset of pleuritic chest pain and mild shortness of breath. His HR is 80 bpm, RR 24 breaths per minute, BP122/75 mmHg, and SaO$_2$ 96% on air. The chest X-ray (CXR) is shown in Figure 1.3. Which is the single most appropriate statement?**

    A. It is mandatory to insert a chest drain immediately

    B. The mediastinal pleura is a part of the visceral pleura

    C. The sensation to the diaphragmatic pleura is through the intercostal nerves

    D. The visceral pleura could be easily separated from the surface of the lungs

    E. The whole of the mediastinal pleura is innervated by the phrenic nerves

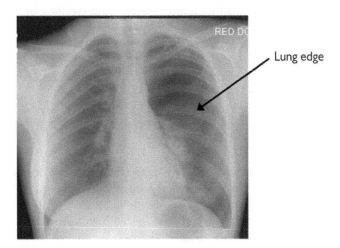

Figure 1.3 CXR.

Reproduced with permission from Jeremy Hull, Julian Forton, and Anne Thomson (eds), *Paediatric Respiratory Medicine* (2 ed.), Figure 38.1. Copyright © 2015 with permission from Oxford University Press.

45. **A 60-year-old man has had sharp pain in the central chest area, which is relieved by sitting forwards and worsened by lying down. His HR is 100 bpm, RR 30 breaths per minute, BP100/75 mmHg, and SaO$_2$ 96% on air. On ultrasound scan, he has pericardial effusion. Which is the single most appropriate statement?**

A. Around 200–250 mL of fluid is necessary to produce cardiomegaly on chest radiograph
B. Most of the blood supply to the pericardium is derived from the aortic root
C. Normally the amount of pericardial fluid is 2–5 mL
D. Pain from the parietal pericardium is transmitted by sympathetic fibres
E. The reduced cardiac output in pericardial effusion is due to compression on the left ventricle

46. **A 68-year-old man who has had endoscopic dilatation of oesophageal stricture attends the ED with severe and sharp pain in the central chest area. He is also short of breath and unable to swallow. His HR is 110 bpm, respiratory rate 30 breaths per minute, BP100/75 mmHg, and SaO$_2$ 90% on air. He is suspected to have an oesophageal rupture. Which is the single most appropriate statement?**

A. Aortic arch crosses oesophagus in the posterior mediastinum
B. The content of oesophagus following it rupture is contained within the posterior mediastinum
C. The left main bronchus crosses the oesophagus about 28 cm from the upper incisor teeth
D. The oesophageal opening lies at the level of T9 vertebral body
E. There are three layers of muscles in oesophagus

47. **A 22-year-old woman has had pain, redness, and swelling in her left breast. She is lactating. A breast abscess is suspected on the upper outer quadrant. Which is the single most appropriate statement?**

A. One-third of the breast sits on the pectoralis major
B. The breast lies between the deep pectoral fascia and chest wall muscles
C. The breast overlies the second to sixth rib in the vertical axis
D. The main blood supply is through perforating branches from intercostal vessels
E. The nipple contains abundant hair follicles, infection in which may result in abscess formation

48. **A 62-year-old man has had chest pain for the last three hours. He is nauseous and feeling dizzy and sweaty. His ECG is shown in Figure 1.4. Which is the single most likely site of blockage?**

A. Circumflex artery
B. Left anterior descending coronary artery
C. Origin of left coronary artery
D. Origin of right coronary artery
E. Posterior descending artery

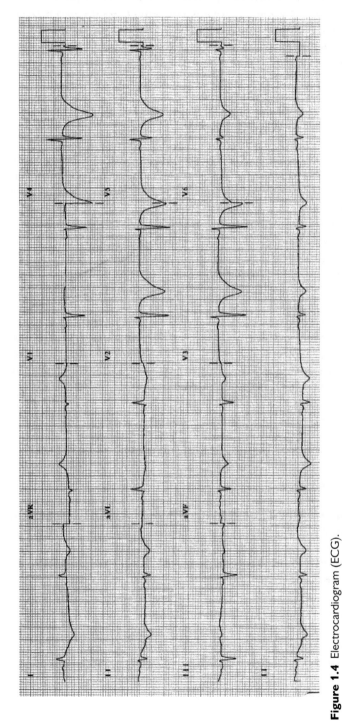

Figure 1.4 Electrocardiogram (ECG).

Reproduced with permission from Saul G. Myerson, Robin P. Choudhury, and Andrew R. J. Mitchell, *Emergencies in Cardiology*, Figure 21.17. Copyright © 2010 with permission from Oxford University Press.

49. **A 45-year-old woman has had pain in the right upper abdomen. She is tender in the right upper quadrant and the Murphy's sign is positive. Acute cholecystitis is suspected. Which single statement is correct regarding the biliary system?**

    A. Calot's triangle is made up of the cystic artery, cystic duct, and the common hepatic duct
    B. Hartmann's pouch is a part of a normal gall bladder
    C. The gall bladder can hold about 50 ml of bile
    D. The venous drainage of the gall bladder is through the cystic vein
    E. The main content of the bile is cholesterol

50. **A 45-year-old man has had pain in the upper-mid abdomen for six hours. It started suddenly and radiated to the back. He is tender in the epigastrium. His serum amylase is 1,250 IU/L. Which is the correct option?**

    A. Secretions from the *Islets of Langerhans* drain into the main duct
    B. The portal vein is formed behind the neck of the pancreas
    C. The splenic vein runs along the upper border of the pancreas
    D. The uncinate process hooks posteriorly to the coeliac axis
    E. The venous drainage from pancreas goes to the inferior vena cava

51. **A 50-year-old man has attended the ED with sudden onset of pain in the right groin developed when he was lifting a heavy weight. He has had an inguinal hernia for some time. He is unable to reduce the swelling himself. The swelling in his right groin is very hard and tender. Which is the single best option regarding hernia?**

    A. The direct inguinal hernia can be controlled by pressure applied above the femoral pulse
    B. The indirect hernia lies above and lateral to the pubic tubercle
    C. The indirect inguinal hernia emerges through the posterior wall
    D. The internal ring lies about 1.2 cm above the femoral pulse
    E. The mid-inguinal point lies halfway between the anterior superior iliac spine (ASIS) and pubic tubercle

52. **A 15-year-old boy has attended the ED with sudden onset of pain in the abdomen for the last 24 hours. His initial pain was around the mid abdomen, but later settled in right lower abdominal area. He is tender in the right iliac fossa. Acute appendicitis is suspected. Which is the correct statement regarding the appendix?**

    A. The afferent nerve from appendix enters the spinal cord at the eleventh thoracic segment
    B. The appendicular artery is an end artery
    C. The attachment of the appendix base to the caecum is variable
    D. The lymphoid follicles in the appendix are present from birth
    E. The histological structure of the caecum and appendix are similar

53. A 25-year-old man has received a kick in his upper abdomen while playing karate in a competition. He has bruising on the left half of the epigastrium. Which single artery may have contributed to the bruising?

A. Deep circumflex iliac artery

B. Inferior epigastric artery

C. Superficial epigastric artery

D. Superior gastric artery

E. Thoracoepigastric artery

54. A 75-year-old man has had sudden abdominal pain, which started centrally and gradually spread to all over the abdomen. He has excruciating pain. He has soft and mildly tender abdomen. He has atrial fibrillation. The diagnosis of mesenteric vascular occlusion is suspected. Which statement is most correct about the blood supply of intestine?

A. Blood through the inferior mesenteric vein eventually drains into the portal vein

B. The inferior mesenteric artery supplies only the colon

C. Superior mesenteric artery supplies the whole of the small intestine

D. The superior mesenteric vein drains into the inferior vena cava

E. The hepatic flexure of transverse colon is prone to ischaemia

55. A 55-year-old man has had sudden abdominal pain, which started in the epigastrium and gradually spread to all over the abdomen. He was previously diagnosed with an ulcer on the posterior wall of the stomach. He is suspected to have a peptic ulcer perforation. In which area will the fluid will be collected initially?

A. Hepatorenal pouch

B. Lesser sac

C. Right subhepatic space

D. Right subphrenic space

E. Splenorenal pouch

56. A 45-year-old man has had sudden pain in his back passage while passing hard stool. He also noticed bright red blood on toilet tissue paper. On examination, he has posterior midline anal fissure. The digital examination is very painful with spasm of sphincter. What is the single best appropriate statement?

A. The anal canal is about 7.5 cm long

B. The anal verge is lined by columnar epithelium

C. Fissure-in-ano extends above the dentate line

D. The external sphincter is relaxed during resting stage

E. Pain sensation is carried through the second to fourth sacral spinal nerves

57. A 25-year-old man has had a fall-astride on the front bar of the bicycle. He has a drop of blood on the external urinary meatus and he is unable to pass urine. What is the single best appropriate statement?

A. The bulbar urethra is the narrowest part of the urethra

B. The membranous urethra is a part of the anterior urethra

C. The extravasated urine cannot travel into the scrotum and penis

D. The extravasated urine may travel to medial side of the thigh, deep to the superficial fascia

E. The most likely site of injury is the bulbar urethra

58. A 65-year-old man has been unable to pass urine since the previous night. He is in pain. He has distension of urinary bladder up to the umbilicus. What is the single best appropriate statement?

A. Sensation of distension is carried by the parasympathetic predominantly

B. The internal sphincter has reach supply of parasympathetic fibres

C. The lining epithelium of the bladder is of columnar type

D. The parasympathetic fibres to bladder arise from lower three thoracic segments

E. The sympathetic component of bladder is supplied by the lower lumbar segments

59. A 14-year-old male has had sudden pain in his left scrotum while in the PE class at school. On examination, the scrotum is red, and the left testis is very tender. A diagnosis of testicular torsion is suspected. Which is the single best appropriate statement regarding torsion of the testis?

A. Fertility is not affected by a single episode of torsion

B. Permanent tissue loss occurs if the torsion is unrelieved within 12 hours

C. The pain is due to tissue ischaemia

D. The Prehn sign is reliable for diagnosing testicular sensation

E. Torsion is always extravaginal

60. A 40-year-old man has had sudden pain in his left loin, which radiates to the groin up to the left scrotum. He has vomited three times over the last four hours since the start of the pain. He is suspected to have left-sided nephrolithiasis. Which is the single most likely area where the stone could be arrested to produce these symptoms?

A. Membranous urethra

B. Neck of the bladder

C. Pelvic brim

D. Pelviureteric junction

E. Vesicoureteric junction

61. **A 70-year-old man has had sudden severe pain in his mid-abdomen and lower back. He is on treatment for hypertension, type 2 diabetes, and ischaemic heart disease. The size of abdominal aorta is 5.5 × 6.5 cm on focused assessment sonography test (FAST) examination. Which single most likely option is true regarding abdominal aorta?**

A. Around 80% of aneurysms occur in the suprarenal segment of the aorta

B. Abdominal aorta begins at the level of the eleventh thoracic vertebra

C. It bifurcates in front of the L5/S1 disc to two common iliac arteries

D. Dorsal branches from the aorta supply blood to the viscera of the abdomen

E. The renal artery arises at the level of L1 vertebral body

62. **A 30-year-old man has had pain and distension in his abdomen for two days. He has vomited many times and has not opened his bowel over the last 24 hours. His abdomen is distended and diffusely tender. The X-ray is shown in Figure 1.5 Which is the single most likely part of the bowel producing the image on the X-ray?**

A. Descending colon

B. Duodenum

C. Jejunum

D. Ileum

E. Sigmoid colon

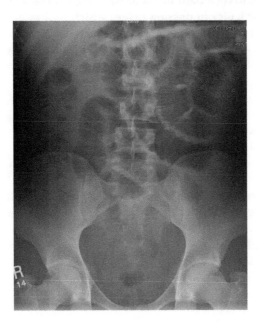

Figure 1.5 X-ray.

63. **A 22-year-old woman has had sudden pain in her left lower abdomen with a few drops of blood spotting through vagina. Her last menstrual period was eight weeks ago. A diagnosis of ruptured ectopic pregnancy is suspected. Which single most likely statement is true?**
    A. All the venous drainage is via internal iliac veins
    B. Ovarian arteries are branches from internal iliac arteries
    C. The main blood supply to the Fallopian tubes is the ovarian arteries
    D. Uterine arteries supply the medial two-thirds of the Fallopian tubes
    E. Uterine arteries arise from the abdominal aorta

64. **A 22-year-old woman has had a severely painful red rash with blisters in the anterior third of her labium majus. A diagnosis of herpes simplex infection is suspected. Which is the single most likely sensory innervations of the affected area in this case?**
    A. Hypogastric nerve
    B. Ilioinguinal nerve
    C. Pelvic splanchnic nerves
    D. Posterior cutaneous nerve of the thigh
    E. Pudendal nerve

65. **A 45-year-old man with known prolapsed intervertebral disc between L5 and S1 has had severe pain in his back, which is radiating down to both legs. He has difficulty in passing urine, which he has never had before. He also feels strange sensation in the perineum. He has reduced tendon reflexes in the ankle joints. A diagnosis of corda equina syndrome is suspected. Which single most likely option is correct in relation to this case?**
    A. Difficulty in micturition is because of involvement of the sympathetic plexus
    B. Loss of anal sphincter function is because of S2–S4 nerve involvements
    C. Loss of ankle jerk is because of a trapped nerve root L4/L5
    D. Loss of perianal sensation is because of S1 nerve root entrapment
    E. Loss of sensation on the medial side of the leg is because of S1 nerve involvement

66. **A 22-year-old male attends the ED with a nosebleed after having been involved in a fight. Which single most likely blood vessel is the source of bleeding?**
    A. Anterior ethmoid artery (a branch of the maxillary artery)
    B. Great palatine artery (a branch of the maxillary artery)
    C. Sphenopalatine artery (a branch of the facial artery)
    D. Superior labial artery (a branch of the ophthalmic artery)
    E. Zygomaticotemporal artery

67. A 36-year-old female has had a headache that is worse when bending forwards. She has recently had a cold. She has a feeling of pressure and tightness in the front of her head. Which is the single most likely location of her pain?

A. The ethmoid sinus

B. The frontal bone

C. The frontal sinus

D. The nasolacrimal duct

E. The sphenoidal sinus

68. An 83-year-old gentleman is brought in by an ambulance with a bleeding head wound sustained following a fall. Direct pressure has been applied to the wound, but after 10 minutes it is still bleeding. The laceration is situated above and at the front of the right ear. Which is the most likely source of bleeding?

A. Occipital artery

B. Posterior auricular artery

C. Superficial temporal artery

D. Supraorbital artery

E. Zygomatico-orbital artery

69. A 38-year-old female has sustained a laceration on the head by a piece of glass after being involved in a fight. The bleeding has now stopped. Which is the single most correct order of structures the glass might have penetrated through in the layers of scalp before striking the skull bone?

A. Aponeurosis, loose areolar tissue, skin, periosteum, connective tissue

B. Aponeurosis, skin, connective tissue, loose areolar tissue, periosteum

C. Skin, aponeurosis, loose areolar tissue, connective tissue, periosteum

D. Skin, connective tissue, aponeurosis, loose areolar tissue, periosteum

E. Skin, connective tissue, loose areolar tissue, aponeurosis, periosteum

70. An 80-year-old gentleman has had a lump on his tongue and difficulty in swallowing. After biopsies he is diagnosed with cancer of the tongue. Which is the single most important reason that tongue cancer is detected early?

A. Curative monotherapy is a highly successful

B. It is extremely painful

C. Progression of the disease can be slowed by lifestyle changes

D. The tongue has bilateral lymph node drainage

E. Weight loss can be significant

71. **A 25-year-old female patient has been brought to the ED by blue light ambulance after an overdose of mixture of medications. Her Glasgow Coma Scale score is 3. To protect her airway, an anaesthetist is about to perform endotracheal intubation. Which is the single most correct statement?**
    A. The aryepiglottic fold is interior to the ventricular fold
    B. The laryngoscope blade should be behind the epiglottis in this case
    C. The oesophageal opening as landmark must be visible
    D. The interarytenoid notch is at the posterior point of the vocal cords
    E. The vallecula is posterior to the epiglottis

72. **A 26-year-old male has a fracture dislocation of his right ankle. He requires procedural sedation for the manipulation of the ankle joint in the ED. On assessment of his airway, to predict any potential airway complication during sedation, it is seen that when he opens his mouth and extends his tongue, the soft and hard palate are visible, but the lower part of his uvula and tonsils are obscured. Which is the single best Mallampati score in this patient?**
    A. 1
    B. 2
    C. 3
    D. 4
    E. Inadequate information given to calculate the score

73. **A 30-year-old male has been brought to the ED with a laceration below the middle of the lower jaw, sustained accidentally. The wound is in the right anterior triangle of the neck. Which is single best correct option with regards to the boundaries of the anterior triangle?**
    A. The floor is the investing fascia
    B. The medial border is the midline
    C. The lateral border is the lateral border of the sternocleidomastoid
    D. The roof is the prevertebral fascia
    E. The superior border is the middle of the jaw

74. **A 30-year-old female has had perioral paraesthesia, muscle twitching, and carpopedal spasm over the last few hours. She has recently had an extensive surgery of the neck. She is suspected to have low calcium due to accidental damage to the parathyroid glands. Which single best statement regarding parathyroid is most likely correct?**
    A. Around 90% of parathyroid glands are aberrant
    B. The numbers of parathyroid glands may vary from seven to ten
    C. The parathyroids are usually unsafe in subtotal thyroidectomy
    D. The superior parathyroid glands are more constant in position than the inferior parathyroid glands
    E. The superior parathyroid gland usually lies at the superior pole of the lobes of the thyroid gland

75. **A 25-year-old male has been brought to the ED with reduced conscious level and extensive facial injury following a fall off a cliff. He has a gurgling noise during breathing. His Glasgow Coma Scale score is 10. Endotracheal intubation could not be accomplished. A decision has been taken to perform emergency cricothyroidotomy. Which is the single most appropriate statement regarding the procedure?**

    A. The cricothyroid membrane is 2 cm wide and 0.2 cm high
    B. The cricothyroid membrane is located about 1 cm above the level of the true vocal cord
    C. The landmark for the site of incision is just above the Adam's apple (laryngeal prominence)
    D. There are few to no vascular structures overlying the cricothyroid membrane
    E. There is a very high chance of injuring the oesophagus

76. **A 25-year-old female with known type 1 diabetes has been brought to the ED with vomiting, abdominal pain, and feeling unwell. Her HR is 130, BP 75/40 mmHg, RR 35 breaths/min, temperature 38.70 °C, and SaO$_2$ 88%. Peripheral intravenous cannulation could not be achieved. Central venous access has been attempted. Which is the single most appropriate statement regarding the procedure?**

    A. It is relatively easier to cannulate the internal jugular vein below the level of the cricoid cartilage
    B. The internal jugular vein is directly visible from the skin surface
    C. The internal jugular vein lies slightly deep and posterior to the common carotid artery in the lower neck
    D. The surface marking of internal jugular vein is from the ear lobe to the lateral margin of the clavicular head of the sternocleidomastoid muscle
    E. Trendelenburg position is not required for subclavian vein access

77. **A 75-year-old female has been brought to the ED with painful swelling on the right cheek area. She has difficulty in chewing and swallowing. She is suspected to have acute parotitis. Which is the single most appropriate statement?**

    A. The arterial supply to the parotid gland is from the internal carotid artery
    B. The branches of facial nerve runs in the superficial fascia under the skin
    C. The opening of the parotid duct is visible opposite the upper first molar tooth
    D. The pain from parotid gland swelling is due to stretching of its capsule
    E. The pain from parotid gland usually is reduced during a meal time

78. **A 40-year-old male has been brought to the ED after an attempt of self-hanging. He did not lose consciousness, neither had any pain. He is alert and orientated. Which is the single most appropriate statement?**

    A. Cervical spine injuries are common in self-hanging
    B. Compression of the airway plays an important role in self-hanging
    C. In judicial hanging, the C2 is fractured through its odontoid peg
    D. In self-hanging, complete arterial occlusion is followed by venous congestion
    E. Morbidity is primarily due to asphyxiation in self-hanging

79. A 35-year-old male has had tooth pain on the right side for the last couple of days. He has swelling and redness near the right mandibular (lower) first premolar. A decision has been taken to anaesthetize the area. Which is the single most appropriate statement about performance of the procedure?

A. Identify the anterior border of the ramus of the mandible from outside the mouth

B. Lingula of the ramus of the mandible is the bony prominence on the medial side of the mandible

C. Palpation of the posterior ramus of the mandible from inside the mouth

D. The inferior alveolar nerve lies 1 cm above the lingula

E. The local anaesthetic is to be injected 1 cm inferior and anterior to the lingula

80. A 20-year-old male has had a sore throat for the past three days. He has painful deglutition and fever with malaise. He is suspected to have acute pharyngitis. Which is the correct option about the boundary of the oropharynx?

A. The anterior boundary is the opening of the mouth

B. The inferior boundary is the tip of the epiglottis

C. Lateral boundaries are pharyngeal pouches

D. The posterior boundary is the soft palate and uvula

E. The superior boundary is the nasopharynx

81. A 28-year-old male has a red and painful right eye. He was working in his garage when he felt something going into his eye. The eye has normal visual acuity, but is watery and has photophobia. Which is the correct option about this clinical situation?

A. Both the eyelids are of same size

B. Both the eyelids contain levator palpebrae superioris muscles

C. Conjunctiva is a single layer of epithelium on the cornea

D. Ducts from the lacrimal gland open in both superior and inferior fornices

E. The most likely place for a foreign body to be stuck is on the bulbar conjunctiva

82. A 20-year-old male has had a tonsillectomy operation earlier this morning. He has attended the ED with bleeding from his operation site. Which single vessel may be the most likely source of severe bleeding?

A. The ascending palatine artery

B. The ascending pharyngeal artery

C. The facial artery

D. The lingual artery

E. The paratonsillar vein

83. **A 40-year-old female has had swelling in the front of the neck, which she only noticed this morning. She has no pain. On examination, the swelling moves up on swallowing. Enlargement of thyroid gland is suspected. Which is the single best correct option?**

    A. A large goitre cannot extend into the superior mediastinum because of fascial attachments
    B. Flexion of the neck makes the goitre readily visible during clinical examination
    C. The enlargement of thyroid gland occurs mostly anteriorly
    D. The thyroid capsule is much denser posteriorly than anteriorly
    E. The upwards movement of the thyroid gland on swallowing is because of a blending of the pretracheal fascia with the larynx

84. **A 19-year-old female has had fever, headache, and neck stiffness. Her computed tomography (CT) scan of the brain is normal. She requires lumbar puncture for further investigation. Which is the correct sequence of layers of tissues the spinal needle may be required to penetrate through?**

    A. Skin, fat, supraspinous ligament, ligamentum flavum, interspinous ligament
    B. Skin, fat, supraspinous ligament, interspinous ligament, ligamentum flavum
    C. Skin, ligamentum flavum, fat, supraspinous ligament, interspinous ligament
    D. Skin, supraspinous ligament, fat, interspinous ligament, ligamentum flavum
    E. Skin, supraspinous ligament, fat, ligamentum flavum, interspinous ligament

85. **A 68-year-old man has had a fall off a ladder from about a height of 2.5 metres. He has neck pain. He is conscious and unable to move his arms, but only just able to move his legs. He has a patchy loss of sensation in both his arms. Which single most likely part of the spinal cord is affected?**

    A. The central part of corticospinal and spinothalamic tracts of the cervical spinal cord
    B. The central part of the corticospinal and spinothalamic tracts of the upper thoracic spinal cord
    C. Disruption of the vascular supply of the grey matter of the spinal cord
    D. The peripheral part of the corticospinal and spinothalamic tracts of the cervical spinal cord
    E. The peripheral part of the corticospinal and spinothalamic tracts of the upper thoracic spinal cord

86. **A 66-year-old man has had sudden onset of weakness to the right upper and lower limbs. He has hyper-reflexia and Babinsky sign. He does not have any sensory loss or dysarthria. Which is the most likely part of the brain affected?**

    A. The anterior limb of the internal capsule
    B. The genu of the internal capsule
    C. The posterior limb of the internal capsule
    D. The thalamus
    E. The thalamus and adjacent posterior limb of internal capsule

87. A 76-year-old man has had sudden onset of dysarthria, limb ataxia on the left side, and has tendency to fall to the left. He is suspected to have a cerebellar stroke. Which cerebellar artery is most likely involved?

A. Left anterior inferior
B. Left lateral superior
C. Left posterior inferior
D. Right anterior inferior
E. Right lateral superior

88. A 72-year-old man has had a feeling of numbness on the left side of his body and face for the last day or so. He has hypertension and type 2 diabetes mellitus. He has no speech problem or weakness in his arms or legs. Which is the single best most likely location of infarct?

A. Basal ganglia
B. Internal capsule
C. Precentral gyrus
D. Temporal lobe
E. Thalamus

89. A 25-year-old man has started passing a high volume of urine. He sustained a head injury a couple of weeks ago. He is suspected to have cranial diabetes insipidus (DI). Which is the most likely correct option?

A. Anterior pituitary is derived from the forebrain
B. Neurohypophysis is an extension of the nervous system
C. The pituitary stalk is highly cellular
D. The posterior pituitary is developed from ectoderm
E. Vasopressin is synthesized in the posterior pituitary

90. A 52-year-old man has had a sudden onset of reduced consciousness, presumably after taking an overdose of unknown tablets. His Glasgow Coma Scale (GCS) score is 3 out of 15. His reflexes are globally depressed; the pupils are bilaterally equal and reacting to light, but the eyes remain in a fixed position within the orbits, and turning with the head in the same direction. Which is the most likely part of the brain affected?

A. Brain stem
B. Cerebellum
C. Corona radiata
D. Globus pallidus
E. Psychogenic

91. An 82-year-old man has been brought to the ED with repeated falls and unsteadiness in gait. He is known to have Alzheimer's disease for the last few years. Which lobe of the brain is primarily affected in Alzheimer's disease?

    A. Frontal
    B. Hypothalamus
    C. Occipital
    D. Parietal
    E. Temporal

92. An 88-year-old man has been brought to the ED as he has been found wandering on a street and being aggressive. According to the neighbour, this is an unusual behaviour. He is having visual hallucinations in the ED. Which is the most likely correct statement regarding delirium?

    A. Both the cerebral cortex and subcortical structures are affected in delirium
    B. Development of disturbances occur over weeks and months
    C. It is an irreversible cerebral dysfunction
    D. Persistent and progressive inattention is the hallmark of delirium
    E. Reduced serotonin levels in the brain is typically associated with delirium

93. A 52-year-old woman has attended the ED after having a sudden onset of severe generalized headache started while watching television about three hours ago. She has had a couple of episodes of vomiting. She is otherwise well. Her right pupil is 6 mm, left 3 mm. The right pupil is unreactive to light. A provisional diagnosis of subarachnoid haemorrhage has been made. Which is the most likely site of the aneurysm?

    A. Anterior cerebral artery
    B. Anterior communicating artery
    C. Middle cerebral artery
    D. Posterior circulation
    E. Posterior communicating artery

94. A 78-year-old man has attended the ED after falling three times in the last 24 hours. He has Parkinson's disease (PD) and recently started treatment. He is not any other medication. Which is the most likely cause of his falls?

    A. Bradykinesia
    B. Disturbance of higher mental function
    C. Dopaminergic stimulation
    D. Loss of postural reflex
    E. Rigidity

95. A 22-year-old woman has had headaches, fever, and malaise, neck stiffness, and vomiting for the last 24 hours. The CT scan of the brain shows dilatation of the ventricular system and reduced differentiation of grey and white matters. Which is the most likely correct statement?

A. Hypothalamus is closely related to the lateral ventricle

B. Increased production of cerebrospinal fluid (CSF) has caused the ventricular enlargement

C. The aqueduct of Sylvius may be blocked

D. The fourth ventricle received the CSF directly from the subarachnoid space

E. There are three pairs of ventricles in the central nervous system (CNS)

96. A 22-year-old man has had a fall from a first floor window and has a head injury. His CT scan of the brain is shown in Figure 1.6 In-between which structures has the haematoma formed?

A. Arachnoid and pia

B. Bone and arachnoid

C. Bone and dura

D. Dura and arachnoid

E. Pia and brain

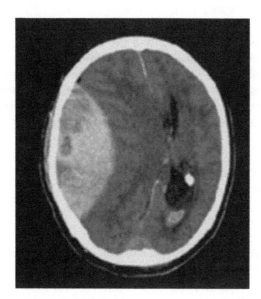

Figure 1.6 Computed tomography (CT) scan.

Courtesy of Dr Rod Gibson.

97. **A 25-year-old woman has had a tonic-clonic seizure lasting for about a minute. She now in a postictal state. She is incontinent of urine and bitten her tongue. She suffers from epilepsy and is on antiepileptic medication. Which is the correct statement regarding generalized seizures?**

A. Excitation of Gama-aminobutyric acid (GABA) receptors precipitates seizures

B. Loss of consciousness and bilateral movements are because of cortical focus

C. Sympathetic stimulation may result in hypoglycaemia

D. Tongue biting is because of repeated jaw muscle contractions

E. Urinary incontinence is because of inhibition of cortical activity on bladder

98. **A 25-year-old man has been brought to the ED following a high-speed motorbike accident. He has flaccid paralysis in the lower limbs, loss of deep tendon reflexes, and urinary retention. He has total loss of sensation below the level of T3. He does not have any other injuries. His HR is 60 bpm, BP 95/55 mmHg, RR 20 breaths per minute, temperature 35.5 °C. Which is the correct statement regarding this clinical situation?**

A. Return of perianal sensation signifies cessation of spinal shock

B. The patient has complete spinal cord injury

C. The patient is in hypovolumic shock

D. The patient is in spinal shock

E. This type of hypotension usually does not cause hypoperfusion

99. **A 32-year-old woman is known to have paraplegia because of multiple sclerosis (MS). She has attended the ED with the sensation of pins and needles in the upper limbs, which are new for her. Her clinical observations are within normal range. The vibration sense and proprioception are lost in the left hand. Which is the most likely correct statement with regards to her presentation?**

A. Cranial nerve involvement is rare in MS

B. Demyelination of the left corticospinal tract has resulted in pins and needles

C. The paraplegia is associated with flaccidity and reduced reflexes

D. The proprioception is carried by the left posterior column

E. The vibration sense is carried by the left spinothalamic tract

100. **A 55-year-old woman has had generalized headache of very sudden onset during intercourse. She felt dizzy and nearly passed out. Which is the most likely statement correct regarding headaches?**

A. Headache in over the age of 50 are mostly of insignificant cause

B. Patients can specifically localize head pains

C. The meninges are insensitive to pain

D. The brain parenchyma is sensitive to pain

E. The vascular headache is mediated through the fifth nerve

101. A 43-year-old male presents to the ED with difficulty smiling and raising one eyebrow. He is diagnosed with a Bell's palsy. Which is the most appropriate statement regarding Bell's palsy?

A. Caused by inflammation of the sixth cranial nerve
B. Causes sensory loss over the mandibular on the affected side
C. Commonly affects both sides of the face at once
D. Linked to Ramsey Hunt syndrome
E. Spares the orbicularis muscle on the affected side

102. A 55-year-old man has had hearing loss and tinnitus in his left ear for the last few weeks, which has become worse. He has unsteady gait and vertigo lasting from a few seconds to a few hours. He does not have any other symptoms or signs. Which is the most likely site of involvement?

A. Cerebellum
B. Labyrinth
C. Middle ear
D. Pons
E. Posterior cranial fossa - acoustic neuroma

103. A 65-year-old female has double vision of sudden onset. The triage nurse notices that when asked to look forwards, her left eye is abducted. Which single muscle is most likely to be causing the abnormalities?

A. Inferior oblique
B. Inferior rectus
C. Lateral rectus
D. Medial rectus
E. Superior rectus

104. A 53-year-old woman has had altered field of vision. She has difficulty in reading and strange vision in the central vision. She does not have any pain. What is the most likely abnormality found with a lesion of the body of the optic chiasm?

A. Binasal hemianopia
B. Bitemporal hemianopia
C. Homonymous hemianopia
D. Total loss of vision in one eye
E. Total loss of vision in both eyes

woman has had injury to her face and nose after a fight
the nightclub. She has swelling of the nose. The bleeding
She feels she is unable to smell. Which?

ry receptors are formed repeatedly during adulthood

eurons cannot be replaced once damaged by injury

epithelial cells are located on all the turbinates in the nasal cavity

epithelial cells are located on all parts of the nasal septum

tions from the Bowman's glands help in olfaction

old woman has had severe electric shock-like pains to the
of the middle of her face. She has been generally fit and well.
t on any medication. There is no preceding history of trauma.
sis of trigeminal neuralgia (TN) is suspected. Which is the
ely statement correct with regards to the distribution of the
ed symptoms?

lar part of the nose is painful when the maxillary division is affected

B. The infraorbital skin is affected when the mandibular division is involved

C. The infraorbital skin is not affected when the maxillary division is involved

D. The lower lip is painful when maxillary division is affected

E. The pain is felt in the upper lip when the mandibular division is affected

107. **A 25-year-old woman has had an injury to her left external auditory canal while cleaning her ears. It bled for a while. Now she has reduced hearing sensation in that ear. Which is the most likely correct statement with regards to this presentation?**

A. Air conduction is heard longer than the bone conduction in Rinne's test

B. Perforation in the superior quadrant of the eardrum may cause significant hearing loss

C. Small perforations in the ear drum may cause profound deafness

D. The mechanism may cause damage to the sensory hair cells

E. The sound localizes to the right ear in Weber's test

108. **A 75-year-old woman has had loss of taste and common sensation in the back of her tongue. She occasionally experiences a choking sensation while having food and drinks. Which is the most likely nerve affected?**

A. Facial

B. Glossopharyngeal

C. Hypoglossal

D. Lingual

E. Vagus

109. **A 33-year-old man has attended the ED following inability to elevate his right shoulder. He had a lymph node biopsy in his neck area a couple of days ago. He has flattening of the right trapezius and drooping of the shoulder. His sternocleidomastoid muscle seems normal. The spinal accessory nerve is suspected to be injured. Which is the most likely location of the lesion?**

    A. Anterior triangle of the neck

    B. Base of the cranium

    C. Nuclear

    D. Posterior triangle of the neck

    E. Retropharyngeal

110. **A 70-year-old man has attended the ED after having difficulty in speaking. He had a carotid endarterectomy a few days ago. The appearance of his tongue is shown in Figure 1.7. Which is the most likely nerve affected?**

    A. Left glossopharyngeal nerve

    B. Left hypoglossal nerve

    C. Left Lingual nerve

    D. Left mandibular nerve

    E. Right lingual nerve

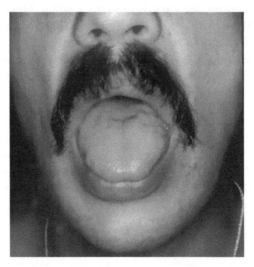

Figure 1.7 Patient's tongue.

111. **An 85-year-old woman has had double vision of sudden onset with headaches. Her eye examination is as shown in Figure 1.8. Which nerve is most likely affected?**
    A. Abducent
    B. Facial
    C. Occulomotor
    D. Ophthalmic division
    E. Trochlear

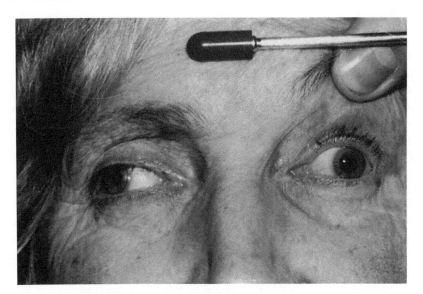

Figure 1.8 Eye examination.

Reproduced with permission from Michael Donaghy (eds), *Brain's Diseases of the Nervous System* (12th Edition), Figure 13.2. Copyright © 2011 with permission from Oxford University Press.

112. **A 70-year-old man has had headaches of sudden onset. He has ptosis, divergent squint, and papillary dilatation on the right side. The third cranial nerve palsy is suspected. Which single statement is most likely correct?**
    A. The divergent squint is due to unopposed action of the inferior oblique and lateral rectus
    B. The loss of accommodation-convergence reflex is due to paralysis of the constrictor pupillae
    C. The loss of light reflex is due to dilator pupillae paralysis
    D. The mydriasis is due to unopposed action of parasympathetic fibres
    E. The ptosis is due to paralysis of the sympathetic fibres

113. **A 32-year-old man has had a tiny laceration to his left cheek when he tripped and fell, striking his face on the sharp corner of a desk. He has drooping of the left corner of the mouth and flattening of the left nasolabial furrow. Which branch of the facial nerve is most likely injured?**
    A. Buccal
    B. Cervical
    C. Mandibular
    D. Temporal
    E. Zygomatic

114. **A 55-year-old man has had hearing loss and tinnitus in his left ear for the last few weeks, which has become worse. He has unsteady gait and vertigo lasting for from seconds to few hours. He does not have any other symptoms or signs. Which is the most likely site of involvement?**
    A. Cerebellum
    B. Labyrinth
    C. Middle ear
    D. Pons
    E. Posterior cranial fossa

115. **A 28-year-old man has been assaulted in a gang fight on the previous night. He has headaches and vomiting. There is bruising behind the left ear. He is suspected to have a basal skull fracture. Which is the most likely correct statement?**
    A. Haemotympanum takes one to three days to develop after the injury
    B. Mastoid bruising develops immediately after the injury
    C. Otorrhea may occur after temporal bone fractures
    D. 'Raccoon eyes' develops within a couple of hours in basal skull fracture
    E. Traumatic carotid cavernous fistula is a common complication after basal skull fracture

1. D. C8.

The skin of the upper limb has a segmental nerve supply, which is systematic and regular. It is derived from nerve roots C4 to T2. The inner surface (ulnar) of the hand is supplied by the C8 segment through the ulnar nerve. C4 supplies skin over the shoulder tip, C5 to the radial side of the upper arm, C6 radial side of the forearm, C7 the skin of the hand, C8 ulnar side of the forearm and hand, T1 ulnar side of the upper arm and T2 skin of the axilla.

Ellis H, Mahadevan V (2013). *Clinical Anatomy: Applied Anatomy for Students and Junior Doctors*, 13th edition (pp. 201–4). Oxford, UK: John Wiley & Sons Ltd.

2. E. Cervicoaxillary opening at the apex of the axilla transmits subclavian artery and brachial plexus from neck into axilla.

- A. Axillary artery becomes brachial artery at the lower border of teres major.
- B. Its shape is irregular and pyramidal.
- C. Axillary artery is divided into three parts by pectoralis minor.
- D. Axillary artery begins at the lateral border of first rib.
- E. Correct answer: The axilla is a zone of transition between the neck and upper limbs. It contains the axillary artery and its branches, axillary vein and tributaries, cords, and branches of brachial plexus, intercostobrachial nerve, and lymph nodes.

Ellis H, Mahadevan V (2013). *Clinical Anatomy: Applied Anatomy for Students and Junior Doctors*, 13th edition (p. 197). Oxford, UK: John Wiley & Sons Ltd.

3. C. Movement of the sternoclavicular joint is reciprocal to the scapular movement.

- A. Abduction is initiated by the supraspinatus muscle followed by the deltoid, which could move the joint up to 90 degrees.
- B. Elevation, depression, rotation, and protraction of the scapula may still be possible even if the shoulder joint is fused.
- C. Correct answer: Movements of the scapula occur with reciprocal movements at the sternoclavicular joint.
- D. The shoulder girdle and the shoulder joint moves smoothly in one smooth motion; it is not possible to divorce both the movements.
- E. The rotation of scapula begins as soon as the abduction starts at the shoulder joint.

Ellis H, Mahadevan V (2013). *Clinical Anatomy: Applied Anatomy for Students and Junior Doctors*, 13th edition (pp. 185–90). Oxford, UK: John Wiley & Sons Ltd.

4. B. The brachial artery bifurcates to the radial and ulnar arteries at the level of the neck of radius.

A. The antecubital fossa (or cubital fossa) is a triangular hollow area in front of the elbow joint.

B. Correct answer.

C. Incorrect, pulsation may be visible on Doppler ultrasound examination.

D. Medial nerve is lateral to the artery in the upper arm crossing to its medial side around the mid arm. In the cubital fossa, it lies medial to the artery.

E. The lateral margin is formed by the brachioradialis muscle. The pronator teres muscle forms the medial boundary. The base is formed by an imaginary line running between medial and lateral epicondyle.

Anaesthesia UK. The cubital fossa. Available at: http://www.frca.co.uk/article.aspx?articleid=100363

Ellis H, Mahadevan V (2013). *Clinical Anatomy: Applied Anatomy for Students and Junior Doctors*, 13th edition (pp. 197–9). Oxford, UK: John Wiley & Sons Ltd.

5. B. The abductor pollicis brevis is innervated by the C8–T1 component of the median nerve.

The muscles of the thenar are the abductor pollicis brevis, flexor pollicis brevis, and opponens pollicis. These three muscles are all supplied by the recurrent branch of the median nerve (C8–T1). The adductor pollicis muscle is supplied by the deep branch of ulnar nerve (C8–T1).

Ellis H, Mahadevan V (2006). *Clinical Anatomy: Applied Anatomy for Students and Junior Doctors*, 13th edition (pp. 193–209). Oxford, UK: John Wiley & Sons Ltd.

Sinnatamby CS (2011). *Last's Anatomy: Regional and Applied*, 12th edition (pp. 37–109). London, UK: Churchill Livingstone.

6. B. FDS.

A. In the palm, the FDP lies deep to the FDS. Then in the fingers, it lies superficial to the partial decussation of the latter before passing distally to be attached to the base of the terminal phalanx. It flexes the terminal IP joint and rolls the fingers and wrist into flexion.

B. Correct answer: FDS. As it crosses the palm, the middle and ring finger tendons lie superficial to those to the index and little finger. It divides into two halves, which spiral round the FDP. Distally it is attached to the middle phalanx. The FDS flexes the proximal IP joint and, secondarily, the metacarpophalangeal (MCP) and wrist joints.

C. Palmer interosseous muscles arise from their own metacarpals. Though the thumb has its own strong adductor muscle, a few fibres may arise from its metacarpal to be inserted to the base of the proximal phalanx, the first palmer interosseous. The second, third, and fourth palmer interossei arise from the middle finger side of the metacarpal bone of the index, ring, and little fingers are inserted into the extensor expansion and the proximal phalanx on the same side. There is no palmer interosseous for the middle finger. The palmer interosseous adducts the fingers relative to the axis of the palm, which is the middle finger and third metacarpal.

D. Palmaris longus—the muscle in the palm splits to form the longitudinally directed fibres of the palmer aponeurosis. It is a weak flexor of the wrist. It does not have function on the fingers.

E. Lumbricals—each of the four FDP tendons gives origin to each of the lumbricals, which then travels on the radial side of the MCP joint to be inserted into the extensor expansion of the dorsum of the first phalanx.

Ellis H, Mahadevan V (2013). *Clinical Anatomy: Applied Anatomy for Students and Junior Doctors*, 13th edition (pp. 171–210). Oxford, UK: John Wiley & Sons Ltd.

Sinnatamby CS (2011). *Last's Anatomy: Regional and Applied*, 12th edition (pp. 37–109). London, UK: Churchill Livingstone.

7. B.   The nail bed is a thin layer of epithelial tissue.

  A. The germinal matrix is responsible for the nail formation. It is the proximal end of the nail bed under the proximal nail fold.
  B. Correct answer: The nail bed is a thin layer of epithelial tissue.
  C. The skin edge at the distal nail margin is called the hyponychium.
  D. Eponychium is the skin that covers the proximal end.
  E. The digital arteries supplying the fingertip are the branches from the ulnar and radial arteries.

Ellis H, Mahadevan V (2013). *Clinical Anatomy: Applied Anatomy for Students and Junior Doctors*, 13th edition (pp. 171–210). Oxford, UK: John Wiley & Sons Ltd.

Sinnatamby CS (2011). *Last's Anatomy: Regional and Applied*, 12th edition (pp. 37–109). London, UK: Churchill Livingstone.

UpToDate (2017). Management of fingertip injuries. Available at: https://www.uptodate.com/contents/management-of-fingertip-injuries

8. E.   The proximal row is made up of the scaphoid, lunate, and triquetrum.

  A. Scaphoid and lunate articulate with the radius.
  B. The carpal bones are organized in two rows, proximal and distal.
  C. The proximal row of carpal bones is mobile because of its connections to the radius and distal row. Each of these bones has its own movements. The transverse arch of the distal row is more rigid.
  D. The scaphoid, because of its articulations with the capitate, trapezium, and trapezoid, contributes to the stability.
  E. Correct answer.

Tibiana R (1998). *Examination of the Hand and Wrist*, 2nd edition (pp. 28–39). London, UK: Martin Dunitz Ltd.

9. B.   Condyloid joint.

  A. Movements among the intercarpal joints add to the flexion of the wrist joint.
  B. Correct answer: The wrist is a condyloid joint allowing flexion, extension, abduction, adduction, and circumduction.
  C. It is not a hinge joint.
  D. As the styloid process of the radius projects distally, the range of abduction is less than that of the adduction.
  E. The articular disc of the inferior radioulnar joint covers the head of the ulna and is attached to the base of the ulnar styloid process.

Ellis H, Mahadevan V (2013). *Clinical Anatomy: Applied Anatomy for Students and Junior Doctors*, 13th edition (pp. 193–4). Oxford, UK: John Wiley & Sons Ltd.

10. D. The superior radioulnar joint is a part of the elbow joint.

A. The capsule of the elbow joint is thin and loose on both anterior and posterior aspects to allow the movements of flexion and extension. The medial and lateral collateral ligaments reinforce the capsules from both sides.

B. The lateral collateral ligament is attached to the annular ligament of the radial head.

C. The medial and lateral condyles are extracapsular.

D. Correct answer: The elbow joint has three articulations: humeroulnar (a hinge joint), humeroradial (a ball-and-socket joint) and superior radioulnar (a pivot joint).

E. The lower margin of the annular ligament is free and below which the synovial tissue protrudes downwards onto the neck of the radius.

Ellis H, Mahadevan V (2013). *Clinical Anatomy: Applied Anatomy for Students and Junior Doctors*, 13th edition (pp. 190–3). Oxford, UK: John Wiley & Sons Ltd.

11. D. The cephalic vein passes through the roof of the 'anatomical snuffbox'.

A. The radial (anterolateral) boundary of the anatomical snuffbox is formed by the tendons of abductor pollicis longus (laterally) and extensor pollicis brevis (immediately medially).

B. The posteromedial/ulnar boundary is formed by the tendon of the extensor pollicis longus.

C. Radial artery pulsation can be palpated deeply on its floor.

D. Correct answer.

E. The floor is formed by the radial surface of the trapezium.

Standring S (2016). Wrist and hand. In: *Gray's Anatomy*, 41st edition (pp. 862–94). London, UK: Elsevier Ltd.

12. E. Triceps.

A. Biceps—C5/6.

B. Brachioradialis C5/6.

C. Long finger flexors C8/T1.

D. Supinator C6.

E. Triceps C6/7.

Sinnatamby CS (2011). *Last's Anatomy: Regional and Applied*, 12th edition (pp. 37–109). London, UK: Churchill Livingstone.

13. B. Intercostobrachial.

The intercostobrachial (ICBN) is a cutaneous branch from the second intercostal nerve and supplies the axillary skin and the medial aspect of the upper arm. The axillary nerve supplies the skin on the outer aspect of the arm near the insertion of deltoid muscle. The radial arm supplies the skin along the posterior surface of the upper arm. The median and ulnar nerve does not give any branch in the arm.

Sinnatamby CS (2011). *Last's Anatomy: Regional and Applied*, 12th edition (pp. 37–109). London, UK: Churchill Livingstone.

14. D. Teres major, which is not a rotator cuff muscle.

The tendons of the supraspinatus, infraspinatus, subscapularis, and teres minor fuse with the lateral part of the capsule of the shoulder joint and are attached to the humerus. Together they stabilize the joint.

Ellis H, Mahadevan V (2013). *Clinical Anatomy: Applied Anatomy for Students and Junior Doctors,* 13th edition (pp. 186–90). Oxford, UK: John Wiley & Sons Ltd.

15. D. Teres major.

The nerve affected in such injuries is the axillary nerve (C5, C6), which arises from the posterior cord of the brachial plexus. It supplies the capsule of the shoulder joint. The deltoid muscle is supplied by both its anterior and posterior branches, but the teres minor is supplied by the posterior branch only. As a result, the external rotation may also be weaker when the axillary nerve is involved.

Sinnatamby CS (2011). *Last's Anatomy: Regional and Applied,* 12th edition (pp. 37–109). London, UK: Churchill Livingstone.

16. A. The cords pass under the clavicle.

The brachial plexus is composed of five roots and three trunks, with six divisions, three cords, and terminal branches. The anterior rami of C5 to T1 after supplying the prevertebral and scalene muscles are called roots. Of these, the upper two (C5 and C6) unite to form the upper trunk and the lower two (C8 and T1) form the lower trunk. The middle one (C7) continues as the middle trunk. The trunks run between the anterior and middle scalene muscles. The three trunks divide into anterior and posterior divisions behind the clavicle. At the outer border of the first rib, below the clavicle, the lateral cord is formed by the upper two anterior divisions. The anterior division runs as the medial cord, while the three posterior division forms the posterior cord.

Sinnatamby CS (2011). *Last's Anatomy: Regional and Applied,* 12th edition (pp. 37–109). London, UK: Churchill Livingstone.

Medscape, brachial plexus anatomy. Available at: http://emedicine.medscape.com/article/1877731-overview#a2

17. C. Lateral aspect of the thigh.

The fascia iliaca block reliably blocks the femoral and lateral femoral cutaneous nerve (LFCN) of the thigh. The LFCN supplies the lateral aspect of the thigh. The femoral nerve (L2–4) is one of the principal branches of the lumbar plexus, the muscular branch of which supplies the muscles of the anterior compartment of the thigh (quadriceps, sertorius, and pectineus). The cutaneous supply is through medial and intermediate cutaneous nerves of the thigh to the medial and anterior aspect of thigh, the medial side of the leg, ankle, and foot. The inguinal area is supplied by the L1 segment. The mid-inguinal point and anterior part of the labia majora are innervated by the ilioinguinal nerve (L1).

Sinnatamby CS (2011). *Last's Anatomy: Regional and Applied,* 12th edition (pp. 111–78). London, UK: Churchill Livingstone.

UpToDate (2017). Lower extremity nerve blocks: Techniques. Available at: https://www.uptodate.com/contents/lower-extremity-nerve-blocks-techniques

18. D. Obturator.

  A. Genitofemoral nerve originates from the ventral rami of L1 and L2 spinal segments. Its motor supply is to the cremasteric muscle and the sensory innervations to the skin of the anterior scrotum or mons pubis and labium majus, and the skin of upper anterior thigh.

  B. Iliohypogastric (L1) is the motor supply to the internal oblique and transversus abdominis, and the sensory innervations to the posterolateral gluteal skin and skin in the pubic region.

C. Ilioinguinal nerve (L1) also has the same motor supply as the iliohypogastric nerve. Skin innervations are to the upper medial thigh, and either the skin over the root of the penis and anterior scrotum, or the mons and labium majus.

D. Correct answer: The obturator nerve (L2–L4) is a branch of the lumbar plexus and runs deep to the internal iliac vessels, to reach the obturator foramen, and enters the thigh by the obturator vessels. Due to its anatomical course, it can be injured in obstetric procedures. The muscular branches supply the obturator externus, adductor, and gracilis muscles, sensations to the medial aspect of the thigh, and articulation of the hip and knee joints.

E. The pudendal nerve (S2–S4) innervates the perineum.

Ellis H, Mahadevan V (2013). *Clinical Anatomy: Applied Anatomy for Students and Junior Doctors*, 13th edition (pp. 272–6). Oxford, UK: John Wiley & Sons Ltd.

Sinnatamby CS (2011). *Last's Anatomy: Regional and Applied*, 12th edition (pp. 111–78). London, UK: Churchill Livingstone.

19. B. L2–L3.

The symptoms are due to the compression of the lateral cutaneous nerve of thigh (L2–L3), which is an exclusively sensory division. It arises directly from lumber plexus and enters in to the thigh deep to inguinal ligament.

Ellis H, Mahadevan V (2013). *Clinical Anatomy: Applied Anatomy for Students and Junior Doctors*, 13th edition (p. 273). Oxford, UK: John Wiley & Sons Ltd.

Sinnatamby CS (2011). *Last's Anatomy: Regional and Applied*, 12th edition (pp. 111–78). London, UK: Churchill Livingstone.

UpToDate (2017). Approach to hip and groin pain in the athlete and active adult. Available at: https://www.uptodate.com/contents/approach-to-hip-and-groin-pain-in-the-athlete-and-active-adult

20. B. The gluteus maximus is a lateral rotator.

A. Gluteus maximus muscle is an extensor with hamstrings, lateral rotator in conjunction with gemellis, quadratus femoris, and gemelli.

B. Correct answer.

C. The hip joint is rotated medially by the tensor fasciae latae and anterior fibres of the gluteus medius and minimus.

D. See answer A. The gluteus medius and minimus are abductors with tensor fasciae latae.

E. The tensor fasciae latae are abductors with the gluteus medius and minimus, and medial rotators with anterior fibres of gluteus medius and minimus.

Ellis H, Mahadevan V (2013). *Clinical Anatomy: Applied Anatomy for Students and Junior Doctors*, 13th edition (pp. 245–8). Oxford, UK: John Wiley & Sons Ltd.

21. D. The right gluteus medius and minimus are affected.

The stability of the hip joint depends on the strength of the muscles and the integrity of the hip joint. When patient is asked to stand on the affected side (right in this case), the gluteus medius, minimus, and tensor fasciae latae contract to maintain the fixation at the hip joint. This may lead to slight tilting of pelvis on the opposite side. If the abductors are weak or paralysed or if there is pathology in the hip joint, the test is positive, as the patient would not be able to stand on the right leg for more than 30 seconds. This particular patient may have a slipped upper femoral epiphysis.

Ellis H, Mahadevan V (2013). *Clinical Anatomy: Applied Anatomy for Students and Junior Doctors*, 13th edition (pp. 245–8). Oxford, UK: John Wiley & Sons Ltd.

McRae R (2004). *Clinical Orthopaedic Examination*, 5th edition (p. 186). London, UK: Churchill Livingstone.

22. B. Disruption of the cervical vessels and retinacular supply of the head are responsible for the necrosis.

- A. The slender acetabular branch from the obturator artery may supply the head through the ligament of head of femur, but the supply is variable and small, almost negligible in adults. However, this source is essential in children when the femoral head is separated by an epiphyseal cartilage from the neck. Hence, in children the avascular necrosis develops due to the interruption of this blood supply.
- B. Correct answer: The blood supply of the head sourced from the extracapsular ring formed around the base of the neck and ascending cervical branches including the retinacular branches travelling along the femoral neck. The major contribution occurs from the medial and lateral femoral circumflex arteries from the posterior and anterior aspects, respectively.
- C. Cruciate anastomosis is formed at the level of the lesser trochanter by contribution from the branches of the median circumflex femoral, lateral circumflex femoral, first perforating the inferior gluteal arteries. This anastomosis can help in blood flow from external iliac artery to popliteal artery if there is a blockage in-between the femoral and external iliac artery. It is not disrupted in such fracture of the neck of the femur.
- D. The extracapsular arterial ring may be contributed small twigs from the superior and inferior gluteal arteries, but the major blood supply sourced from the arteries mentioned in B.
- E. Please see answer A.

Ellis H, Mahadevan V (2013). *Clinical Anatomy: Applied Anatomy for Students and Junior Doctors*, 13th edition (pp. 236–9). Oxford, UK: John Wiley & Sons Ltd.

Sinnatamby CS (2011). *Last's Anatomy: Regional and Applied*, 12th edition (pp. 111–78). London, UK: Churchill Livingstone.

23. A. Loss of the dorsalis pedis pulse is a likely clinical finding.

- A. Correct answer: As the sharp edge of the distal fragment may injure the popliteal artery, loss of the dorsalis pedis pulsation may occur.
- B. The distal fragment is angulated by gastrocnemius because of its attachment to the back of the condyles; the two heads are attached to the two condyles providing the strong pull.
- C. The hamstrings are attached to the tibia (semimembranosus and semitendinosus) and fibula (biceps femoris), hence it would not be pulled up by the hamstrings.
- D. The great saphenous vein runs on the medial side of the knee under the skin in the superficial fascia, hence likelihood of injury to vein is very minimal.
- E. Injury to the tibial nerve is uncommon injury in such a fracture.

Ellis H, Mahadevan V (2013). *Clinical Anatomy: Applied Anatomy for Students and Junior Doctors*, 13th edition (p. 240). Oxford, UK: John Wiley & Sons Ltd.

24. C. Semimembranosus and semitendinosus muscles lie on the medial aspect.

- A. All hamstring muscles cause extension of the hip and flexion of the knee joints. In the semiflexed knee, the biceps femoris causes lateral rotation, but semimembranosus and semitendinosus cause medial rotation.

B. Semimembranosus originates from the ishchial tuberosity and enters the medial condyle of the tibia.

C. Correct answer.

D. Semimembranosus at its insertion contribute to the formation of the ligaments and fascia around the joint.

E. The biceps femoris is inserted in to the head of the fibula.

Sinnatamby CS (2011). *Last's Anatomy: Regional and Applied*, 12th edition (pp. 111–78). London, UK: Churchill Livingstone.

25. A. Associated with disruption of the medial patellofemoral ligament and medial retinaculum.

A. The lateral dislocation of the patella is a common condition and results following disruption of the medial patellofemoral ligament and medial retinaculum.

B. If keeping the foot fixed on the ground when a twisting force with internal rotation is applied to the flexed knee in valgus, the patella may dislocate laterally.

C. When the leg is in extension, the knee extensors (vastus medialis, intermedius and lateralis, and quadriceps femoris) tend to place an oblique force laterally, which is markedly increased during flexion.

D. The forwards prominence of the lateral condyle of the femur prevents lateral dislocation.

E. The patellar ligament is vertical, but the pull of the quadriceps tendon is oblique in the axis of the shaft of the femur, which tend to draw the patella laterally.

Ellis H, Mahadevan V (2013). *Clinical Anatomy: Applied Anatomy for Students and Junior Doctors*, 13th edition (p. 240–2). Oxford, UK: John Wiley & Sons Ltd.

26. A. The fat in the fossa may bulge in full extension of the knee, giving the appearance of a swelling.

A. Correct answer. The hamstring tendons butt against the femoral condyles during full extension of the knee and the popliteal fat bulges from the roof of the fossa.

B. The floor of the fossa is formed by the popliteal surface of the femur, the capsule of the knee joint, popliteal ligament, and the popliteus muscle covered by its fascia.

C. The fossa is a diamond space hollow cavity behind the knee joint. Its boundary is constituted by semimembranosus and the semitendinosus on the medial side, and the biceps femoris on the lateral side.

D. The two heads of the gastrocnemius makes the boundary of the lower part of the space.

E. The roof of the fossa is covered by a layer of fascia lata covered by skin.

Sinnatamby CS (2011). *Last's Anatomy: Regional and Applied*, 12th edition (pp. 111–78). London, UK: Churchill Livingstone.

27. B. The deep peroneal nerve.

A. The common peroneal or fibular nerve travels medial to the biceps femoris downwards and disappears in the substance of peroneus longus.

B. Correct answer: The deep peroneal nerve is a branch of common peroneal (fibular) nerve after the later curves round the fibular neck and enters the substance of peroneus longus.

C. The posterior cutaneous nerve of the thigh passes through the roof of the fossa to continue inferiorly with the small saphenous vein to supply the skin of the upper half of the back of the leg.

D. The superior genicular nerve is a branch from common peroneal nerve and supplies the capsule of the knee joint.

E. The small saphenous vein perforates the roof of the fossa and drains into the popliteal vein.

Ellis H, Mahadevan V (2013). *Clinical Anatomy: Applied Anatomy for Students and Junior Doctors*, 13th edition (p. 276–9). Oxford, UK: John Wiley & Sons Ltd.

Sinnatamby CS (2011). *Last's Anatomy: Regional and Applied*, 12th edition (pp. 111–78). London, UK: Churchill Livingstone.

28. D.   The medial ligament may be torn when a violent abduction strain is applied.

A. In the valgus stress test, if a gap is produced on the medial side of the knee joint during abduction of the leg, the patient usually has a major medial and posterior ligament rupture. In minimal sprain, tenderness may be elicited with such test at the site of medial collateral ligament.

B. The collateral ligaments are likely to be injured when the knee is in full extension, as they are taut in this position.

C. The medial collateral ligament injuries are the most common knee injuries.

D. Correct answer: When a violent abduction force is applied to the lateral aspect of the knee join or an indirect stress through abduction or rotation of the leg. The medial collateral ligament (MCL) is about 8–10 cm long. It is proximally attached to the medial femoral condyle and distally to the anterior medial tibia.

E. The stability of the knee joint depends more on the strength of its muscles than the ligaments.

Ellis H, Mahadevan V (2013). *Clinical Anatomy: Applied Anatomy for Students and Junior Doctors*, 13th edition (p. 250–3). Oxford, UK: John Wiley & Sons Ltd.

Sinnatamby CS (2011). *Last's Anatomy: Regional and Applied*, 12th edition (pp. 111–78). London, UK: Churchill Livingstone.

UpToDate (2017). Medial collateral ligament injury of the knee. Available at: https://www.uptodate. com/contents/medial-collateral-ligament-injury-of-the-knee

29. D.   The ACL may be torn in violent hyperextension of the knee.

A. The distal attachment of the ACL is on the anterior part of the tibial plateau in-between the attachments of the anterior horns of the medial and lateral meniscus.

B. Its proximal attachment is to the posterolateral aspect of the lateral femoral condyle.

C. The PCL is stronger and shorter than the ACL.

D. Correct answer. The ACL may be torn in both contact and non-contact sports. It is taut in extension and a direct blow causing hyperextension or valgus rotation of the knee may result in ACL injury. Non-contact injuries are more common (70% of ACL tears are non-contact). It occurs in athletes when, during running or jumping, they suddenly change direction causing rotation or valgus stress on the knee. Injury during skiing occurs with the similar mechanism.

E. The cruciate ligaments are intracapsular, but extrasynovial. The ligaments are covered by synovial membrane from the front and sides, but not from the posterior aspect.

Ellis H, Mahadevan V (2013). *Clinical Anatomy: Applied Anatomy for Students and Junior Doctors*, 13th edition (p. 250–3). Oxford, UK: John Wiley & Sons Ltd.

Sinnatamby CS (2011). *Last's Anatomy: Regional and Applied*, 12th edition (pp. 111–78). London, UK: Churchill Livingstone.

UpToDate (2017). Anterior cruciate ligament injury. Available at: https://www.uptodate.com/contents/anterior-cruciate-ligament-injury

30. A. Common peroneal nerve.

A. Correct answer: The common peroneal nerve, a branch from the sciatic nerve, is more commonly compressed when it wraps round the neck of fibula, resulting in acute foot drop. Because of the compression neuropathy, the patients have weakness of foot dorsiflexion and foot eversion because of involvement of the deep and superficial peroneal nerve. The dorsum of the foot and the lateral surface of the lower leg have the sensory impairment. The tendon reflexes are not affected.

B. In diabetic neuropathy, clinically the patients have pain followed by weakness in proximal leg. The symptoms/signs are not limited to one particular nerve, but involve lumbosacral nerve roots and peripheral nerves. There may be associated autonomic neuropathy.

C. The femoral nerve is rare but may occur following hip or pelvic fractures. Clinically the patient may have weakness of the quadriceps and iliopsoas muscles. In addition, the sensation is affected to the anterior and medial part of the thigh.

D. The LFCN is a sensory nerve emerged directly from the lumbar plexus. Compression of the nerve may cause the features of meralgia paraesthesia (i.e. impaired sensation on the lateral aspect of the thigh).

E. Posterior tibial nerve: The compression may occur on the medial aspect of the ankle joint as the nerve travels under the flexor retinaculum. It is also called tarsal tunnel syndrome. The patient usually has sensory impairment on the sole and the toes of the foot, which may be worse at night or on standing.

Ellis H, Mahadevan V (2013). *Clinical Anatomy: Applied Anatomy for Students and Junior Doctors*, 13th edition (p. 233–4). Oxford, UK: John Wiley & Sons Ltd.

UpToDate (2017). Overview of lower extremity peripheral nerve syndromes. Available at: https://www.uptodate.com/contents/overview-of-lower-extremity-peripheral-nerve-syndromes

31. A. Anterior talofibular ligament.

A. Correct answer: Lateral ankle sprain is very common injury occurs when the joint is in inversion with the foot in a planter-flexed position. The lateral ligament complex constitutes anterior talofibular, calcaneofibular, and posterior talofibular ligaments. The anterior talofibular ligament is injured first with such a mechanism, which is followed by injury to the calcaneofibular ligament with increasing force. The isolated calcaneofibular ligament injury is uncommon. The ankle joint is unstable when all the three ligaments are injured. There are three grades of ankle sprains: Grade 1: Mild swelling and tenderness with only stretching of the ligament. There is no joint instability. In Grade II there is partial tear of the ligament, in which the patients will have moderate swelling and tenderness. There may be mild joint instability. Grade III will involve complete tear of a ligament, with all the discussed features of severe degrees. The joint is unstable.

B. Anterior tibiofibular ligament is a part of syndesmotic sprain, which may occur in dorsiflexion and/or eversion of the ankle joint. The syndesmotic structures include anterior tibiofibular, posterior tibiofibular, transverse tibiofibular ligaments, and interosseous membrane, which are essential for ankle stability.

C. See answer A.

D. The deltoid ligament complex is situated on the medial side of the joint and is the strongest ligament around the ankle. As a result, often forced eversion causes an avulsion fracture of the tip of the medial malleolus rather than rupture of the ligament.

E. See answer B.

Ellis H, Mahadevan V (2013). *Clinical Anatomy: Applied Anatomy for Students and Junior Doctors*, 13th edition (p. 253–5). Oxford, UK: John Wiley & Sons Ltd.

UpToDate (2017). Ankle sprain. Available at: https://www.uptodate.com/contents/ankle-sprain

32. A. The great saphenous vein drains the medial part of the dorsal foot.

    A. Correct answer: The great saphenous vein drains the venous plexus from the medial part of the dorsum of the foot and travels in front of the medial malleolus upwards. It crosses the posterior part of the medial tibial and femoral condyles. It pierces the deep fascia at the saphenous opening 2.5 cm below the inguinal ligament to enter the femoral vein.

    B. See A.

    C. The short (small) saphenous vein drains the blood from the lateral side of the foot, and travels behind the lateral malleolus. It courses over the back of the calf and terminates in popliteal vein in the popliteal fossa. It is accompanied by sural nerve, a sensory branch of the tibial nerve.

    D. The position of the great saphenous vein is constant immediately in front of the medial malleolus.

    E. The saphenous nerve accompanies the great saphenous vein with its tributaries in front and behind. It can be caught up by a ligature during cannulation and cause severe pain.

Ellis H, Mahadevan V (2013). *Clinical Anatomy: Applied Anatomy for Students and Junior Doctors*, 13th edition (p. 269–71). Oxford, UK: John Wiley & Sons Ltd.

33. A. Left anterior descending artery.

ST elevation in the anterolateral leads with reciprocal depression is typical for a lateral Myocardial Infarct. The lateral wall of the left ventricle is predominantly supplied by the left anterior descending artery, although it does have some supply from the left circumflex artery.

The right coronary artery and its branches supply the right ventricle and varying portions of the atria.

Sinnatamby CS (2011). *Last's Anatomy: Regional and Applied*, 12th edition (pp. 37–109). London, UK: Churchill Livingstone.

34. D. The ribs attach to the sternum via its costal cartilage.

The sternum is made up of three parts: the manubrium, the body, and the xiphoid process or xiphisternum. The angle of Louis is the joint between the manubrium and body of the sternum and is at the level of T4. The xiphoid process has no ribs attached to it. The first rib articulates with the manubrium.

Sinnatamby CS (2011). *Last's Anatomy: Regional and Applied*, 12th edition (pp. 37–109). London, UK: Churchill Livingstone.

35. B. T4.

Shingles is a reactivation of dormant varicella zoster virus. It affects a single nerve route and therefore has a dermatomal distribution that does not cross the midline.

T4 is the dermatome that involves the nipples.

The T8 and T10 dermatomes cover the xiphoid process and umbilicus, respectively.

Drake R (2004). *Gray's Anatomy for Students*. London, UK: Churchill Livingstone.

36. B. The eleventh and twelfth ribs are sometimes called floating ribs.

The eleventh and twelfth ribs can be called floating ribs, as they have no anterior connection to the sternum. Most of the ribs articulate both with their own vertebra but also the one above it. Exceptions are the first, eleventh, and twelfth ribs, which own articulate with one vertebra. There are 12 ribs bilaterally. The false ribs are numbers 8–10. They do attach to the sternum, but not directly, and instead are joined via a ligament. The ribs ossify from back to front to allow the anterior aspect to remain cartilage.

Standring S (2016). *Gray's Anatomy*, 41st edition. London, UK: Elsevier Ltd.

37. D.   The neurovascular bundle lies between the internal and innermost intercostal muscle layers.

A. The blunt dissection during the chest drain insertion goes through three layers of muscles: the external, internal, and innermost intercostal muscle layers. These are thin layers of muscular and tendinous fibres occupying the intercostal spaces.

B. The skin of the thorax is supplied by the cutaneous branches of cervical and thoracic nerves consecutively. The ventral rami of the first to eleventh nerves travels into the appropriate intercostal space giving off a lateral cutaneous branch, which arises beyond the angle of the rib and divides into anterior and posterior branches. It terminates near the sternum as the anterior cutaneous branch.

C. The neurovascular bundle is organized as vein, artery, and nerve.

D. Correct answer: The neurovascular bundle lies in-between the internal and innermost intercostal muscle layers.

E. The neurovascular bundle lies just below each rib in a groove (costal groove). Hence it is advised to dissect the plane of muscle layers just above the rib below (the sixth rib in this case) to avoid damage to these structures.

Standring S (2016). Chest wall and breast. In: *Gray's Anatomy*, 41st edition (Chapter 53; pp. 931–52). London, UK: Elsevier Ltd.

38. D.   The sensation from the central diaphragm is carried by the phrenic nerve.

A. The blunt dissection during the chest drain insertion goes through three layers of muscles: the external, internal, and innermost intercostal muscle layers. These are thin layers of muscular and tendinous fibres occupying the intercostal spaces.

B. The skin of the thorax is supplied by the cutaneous branches of cervical and thoracic nerves consecutively. The ventral rami of the first to eleventh nerves travels into the appropriate intercostal space giving off a lateral cutaneous branch, which arises beyond the angle of the rib and divides into anterior and posterior branches. It terminates near the sternum as anterior cutaneous branch.

C. The neurovascular bundle is organized as vein, artery, and nerve.

D. Correct answer: The neurovascular bundle lies in-between the internal and innermost intercostal muscle layers.

E. The neurovascular bundle lies just below each rib in a groove (costal groove). Hence it is advised to dissect the plane of muscle layers just above the rib below (the sixth rib in this case) to avoid damage to these structures.

Ellis H, Mahadevan V (2013). *Clinical Anatomy: Applied Anatomy for Students and Junior Doctors*, 13th edition (p. 269–71). Oxford, UK: John Wiley & Sons Ltd.

Standring S (2016). Chest wall and breast. In: *Gray's Anatomy*, 41st edition (Chapter 53; pp. 931–52). London, UK: Elsevier Ltd.

40. E.   The right main bronchus is shorter and wider than the left main bronchus.

A. The foreign body has tendency to go to the right main bronchus because it has greater width and runs more vertical course. For the same reason, the aspirated contents also travel through the right main bronchus to the right middle and lower lobes of the right lung.

B. The left main bronchus does not give off any branch outside the hilum of the lungs.

C. The left main bronchus enters the hilum of the lungs at the level of T6.

D. The right main bronchus enters the hilum of the lung opposite T5.

E. Correct answer: The right main bronchus is about 1 inch (2.5 cm) long and passes directly to the root of the lung. The left main bronchus is 2 inches (5 cm) long and enters the hilum opposite T6.

Ellis H, Mahadevan V (2013). *Clinical Anatomy: Applied Anatomy for Students and Junior Doctors*, 13th edition (p. 25). Oxford, UK: John Wiley & Sons Ltd.

41. B. The right middle lobe.

A. The consolidation in the right lower lobe would obliterate the margin of the right hemidiaphragm. As the hemidiaphragm is clearly visible, the consolidation is not in the lower lobe.

B. Correct answer: As the right border of the heart is obliterated, the consolidation is in the right middle lobe.

C. A consolidation in the right middle and lower lobes would obliterate both the right heart border and the right hemidiaphragm.

D. The subdiaphragmatic lesion may produce an effusion in the pleural cavity, but may also cause elevation of the right hemidiaphragm, lungs abscesses, and so on.

E. The consolidation in the upper lobe would show opacity in the apical and upper lobe area of the lungs. In this case there is no abnormality in the upper lobe.

Matone L (2016). Pulmonary infections. In: Hani A (Ed.), *Emergency Radiology*. Oxford, UK: Oxford University Press.

42. E. Only 15% of patients with PE have signs of DVT.

A. Hypoxaemia is not only because of pulmonary arterial obstruction, but also contributed by the alveolar collapse, inflammatory reactions resulting in further vasoconstriction.

B. In most PEs, the thrombus is lodged in the main lobar, segmental or subsegmental pulmonary artery. PE are typically multiple with the lower lobes being involved in majority of cases.

C. In PE pulmonary vascular resistance is increased due to the physical obstruction and hypoxaemic vasoconstriction of the vessels. The whole process impedes right ventricular outflow resulting in right ventricular dilatation, which in turn diminishes left ventricular preload and reduced cardiac output may result in death. Sudden death may occur due to acute right ventricular failure.

D. The pleuritic chest pain is because of the peripheral lung infarction and associated inflammatory reaction of the adjacent pleura.

E. Correct. The common source is deep vein thrombosis of lower limbs, which can be found in 70–80% of patients with PE if sensitive diagnostic methods are used. However, obvious clinical signs of DVT are found only in 15% of patients.

Katritsis KD, Gersh BJ, Camm AJ (2016). Pulmonary embolism. In: Camm J, Gersh BJ, Katritsis DG (Eds.), *Clinical Cardiology: Current Practice Guidelines* (Chapter 76). Oxford, UK: Oxford University Press.

National Institute for Health and Care Excellence (NICE) (2015). Clinical Knowledge Summaries. Pulmonary embolism. Available at: https://cks.nice.org.uk/pulmonary-embolism

UpToDate (2017). Overview of acute pulmonary embolism in adults. Available at: https://www.uptodate.com/contents/overview-of-acute-pulmonary-embolism-in-adults

42. A. Crack cocaine may be a high-risk condition for aortic dissection.

A. Correct answer: The following conditions are associated with aortic dissection: a) hypertension; b) collagen disorders (Ehlers–Danlos syndrome, Marfan syndrome, and so on); c) pre-existing aortic aneurysm; d) bicuspid aortic valve; e) aortic surgery; f) aortic coarctation; g) Turner syndrome; h) pregnancy and delivery; i) inflammatory diseases (giant cell arteritis, syphilitic aortisits, and so on); j) traumatic. Crack cocaine may cause transient rise in BP due to catecholamine release, may result in aortic dissection.

B. Around 50–65% of aortic tears originate in ascending aorta. About 20–30% originate near left subclavian artery and extend into the descending aorta.

C. Pulse deficit may occur because of the intimal flap or compression by haematoma. Pulse deficit is common in aortic arch and/ or thoracoabdominal aorta involvement (19–30%) compared with 9–21% in descending aortic involvement.

D. There is increased mortality in patients with pulse deficits.

E. The primary event in aortic dissection is intimal tear. Blood travels through the tear into the media separating intima from the surrounding media and/or adventitia creating a false lumen.

UpToDate (2017). Clinical features and diagnosis of acute aortic dissection. Available at: https://www.uptodate.com/contents/clinical-features-and-diagnosis-of-acute-aortic-dissection

43. A. Airflow obstruction is contributed by smooth muscle spasm, oedema, and mucus production.

A. Correct answer: Following exposure to allergic or non-allergic stimuli, the bronchoconstriction occurs because of release of mediators from inflammatory cells resulting in oedema, inflammation, mucus production, and airway smooth muscle spasms.

B. The trachea and extrapulmonary airways contain incomplete cartilaginous rings joined by fibrous tissue and smooth muscles. The intrapulmonary airways have discontinuous islands of such cartilages in their walls. There is no cartilage in the bronchioles and they do not contribute to airflow obstruction.

C. Numerous mast cells are present in the connective tissue of respiratory tree, especially towards the bronchioles. The histamine-containing granules are released after exposure to irritants, allergens, and so on.

D. The smooth muscles are present in the extrapulmonary airways. In the intrapulmonary airways, it gradually becomes thinner towards the periphery and finally disappears at the level of alveoli. The alveoli are thin-walled pouches with two types of epithelial cells on delicate connective tissue within which a network of capillaries exists for smooth gas exchange.

E. The epithelia of trachea, bronchi, and bronchioles are like each other. The larger intrapulmonary and extrapulmonary airways are lined by ciliated pseudostratified epithelium. There are fewer cilia in the terminal and respiratory bronchioles. The cell heights are reduced form columnar to cuboidal. In the alveoli, the cells are cuboidal and non-ciliated.

Standring S (2016). Pleura, lungs, trachea and bronchi. In: Sandring, S. (Ed.), *Gray's Anatomy*, 41st edition (Chapter 54; pp. 953–69). London, UK; Elsevier.

44. E. The whole of the mediastinal pleura is innervated by the phrenic nerves.

A. A spontaneous pneumothorax may not always need tube thoracostomy. The primary small pneumothoraces may be left alone to be resolved spontaneously. Some requires aspirations. The secondary spontaneous pneumothoraces may require tube thoracostomy following the Seldinger technique.

B. The mediastinal pleura are a part of parietal pleura. The other parts of parietal pleura are the costovertebral pleura (lining the internal thoracic wall and vertebral bodies), the diaphragmatic pleura (covering the muscular surface of the diaphragm), and the cervical pleura (covering the pulmonary apices).

C. The peripheral diaphragmatic pleura are innervated by the intercostal nerves. The mediastinal and central parts of the diaphragm are innervated by the phrenic nerves.

D. The visceral pleura is an integral part of the lungs and cannot be separated from except at the hilum and along a line descending from the root which denotes the attachment of the pulmonary ligament.

E. Correct answer: see also answer C. Standring S (2016). Pleura, lungs, trachea and bronchi. In: *Gray's Anatomy*, 41st edition (Chapter 54; pp. 953–69). London, UK; Elsevier.

45. A. 200–250 mL of fluid is necessary to produce cardiomegaly on chest radiograph.

A. Correct answer.

B. About 80% of blood supply to pericardium is through both sided internal thoracic arteries via pericardiophrenic branches. The intercostal and superior phrenic arteries may supply small branches to the pericardium inferiorly.

C. Normally the pericardial cavity contains 15–20 mL of serous plasma ultrafiltrate.

D. Pain from parietal pericardium is mainly transmitted by the phrenic nerves, while pain from serous pericardium is carried by sympathetic fibres. Vagus also supplies the pericardium via the oesophageal plexus and recurrent laryngeal nerve.

E. Pericardial effusion causes compression of the right atrium, reducing the venous return, and therefore the cardiac output.

Jouriles N (2010). Pericardial and myocardial disease. In: Hockberger RS, Walls RM (Eds.), *Rosen's Emergency Medicine*, 7th edition (Chapter 80, pp. 1054–9). Philadelphia, PA: Mosby Elsevier.

Standring S (2016). Heart. In: *Gray's Anatomy*, 41st edition (Chapter 57; pp. 994–1023). London, UK; Elsevier.

46. C. The left main bronchus crosses the oesophagus about 28 cm from the upper incisor teeth.

A. Aortic arch lies in the superior mediastinum and the distal part of the arch crosses the oesophagus in this part.

B. Following the rupture of oesophagus, the content may escape to the neck through the superior mediastinum and to the abdomen through various openings in the diaphragm (oesophageal aperture, aortic aperture, apertures within the diaphragmatic crura and the apertures deep to the medial lumbosacral arches.

C. Correct answer: In addition to this, the oesophagus is constricted at 15 cm, 23 cm as the aortic arch crosses, and 40 cm when it passes through the diaphragm from the incisor teeth.

D. The oesophageal opening lies at the level of T10 vertebral body.

E. There are two layers of muscles: the external longitudinal and the inner circular muscles, striated in the upper two-thirds and smooth in the lower one-third.

Ellis H, Mahadevan V (2013). *Clinical Anatomy: Applied Anatomy for Students and Junior Doctors*, 13th edition (pp. 46–50). Oxford, UK: John Wiley & Sons Ltd.

Standring S (2016). Mediastinum. In: *Gray's Anatomy*, 41st edition (Chapter 56; pp. 976–93). London, UK; Elsevier.

47. C.   The breast overlies the second to sixth rib in the vertical axis.

A. Two-thirds of the breast sits on the pectoralis major and one-third on the serratus anterior.

B. The breast tissue lies between the superficial fascia and deep pectoral fascia overlying the pectoral muscles.

C. Correct answer: It overlies from the second to sixth ribs on vertical axis and sternal edge. In the horizontal axis, it extends between the sternal edge and the midaxillary line.

D. The principal blood supply is from the internal mammary artery (hence the name). Approximately one-third of the blood supply (mainly to the upper outer quadrant) is provided by the axillary artery via lateral thoracic and acromiothoracic arteries. The intercostal arteries provide some blood supply through the lateral perforating branches, an unimportant source.

E. The nipple does not contain any hair follicles. It has abundant sensory nerve endings, and sebaceous and apocrine glands. The skin of the breast contains hair follicles, and the two types of glands.

Ellis H, Mahadevan V (2013). *Clinical Anatomy: Applied Anatomy for Students and Junior Doctors*, 13th edition (pp. 210–14). Oxford, UK: John Wiley & Sons Ltd.

UpToDate (2017). Breast development and morphology. Available at: https://www.uptodate.com/contents/breast-development-and-morphology

48. B.   Left anterior descending coronary artery.

The ECG shows the deep T-wave insertion across the anterior leads. This is caused by the stenosis of the left anterior descending coronary artery (see Table 1.1 for the territories of the coronary arteries and ECG changes associated with involvement of each artery)

A. Circumflex artery runs posteriorly in the left atrioventricular (AV) groove and gives obtuse marginal branches to the lateral wall of the left ventricle (LV) supplying the posterior wall of LV. When occluded, the ECG changes occur as mirror images in V1–V2 or V3 (i.e. ST segment depression ± inferior changes: tall R in V1).

B. Correct answer: The left anterior descending artery runs in the anterior interventricular groove supplying the anterior wall of the heart. It gives off septal branches that supply blood to the anterior two-thirds of the interventricular septum and left bundle branch. The changes in the ECG are in the leads V4–V6, I, VL for anterolateral, and V1–V4 and left bundle branch block (LBBB) in anteroseptal.

C. The left main stem arises from the left aortic sinus and soon gives rise to the left anterior descending and circumflex coronary arteries.

D. The right coronary artery normally has separate origin from the right coronary sinus. It runs in the right AV groove and gives branches to the sinoatrial (SA) node, AV node, and right ventricle (RV). On reaching to the posterior interventricular groove, it gives rise to the posterior descending artery which supplies the inferior wall of the LV and the inferior one-third of the interventricular septum. When affected, the ECG changes are noticed in II, III, and aVF, and ST elevation in V4R and V6R.

E. See D.

Myerson SG, Choudhury RP, Mitchell AR (2010). *Emergencies in Cardiology*, 2nd edition. Oxford, UK: Oxford University Press.

Table 1.1 Coronary artery territories with changes which may occur during a myocardial infarction

Site of arterial occlusion	Myocardial territory	ECG changes
LAD	Anterolateral	V4–V6, I, VL
	Anteroseptal	V1–V4
		LBBB
LCX	Posterior	Mirror image changes in V1–V2 or V3 (i.e. ST segment depression ± inferior changes; tall R in V1). May be electrically silent on standard 12-lead ECG
RCA	Inferior wall of LV	II, III, aVF
	RV	ST elevation V4R to V6R

49. C. The gall bladder can hold about 50 mL of bile.

A. The Calot's triangle is formed by the common hepatic duct, the cystic duct, and the liver. The cystic artery is the content of the triangle.

B. Hartmann's pouch is a small sac type structure, which is found in a dilated pathological gall bladder on its ventral side just proximal to the neck. Gallstones may be lodged in the pouch.

C. Correct answer: The gall bladder can hold about 50 mL of bile. It acts as concentrator and reservoir.

D. There is no vein called cystic vein. The venous drainage from the gall bladder occurs through small veins travelling from the gall bladder directly to liver bed, and then to tributaries of right portal vein.

E. The main content of bile is cholesterol and bile acids.

Ellis H, Mahadevan V (2013). *Clinical Anatomy: Applied Anatomy for Students and Junior Doctors*, 13th edition. Oxford, UK: John Wiley & Sons Ltd.

50. B. The portal vein is formed behind the neck of the pancreas.

A. The *Islets of Langerhans* situated in-between the alveoli secrete insulin into blood stream: the endocrine function.

B. Correct answer: The portal vein is formed behind the neck of pancreas by joining of splenic vein and the superior mesenteric vein.

C. The tortuous splenic artery, one of the three main branches of coeliac axis runs along the upper border of the pancreas. The splenic vein runs behind the gland.

D. The uncinate process hooks posteriorly to the superior mesenteric vessels.

E. The veins from pancreas drain into portal system.

Ellis H, Mahadevan V (2013). *Clinical Anatomy: Applied Anatomy for Students and Junior Doctors*, 13th edition. Oxford, UK: John Wiley & Sons Ltd.

51. D. The internal inguinal ring lies about 1.2 cm above the femoral pulse.

A. A direct inguinal hernia pushes through the posterior wall of the inguinal canal. As it is medial to the internal inguinal ring, it cannot be controlled by finger pressure applied immediately above the femoral pulse.

B. An indirect inguinal hernia emerges through the external inguinal ring, and lies above and medial to the pubic tubercle.

C. The direct inguinal hernia emerges through the posterior wall. The indirect inguinal hernia through the internal ring.

D. Correct answer: The patient's hernia is irreducible or obstructed because of inability to reduce through the narrow internal ring. The constriction at the internal ring further compromises the blood supply, resulting in swelling of the gut and congestion of the vascular drainage leading to gangrene of the bowel in the herniated sac. Therefore, such situations are treated as an emergency.

E. The mid-inguinal point lies between the anterior superior iliac spine and the symphysis pubis.

Ellis H, Mahadevan V (2013). *Clinical Anatomy: Applied Anatomy for Students and Junior Doctors*, 13th edition. Oxford, UK: John Wiley & Sons Ltd.

52. B. The appendicular artery is an end artery.

A. The afferent nerve from appendix enters the spinal cord at the tenth thoracic segment. Distension and inflammation of appendix results in afferent signals, which are responsible for the initial symptoms of colicky pain with or without vomiting. The initial pain is referred to the mid abdomen (around umbilicus) because of its origin from midgut, and poorly localized. Localization of pain in the right iliac fossa (RIF) is due to stimulation of somatic nociceptors.

B. Correct answer: Though the base of the appendix has a rich arterial anastomosis, but the appendicular artery is an end artery. As the artery is near the appendicular wall, during appendicitis it is susceptible to thrombosis. Hence there is a high frequency of gangrenous perforation in acute appendicitis.

C. The attachment of the base of appendix to caecum is constant on its posteromedial wall below the ileocolic junction. The appendix usually situated in the RIF, but its tip lies in variable positions. The most common position of the tip is retrocaecal, retrocolic, or pelvic. These normal variances may make the diagnosis of appendicitis difficult. The surface marking of the base of the appendix is described as McBurney's point, which is a point a third of the way along a line drawn between umbilicus and ASIS. The position is variable.

D. There are no lymphoid follicles at birth. They start accumulating in the first 10 years of life to become prominent.

E. The appendix has B and T lymphoid cells in its mucosa and submucosa, which is absent in the caecum. It operates as a part of gut-associated lymphoid tissue system. The large lymphoid aggregates may narrow or obstruct the appendicular lumen and lead to appendicitis.

Lunniss PJ (2016). Large intestine. In: *Gray's Anatomy*, 41st edition (Chapter 66). London, UK: Elsevier.

UpToDate, Acute appendicitis in adults: Clinical manifestations and differential diagnosis. Available at: https://www.uptodate.com/contents/acute-appendicitis-in-adults-clinical-manifestations-and-differential-diagnosis

53. D. Superior gastric artery.

A. The deep circumflex iliac artery, a branch from the external iliac artery, travels into the lower part of the abdomen and supplies the lateral and lower part of the abdomen.

B. The inferior epigastric artery, also called the deep inferior epigastric artery, arises from the external iliac artery. It ascends along the medial border of the deep inguinal ring. It anastomoses with the superior gastric artery above the level of the umbilicus. This artery is forms the lateral border of Hesselbach's triangle. The base of the triangle is formed by the inguinal ligament and the medial border is by the lateral margin of the rectus abdominis muscle.

C. Superficial epigastric artery, a branch from femoral artery, also supplies the lateral aspect of the abdomen.

D. Correct answer: Superior epigastric artery is the terminal branch from internal thoracic artery. It enters the rectus sheath from above after descending between the xiphoid and costal slips of the diaphragm. Blunt injury in the upper abdomen may result in bleeding from this vessel.

E. Thoracoepigastric artery: This is a very rare branch from the axillary artery. There is no constant artery in this name. The thoracoepigastric vein drains blood from the anterolateral part of the anterior abdominal wall and to lateral thoracic vein ending into axillary vein.

Standring S (2016). Anterior abdominal wall. In: *Gray's Anatomy*, 41st edition (Chapter 61; pp. 1069–82). London, UK: Elsevier Ltd.

54. A. Blood through inferior mesenteric vein drains eventually into portal vein.

A. Correct answer: The inferior mesenteric vein joins the splenic vein, but occasionally it may drain into the superior mesenteric vein. Eventually it drains into portal vein.

B. The inferior mesenteric artery supplies the colon, which also receives supply from the superior mesenteric artery (SMA). The rectum receives its blood supply from the superior rectal artery, which is the terminal continuation of the inferior mesenteric artery.

C. The superficial mesenteric artery supplies the whole of small intestine except the proximal duodenum. It also supplies the proximal colon.

D. The superior vein travelling right to the artery crosses the third part of the duodenum and is joined by the splenic vein to form portal vein behind the neck of the pancreas.

E. The splenic flexure is the area prone to ischaemia, because the marginal artery of Drummond is very small in this area. The rectosigmoid junction is also a weak area prone to ischaemia, called Sudek's point, the anastomotic area between the left colic artery and superior colic artery.

Standring S (2016). Small intestine. In: *Gray's Anatomy*, 41st edition (Chapter 65; pp. 1069–82). London, UK: Elsevier Ltd.

UpToDate (2017). Overview of intestinal ischemia in adults. Available at: https://www.uptodate.com/contents/overview-of-intestinal-ischemia-in-adults

55. B. The lesser sac.

A. Hepatorenal pouch (right subhepatic space). The space, a part of greater sac, is between the inferior surface of the right lobe of the liver and right kidney. In the supine position, it is the more dependent part than the right paracolic gutter. Fluid may be collected in this space by travelling from below through the paracolic gutter or escaping from the lesser sac via the foramen of Winslow.

B. Correct answer: The lesser sac (Omental bursa) is a peritoneal cavity behind the stomach. Through the epiploic foramen (of Winslow) it opens into the greater sac. The anterior wall is formed by the posterior layer of lesser omentum, the posterior surface of the stomach and the posterior of the two layers of the greater omentum. Hence, fluid will initially escape to the lesser omentum if there is perforation of the posterior surface of the stomach.

C. The right subhepatic space is situated behind the right lobe of liver and in front of the right kidney. This space is closed above by inferior layer of coronary ligament and the small right triangular ligament. To the right, it is bounded by the diaphragm. On the left, it communicates with the lesser sac through the epiploic foramen. Inferiorly it is continuous with the right paracolic gutter. The fluid may escape from the lesser omentum to this space through the epiploic foramen and be detected by the FAST scan.

D. The right subphrenic space is situated between the diaphragm and the anterior, superior, and right lateral surface of the liver. As the peritoneal fluid flows clockwise in the abdomen, the fluid from the perforation of appendix or duodenal ulcer may be collected in this space.

E. The splenorenal recess is located between the spleen and fascia in front of the left kidney. It is an anatomical site commonly used to diagnose fluid accumulation in supine position by FAST scan.

Standring S (2016). Small intestine. In: *Gray's Anatomy*, 41st edition (Chapter 65; pp. 1069–82). London, UK: Elsevier Ltd.

56. E. Pain sensation is carried through the second to fourth sacral spinal nerves.

A. The anal canal is about 2–5 cm long in adults. The posterior wall is slightly longer than the anterior. Functionally it represents a zone of high pressure.

B. Anal verge is the external end of anal canal. At the anal verge, the squamous epithelium lining the lower anal canal is continuous with the skin of the perineum. The upper part of the anal canal is lined by the columnar epithelium.

C. Fissure-in-ano, most common in the posterior midline position, is below the dentate line. It occurs because the stretching of the mucosa goes beyond its normal capacity. The exposed internal sphincter goes into spasm following the occurrence of the fissure.

D. In the resting phase, the external anal sphincter (like the levator ani and internal anal sphincter) is tonically contracted (the postural reflex).

E. Correct answer: The external sphincter is innervated by the inferior rectal branch of the pudendal nerve, which contains the contribution from the second, third, and the fourth sacral spinal nerves. This nerve also carries the afferent fibres from the lining of the anal canal and perianal skin.

Standring S (2016). Small intestine. In: *Gray's Anatomy*, 41st edition (Chapter 65; pp. 1069–82). London, UK: Elsevier Ltd.

57. E. The most likely site of injury is the bulbar urethra.

A. The bulbar urethra is the widest part of the urethra. It starts below the perineal membrane and is surrounded by bulbospongiosus.

B. The membranous along with the preprostatic and prostatic urethra is a part of posterior urethra.

C. In such injuries, one of the features is that the urine may be extravasated between the perineal membrane and the membranous part of the superficial fascia (Colles' fascia). The urine may track anteriorly into the loose connective tissue of scrotum and penis, subsequently to anterior abdominal wall.

D. As the Colles' fascia is attached to the pubic and ischial rami, the urine cannot pass laterally. As the two layers are continuous around the superficial transverse perineal muscles, the extravasated urine cannot pass posteriorly.

E. Correct answer: The most likely site of injury is the bulbar urethra or at the junction of membranous and bulbar urethra.

Standring S (2016). Bladder, prostate and urethra. In: *Gray's Anatomy*, 41st edition (Chapter 75; pp. 1255–71). London, UK: Elsevier Ltd.

58. A.　Sensation of distension is carried by the parasympathetic predominantly.

A.　Correct answer: The sensation of pain and distension or spasm is due to stone travel through both the sympathetic and parasympathetic fibres, but predominantly the latter. The parasympathetic source is sacral nerves S2 to S4 and the sympathetic source is lumbar 1 and 2 segment, and lower thoracic segments.

B.　The internal sphincter has a rich supply of sympathetic fibres (noradrenargic), almost devoid of parasympathetic nerves (cholinergic). For most of the bladder, the sympathetic fibres are vasomotor and at the muscle of the bladder neck.

C.　The lining epithelium is transitional epithelium (urothelium), 4–7 cells thick.

D.　See answer A.

E.　See answer A.

Standring S (2016). Bladder, prostate and urethra. In: *Gray's Anatomy*, 41st edition (Chapter 75; pp. 1255–71). London, UK: Elsevier Ltd.

59. C.　The pain is because of tissue ischaemia.

A.　Fertility can be affected by a single episode of torsion.

B.　Permanent tissue loss can occur if the torsion is not relived by four to six hours. The testicular artery is a branch from the abdominal aorta. It runs with the spermatic cord through deep inguinal ring and reaches posterior aspect of the testis. Testicular veins form the pampiniform plexus in the spermatic cord. The veins (three to four in number) enter through the deep ring into the abdomen and ultimately as a single vein drains to the inferior vena cava (IVC) on the right and left renal vein on the left.

C.　Correct answer: The testis is innervated by sympathetic nerves at the T10 and T11 segment of the spinal cord. The fibres run along the testicular artery from celiac ganglia. The sensory fibres share the same sensory pathway.

D.　The Prehn sign is not a reliable sign to diagnose testicular torsion. The Prehn sign is when the scrotum is elevated, the pain in patients with epididymitis is relieved but remains unchanged in patients with testicular torsion.

E.　The torsion may be extravaginal or intravaginal. The tunica vaginalis is the layer covering testis and scrotal wall from inside contains a potential space called cavity of tunica vaginalis has a thin layer of fluid normally. If the rotation of testis involves both tunica vaginalis and testis, it is called intravaginal torsion. It the testis alone is rotated, it is extravaginal. The tunica vaginalis is intact in the later. In both the situation, the blood supply is affected resulting in testicular ischaemia.

Standring S (2016). Male reproductive system. In: *Gray's Anatomy*, 41st edition (Chapter 72; pp. 1271–87). London, UK: Elsevier Ltd.

UpToDate (2017). Evaluation of scrotal pain or swelling in children and adolescents. Available at: https://www.uptodate.com/contents/evaluation-of-scrotal-pain-or-swelling-in-children-and-adolescents

60. E.　The vesicoureteric junction.

The stone descending from the kidney could be arrested at one of the areas in the ureter, pelviureteric junction, pelvic brim (where it crosses common iliac artery), or the vesicoureteric junction. The latter, being the narrowest of all of them, may cause obstruction even with a stone of 2–3 mm size stone.

The pain is caused by the excessive distension of the ureter or muscle spasm. If the stone is obstructed in renal pelvic area, the pain could be located in the loin. The pain radiates to the groin/scrotum or labium majus when the stone is arrested in the lower ureter. The pain may be referred to the cutaneous areas supplied by T11 to L2, which also supplies the ureter.

A differential diagnosis of dissecting aneurysm and acute abdomen should be kept in mind if the pain has a variable location.

Standring S (2016). Kidney and ureter. In: *Gray's Anatomy*, 41st edition (Chapter 74; pp. 1237–54). London, UK: Elsevier Ltd.

UpToDate (2017). Diagnosis and acute management of suspected nephrolithiasis in adults. Available at: https://www.uptodate.com/contents/diagnosis-and-acute-management-of-suspected-nephrolithiasis-in-adults

61. E.   Renal artery arises at the level of L1 vertebral body.

  A. About 80% of abdominal aortic aneurysm occurs in the infrarenal segment of the aorta.
  B. Abdominal aorta enters the abdomen through the aortic hiatus in diaphragm in front of the twelfth thoracic vertebra. It descends in front of the bodies of lumbar vertebrae.
  C. It bifurcates in front of the body of the fourth lumbar vertebra or the L4/L5 disc into two common iliac arteries.
  D. Dorsal branches (inferior phrenic, lumbar and median sacral arteries) supply the body wall, vertebral column, vertebral canal and its content. The viscera of the abdomen are supplied by the anterior (Coeliac trunk, superior mesenteric and inferior mesenteric) and lateral branches (suprarenal, renal, and gonadal arteries).
  E. Renal arteries, the largest branches of aorta, originate below the superior mesenteric artery at about the level of the body of the L1 vertebra.

Standring S (2016). Posterior abdominal wall and retroperitoneum. In: *Gray's Anatomy*, 41st edition (Chapter 62; pp. 1083–97). London, UK: Elsevier Ltd.

62. C.   The jejunum.

This is a typical supine film of the abdomen in acute small bowel obstruction. In such cases, the proximal bowel is distended more than 2.5 cm and the distal bowel (distal to the obstruction) is collapsed. The small intestine is comprised of duodenum, jejunum, and ileum.

  A. The descending colon is situated along the left side of the abdomen. In this X-ray, the colon is not visible as there is no intraluminal gas could go into the colon because of the obstruction.
  B. Duodenum is the proximal part of the small intestine situated in the upper abdomen. Its initial 2.5 cm is intraperitoneal and the rest is retroperitoneal. The total length is about 10 cm. It forms the C-loop around the head of the pancreas at about the level of the L2 vertebra. The first part is at the level of L1, the third part at the level of L3, and the last part at L2. The duodenum is not clearly visible on the X-ray.
  C. Correct answer: The jejunum is situated in the upper left infracolic compartment. On supine films, it lies in the left upper abdomen. It has circular folds of mucosa called plicae circulares or valvulae conniventes, visible on X-ray film as concertina effects.
  D. On the supine abdominal films, the ileum tends to lie on the right lower abdomen and pelvis. On obstruction distal to the ileum, the distended ileum takes up the distended tube, which

does not have any conniventes. It appears plain and is often called 'characterless'. The ileum is not visible on this film.

E. The sigmoid colon is normally situated in the pelvic cavity. The large bowel in general has haustra, which runs only halfway through across the wall of the colon. These are visible on the distended colon. This organ is not visible as there is no gas going through the small bowel bypassing the obstruction.

Standring S (2016). Small intestine. In: *Gray's Anatomy*, 41st edition (Chapter 65; pp. 1124–35). London, UK: Elsevier Ltd.

63. D. Uterine arteries supply the medial two-thirds of the Fallopian tubes.

A. The venous drainage from uterine tubes goes through the ovarian and uterine veins. The right ovarian vein drains to the IVC directly, but the left ovarian vein drains to left renal vein. The venous drainage through uterine veins follows the uterine arteries and drains into the internal iliac veins.

B. Ovarian arteries arise from the abdominal aorta.

C. Usually the ovarian arteries supply the lateral third of the uterine tubes.

D. Correct answer: The uterine arteries generally supply the medial two-thirds of the uterine tubes.

E. The uterine arteries are the branches of internal iliac arteries.

Standring S (2016). Female reproductive system. In: *Gray's Anatomy*, 41st edition (Chapter 77; pp. 1288–313). London, UK: Elsevier Ltd.

64. B. Ilioinguinal nerve (L1).

A. Hypogastric nerves (right and left) originate from the superior hypogastric plexus, which consists of sympathetic fibres. It runs down to join the inferior hypogastric plexuses, which in turn joins the uterovaginal plexus, and is responsible for contraction of uterine tube, uterus, and upper vagina.

B. Correct answer: The sensory innervation of the anterior and posterior parts of the labium majus is different. The anterior third is supplied by the ilioinguinal nerve and the posterior two-thirds are supplied by the pudendal nerve (S2) (thorough the posterior labial branches of the perineal nerves). The lateral aspect is innervated by the perineal branches of the posterior cutaneous nerve of thigh (S2).

C. The pelvic splanchnic nerves originate from lateral horn of sacral segments 2 to 3 or 4, join the inferior hypogastric plexus, and provide parasympathetic innervation to the uterine tube and uterus.

D. See answer B.

E. See answer B. The pudendal nerve, a branch from sacral plexus (S2, 3, 4) innervates the skin of the external genitalia. When the nerve travels through the lateral wall of the ischioanal fossa, it lies in a canal called the pudendal canal (of Alcock) with the pudendal vessels. The nerves could be blocked providing regional anaesthesia during obstetric forceps delivery.

Ellis H, Mahadevan V (2013). *Clinical Anatomy: Applied Anatomy for Students and Junior Doctors*, 13th edition. Oxford, UK: John Wiley & Sons Ltd.

Standring S (2016). Female reproductive system. In: *Gray's Anatomy*, 41st edition (Chapter 77; pp. 1288–313). London, UK: Elsevier Ltd.

65. B. Loss of anal sphincter function is due to entrapment of the S3–S5 nerve roots.

The spinal cord extends from the base of the skull to the lower border of the L1 vertebral body, distal to which the cauda equina is formed by combining the lumbar, sacral, and coccygeal spinal nerve roots.

A. The autonomic bladder control is mainly by the parasympathetic. The innervation of the bladder is received from the S2–S3 spinal segments through the sacral plexus and pelvic nerves, which contain both the sensory and the motor components. Normally the stretch sensation from the bladder wall and the posterior urethra initiates the reflex causing the bladder emptying. The motor nerves transmitted to the bladder are parasympathetic which causes contraction of the detrusor. The external bladder sphincter receives its innervation through the pudendal nerve and the somatic nerve fibres, which control the voluntary function of the sphincter. From the L2 segment of the spinal cord, the bladder receives its sympathetic innervation through hypogastric nerves. The sympathetic fibres mainly stimulate the blood vessels and have little to do with bladder contractions. However, some sensory fibres are transmitted via sympathetic system and may be important in sensation of fullness and some pain. Injury to the S2–S4 spinal nerves due to disc prolapse may interrupt the bladder reflex circuit. Instead of emptying periodically, the bladder fills to capacity and overflows a few drops at a time—overflow incontinence. If the cord lesion is above the S2 level of the cord interrupting the descending fibres, it produces an 'automatic bladder'. The bladder empties reflexively when expanded to a certain degree, as it is no longer controlled by the brain.

B. Correct answer: Anal sphincter paralysis usually is caused by damage to the S2–S4 sacral nerve roots. The external anal sphincter, which has innervation from pudendal nerves (S2–S4), is under voluntary control. The internal anal sphincter is supplied by the sympathetic and parasympathetic nerves. Stimulation of the parasympathetic fibres causes the internal anal sphincter to relax and longitudinal anal muscle contraction, whereas stimulation of the sympathetic nerves causes contraction of both the internal sphincter and longitudinal muscles.

C. The ankle jerk is mediated via the S1 nerve root. The nerve root between L4/L5 is L4, which is the proximal to the area of the insult. The loss of ankle jerk in this case is because of involvement of the S1 nerve root by the central prolapse of the L5 disc.

D. The skin's sensation in the perianal area is supplied by the S2–S4 nerve roots. A central disc prolapse may cause damage to these nerve roots, causing loss of sensation in the perianal area.

E. The sensory afferent fibres from the medial side of the leg are carried to the L4 segment of the spinal cord, which is not affected in this case.

Hall JE (2010). *Guyton and Hall: Textbook of Medical Physiology*, 12th edition (p. 310). Philadelphia, PA: Saunders Elsevier Ltd.

UpToDate (2017). Anatomy and localization of spinal cord disorders. Available at: https://www.uptodate.com/contents/anatomy-and-localization-of-spinal-cord-disorders

66. B. The great palatine artery is a branch of the maxillary artery.

The most common site of bleeding in epistaxis is from Little's area. This area of the nasal septum contains the anastomosis of four arteries:

- Anterior ethmoid artery (a branch of the ophthalmic artery)
- Great palatine artery (a branch of the maxillary artery)
- Sphenopalatine artery (a branch of the maxillary artery)
- Superior labial artery (a branch of the facial artery)

Standring S (2016). Nose, nasal cavity and paranasal sinuses. In: *Gray's Anatomy*, 41st edition (Chapter 33; pp. 556–70). London, UK: Elsevier Ltd.

67. C. The frontal sinus.

The likely diagnosis is acute sinusitis. This usually occurs after an upper respiratory tract infection when the cilia fail to work as efficiently and drainage through the ostium of the sinuses slows. This results in an accumulation of fluid in the frontal and maxillary sinuses and causes pain, which is typically worse on bending forwards.

Warner G, Burgess A, Patel S, et al. (2009). *OSH Otolaryngology and Head and Neck Surgery*. Oxford, UK: Oxford University Press.

68. C. The superficial temporal artery.

A. The occipital artery ascends in the neck from the external carotid artery. The branches supply the occipital belly of occipitofrontalis and the skin and pericranium associated with the scalp up to the vertex.

B. The posterior auricular artery is also a branch from external carotid artery and ascends between the auricle and the mastoid process. It supplies the cranial surface of the auricle, the occipital belly of occipitofrontalis, and the scalp behind and above the auricle.

C. Correct answer: The superficial temporal artery is the terminal branch of the external carotid artery. It arises in the parotid gland behind the neck of the mandible. The artery supplies the side of the face, the scalp, the parotid gland, and the temporomandibular joint.

D. The supraorbital artery is a branch of the ophthalmic artery, which leaves the orbit via supraorbital notch or foramen. It supplies the skin of the forehead, the skin and the muscles of the upper eyelid, and the scalp.

E. Zygomatico-orbital artery, a branch from superficial temporal artery, supplies the orbicularis oculi.

Standring S (2016). Face and scalp. In: *Gray's Anatomy*, 41st edition (Chapter 30; pp. 475–506). London, UK: Elsevier Ltd.

69. D. Skin, connective tissue, aponeurosis, loose areolar tissue, periosteum.

The layers of the scalp are best remembered as the acronym SCALP:

- **S**kin
- **C**onnective tissue
- **A**poneurosis
- **L**oose areolar tissue
- **P**eriosteum

Ellis H, Mahadevan V (2013). The head and neck. In: *Clinical Anatomy: Applied Anatomy for Students and Junior Doctors*, 13th edition (p. 342). Oxford, UK: John Wiley & Sons Ltd.

70. D. The tongue has bilateral lymph node drainage.

A. Chemotherapy is not used as a curative monotherapy for tongue cancer currently. It is used for symptoms control in palliation and in conjunction with radiotherapy and surgery to be curative.

B. The early stages of tongue cancer are usually painless. It may become painful in advanced stages of the disease.

C. Lifestyle choices such as smoking are thought to be a major risk factor for developing tongue cancer, but once the disease is present stopping these choices is unlikely to affect the cancer.

D. Correct answer: The tongue is a midline structure; hence, it has bilateral midline lymph drainage. Therefore, the spread of the cancer, if not caught early enough, may be substantial to both sides of the neck. Once the cancer has spread bilaterally, surgery becomes more technically difficult and outcomes are worse.

E. Although weight loss is important with any tongue problem, this is regardless of the diagnosis and can be treated with alternative feeding options such as nasogastric tube or percutaneous endoscopy gastrostomy tube feeding.

UpToDate (2017). Treatment of stage I and II (early) head and neck cancer: The oral cavity. Available at: https://www.uptodate.com/contents/treatment-of-stage-i-and-ii-early-head-and-neck-cancer-the-oral-cavity

71. D. The interarytenoid notch is at the posterior point of the vocal cords.

During laryngoscopy, it is most common in adult patients to place the tip of the blade into the vallecula, the space anterior to the epiglottis, and pull upwards to move the epiglottis out of the way. It does, however, keep it in view. During the intubation of young children, a different technique is used, and the blade can be put posterior to the epiglottis to move it from the view of the cords.

The oesophagus lies posterior to the trachea and the vocal cords.

The aryepiglottic fold is the outermost ring with the ventricular folds sitting interior that that and then the vocal cords.

The oesophageal opening is not considered to be a landmark during this procedure.

Standring S (2016). Larynx. In: *Gray's Anatomy*, 41st edition (Chapter 35; pp. 586–604). London, UK: Elsevier Ltd.

Yealy DM, Callaway C (2013). *Emergency Department Critical Care*. Oxford, UK: Oxford University Press.

72. B. 2

Mallampati scoring is used to predict the difficulty of intubation, with low scores being easier than high scores. It is done by sitting directly opposite the patient, at the same level, and asking them the open their mouth and stick out their tongue. The score is then made dependent upon which structures can be seen.

Mallampati 1—The tonsils, uvula, soft palate, and hard palate are visible. This is reassuring and generally associated with a good view at laryngoscopy.

Mallampati 2—The soft palate and hard palate are visible, but the lower parts of the tonsils and uvula are obscured. This is usually reassuring.

Mallampati 3—The soft and hard palate are visible, but only the base of the uvula can be seen. This can be associated with difficult views at the direct laryngoscopy.

Mallampati 4—Only the hard palate is visible, no soft palate is visible at all. This is worrying and is associated with poor view at laryngoscopy.*

*Source: data from *Canadian Anaesthetists' Society Journal, 32*, 4, Mallampati SR, Gatt SP, Gugino LD, et al. A clinical sign to predict difficult tracheal intubation: A prospective study, 429–34, 1985.

Greig P, Crabtree N (2014). Planning for general anaesthesia. In: *Introducing Anaesthesia*. Oxford, UK: Oxford University Press.

73. B. The medial border is the midline.

The borders of the anterior triangle of the neck are:

- The medial border is the midline
- The lateral border is the anterior border of the sternocleidomastoid
- The superior border is the lower edge of the jaw
- The roof is the investing facia
- The floor is the prevertebral facia

Ellis H, Mahadevan V (2013). The head and neck. In: *Clinical Anatomy: Applied Anatomy for Students and Junior Doctors*, 13th edition (pp. 287–90). Oxford, UK: John Wiley & Sons Ltd.

74. D. The superior parathyroid glands are more constant in position than inferior.

A. Ten per cent (10%) of parathyroid glands are aberrant, 90% of the time; they are in close relationship to the thyroid gland.

B. The numbers of parathyroid glands may vary between two to six.

C. The parathyroid glands are usually safe in subtotal thyroidectomy.

D. Correct answer.

E. The superior parathyroid glands usually lie at the middle of the posterior border of the thyroid lobe, above the level where the inferior thyroid artery crosses the recurrent laryngeal nerve. The inferior parathyroid glands are usually situated below the inferior thyroid artery, close to the lower pole of the thyroid gland.

Ellis H, Mahadevan V (2006). The head and neck. In: *Clinical Anatomy: Applied Anatomy for Students and Junior Doctors*, 11th edition (pp. 294–5). Oxford, UK: John Wiley & Sons Ltd.

75. D. There are no vascular structures overlying the cricothyroid membrane.

A. The cricothyroid membrane is 2–3 cm wide and 9–10 mm in height.

B. The membrane is located about 1 cm below the level of the true vocal cord. It connects the thyroid, and cricoid and arytenoid cartilages.

C. The landmark is just below the Adam's apple. Palpate the laryngeal prominence with the tip of the index finger strictly in the midline. Then slide down the finger, which will then fall into a hollow area, which is the location of the membrane and the site of the incision. The structure below this hollow area is a firm cartilaginous ring of cricoid cartilage.

D. Correct answer.

E. As the cricothyroid membrane is in the upper part of the neck, there is less chance of injuring the oesophagus. The anatomical landmarks are superficial, and easily seen and palpated. There is no important structure in front of the membrane, so it is easily accessible. The procedure can be performed with little training and no surgical support.

Ellis H, Mahadevan V (2006). The head and neck. In: *Clinical Anatomy: Applied Anatomy for Students and Junior Doctors*, 11th edition (pp. 300–62). Oxford, UK: John Wiley & Sons Ltd.

Nagy K (2004). Cricothyroidotomy. In: *Emergency Medicine Procedures* (pp. 101–17). New York, NY: McGraw-Hill.

76. A. It is relatively easier to cannulate the internal jugular vein below the level of the cricoid cartilage.

A. Correct answer. The internal jugular vein's diameter increases as it descends into the neck and thorax as it is joined by its tributaries. Hence, it is easier to cannulate below the level of the cricoid cartilage.

B. The internal jugular vein is not directly visible from the surface of the skin.

C. The internal jugular vein lies slightly lateral and anterior to the common carotid artery, which is an important landmark in locating the vein.

D. The internal jugular vein runs from the ear lobe to the medial clavicle between the sternal and clavicular heads of the sternocleidomastoid muscle.

E. To prevent an air embolism, the patient should be positioned in at least a 10-degree Trendelenburg position with subclavian vein cannulation. A 15-degree Trendelenburg position would be preferable for internal jugular vein access.

Feldman R (2004). Central venous access. In: *Emergency Medicine Procedures* (pp. 314–37). New York, NY: McGraw-Hill.

Standring S (2016). Neck. In: *Gray's Anatomy*, 41st edition (Chapter 29; p. 442–74). London, UK: Elsevier Ltd.

77. D. The pain from parotid gland swelling is due to the stretching of its capsule.

A. The arterial supply is sourced from the external carotid artery, which traverses the gland through its posteromedial surface and divides into the maxillary artery and superficial temporal artery.

B. The facial nerve enters the gland through the posteromedial surface and branches into superior (temporofacial) and inferior (cervicofacial) trunks.

C. The opening of the parotid duct is usually visible opposite the upper third molar tooth.

D. Correct answer. The pain from the parotid gland swelling is because of the stretching of the capsule and irritation of the greater auricular nerve.

E. The pain and swelling in the parotid gland is increased during mealtime, when the gustotary stimulus further increases the turgor within the capsule.

Standring S (2016). Face and scalp. In: *Gray's Anatomy*, 41st edition (Chapter 30; pp. 475–506). London, UK: Elsevier.

78. E. Morbidity is primarily due to asphyxiation in self-hanging.

A. Cervical spine injuries are uncommon in self-hanging, which is usually referred as incomplete hanging because of partial suspension of the victim's body with some contact with the ground. In judicial hanging, the victim is dropped from a height and is suspended freely.

B. The compression of the airway does not play as important a role in self-hanging as vascular occlusion.

C. In judicial hanging, the axis is fractured through its both pedicles with complete transection of the cord and death.

D. The initial step is venous congestion with stasis of cerebral blood flow leading to unconsciousness. Complete arterial occlusion follows, resulting in brain injury and death.

E. Correct answer.

Newton K, Claudius I (2014). Neck. In: *Rosen's Emergency Medicine*, 8th edition (Chapter 44; pp. 421–30). Philadelphia, PA: Elsevier Ltd.

79. B. The lingula on the ramus of the mandible is the bony prominence on the medial side of the mandible.

The procedure is as follows:

1. Landmarks: The anterior border of the ramus of the mandible is identified from within the mouth and the posterior border externally. Equidistance from these two points lies the lingual nerve and the inferior alveolar nerves. The lingula, a bony projection on the medial side of the mandible, can be identified by palpation.

2. Needle insertion:

    a) Position the patient in a dental chair with headrest, and ask the patient to keep the mouth open.

    b) Place the thumb of the non-dominant hand on the anterior border of the ramus.

    c) Feel the posterior border with the index finger of the non-dominant hand externally.

    d) Now feel the lingula by sliding down the thumb on the non-dominant hand posteromedially of the anterior border of the ramus.

    e) Pull the cheek outward using the non-dominant thumb as a lever.

    f) Use a 3-mL syringe and 27-gauge needle.

    g) The needle tip should be aligned towards the lingula with the syringe between the contralateral first and second premolars.

    h) Insert the needle just superior and posterior to the lingula.

    i) The tip of the needle should be advanced until it contacts with the ramus.

    j) Aspirate to check the needle tip is not in a blood vessel. Once confirmed, inject about 2 ml of local anaesthetic into this area.

Reichman EF, Kern KP (2004). Dental anaesthesia and analgesia. In *Emergency Medicine Procedures* (Chapter 154; pp. 1353–2467). New York, NY: McGraw-Hill.

80. B. The inferior boundary is the tip of the epiglottis.

A. Anteriorly, the oropharynx opens into the mouth through the oropharyngeal isthmus, which is demarcated by the palatoglossal arch.

B. Correct answer.

C. The lateral wall is formed by the palatopharyngeal arch and palatine tonsils.

D. The bodies of the second and upper part of the third cervical vertebrae with prevertebral fascia in front of them form the posterior boundary.

E. Superiorly, it is bounded by the soft palate and uvula.

Ellis H, Mahadevan V (2006). The head and neck. In: *Clinical Anatomy: Applied Anatomy for Students and Junior Doctors*, 11th edition (pp. 304–8). Oxford, UK: John Wiley & Sons Ltd.

Standring S (2016). Pharynx. In: *Gray's Anatomy*, 41st edition (Chapter 34; pp. 571–85). London, UK: Elsevier.

81. C. Conjunctiva is a single layer of epithelium on the cornea.

A. The upper eyelid is larger than the lower and more mobile.

B. The levator palpabrae superioris muscle is only present in the upper eyelid and helps in elevating the lid. The thickness of the layer of cells varies from one part to the other in the various parts of the eye.

   C. Correct answer: The conjunctiva is composed of an epithelial layer with an underlying fibrous layer (substantia propria).

   D. Between 8 to 12 ducts from the lacrimal glands, situated in the lacrimal fossa, drain to the lateral part of the superior conjunctival fornix.

   E. The most likely place for a foreign body to be stuck in the scenario discussed is on the corneal epithelium. The presence of photophobia with acute pain and increased lacrimation is an indicator of the foreign body's location.

Ellis H, Mahadevan V (2006). The nervous system. In: *Clinical Anatomy: Applied Anatomy for Students and Junior Doctors*, 11th edition (pp. 427–8). Oxford, UK: John Wiley & Sons Ltd.

Standring S (2016). Orbit and accessory visual apparatus. In: *Gray's Anatomy*, 41st edition (Chapter 41; pp. 666–85). London, UK: Elsevier.

82. E. The paratonsillar vein.

The arterial supply is derived from external carotid artery. The tonsillar artery is a branch of the facial, dorsal lingual branches from the lingual artery, ascending the pharyngeal artery, and descending the palatine artery. The venous drainage passes to the pharyngeal plexus. The important constant vein, the paratonsillar vein, descends from the soft palate across the lateral aspect of the tonsillar capsule. It is nearly always damaged in tonsillectomy surgery, resulting in troublesome bleeding.

Ellis H, Mahadevan V (2006). The head and neck. In: *Clinical Anatomy: Applied Anatomy for Students and Junior Doctors*, 11th edition (pp. 306–8). Oxford, UK: John Wiley & Sons Ltd.

83. E. The upward movement of goitre on swallowing is due to blending of the pretracheal fascia with larynx.

   A. Because of the attachment of the fascial compartment, a large goitre may also extend into superior mediastinum.

   B. During clinical examination, extension of the neck makes the thyroid gland more visible.

   C. The thyroid gland is enclosed in the pretracheal fascia, which is one of the four parts of deep fascia in the neck. The other three are the investing layer of deep cervical fascia, prevertebral fascia, and carotid sheaths (right and left). The capsule of the thyroid gland is much denser in the front than behind, due to which an enlarging gland tends to push backwards around the sides of trachea and oesophagus.

   D. See the answers to A, B, and C.

   E. Correct answer: Superiorly, as the pretracheal fascia blends with the larynx, the thyroid gland moves upwards with each action of swallowing.

Ellis H, Mahadevan V (2006). The head and neck. In: *Clinical Anatomy: Applied Anatomy for Students and Junior Doctors*, 11th edition (pp. 300–62). Oxford, UK: John Wiley & Sons Ltd.

84. B. Skin, fat, supraspinous ligament, interspinous ligament, ligamentum flavum.

The correct order is skin, fat, supraspinous ligament, interspinous ligament, and finally the ligamentum flavum before the tip of the needle enters the dura of the spinal canal.

Lumbar punctures are typically performed around the L3–4 region, so that the cord has ended so there is minimal risk of doing any damage to it.

Sinnatamby CS (2011). Head and neck and spine. In: *Last's Anatomy Regional and Applied Anatomy*, 12th edition (pp. 329–454). London, UK: Elsevier Ltd.

85. A. It is a central part of the corticospinal and spinothalamic tracts of the cervical spinal cord.

The patient has central cord syndrome (CCS), which often occurs following a hyperextension injury to the cervical spine. This is more common after the age of 50 in longstanding, degenerative spinal disease.

It is believed to cause contusion of the cord with stasis of axoplasmic flow in axons with relative preservation of grey area.

The upper limb motor function is more affected than the lower limbs, because of the pattern of lamination of the corticospinal and spinothalamic tracts. Sacral segments are the most lateral with lumbar, thoracic, and cervical components arranged somatotopically proceeding medially towards the central canal.

Medscape (2018). Central cord syndrome. Available at: http://emedicine.medscape.com/article/321907-overview#a5

86. C. The posterior limb of the internal capsule.

A. The main symptoms are dysarthria and clumsiness (i.e. weakness) of the hand.

B. The genu transmits corticobulbar tracts, infarction of which may cause mild paralysis of the facial muscles as they are innervated bilaterally. However, a lesion to the upper motor neurone for the facial nerves will result in spastic paralysis of the muscles in the contralateral lower quadrant of the face. A lesion to the upper motor neurones for hypoglossal nerve will result in spastic paralysis of contralateral side of the genioglossus, resulting in the deviation of the tongue to the contralateral side.

C. Correct answer: Pure motor stroke/hemiparesis occurs in the posterior limb of the internal capsule.

D. The contralateral thalamus when affected causes persistent or transient numbness, tingling on one side of the body, and/or burning sensations.

E. Causes mixed sensorimotor stroke—hemiparesis/ hemiplegia with contralateral sensory involvement.

Stanford Medicine: Introduction to the Exam for Internal Capsular Stroke. Available at: http://stanfordmedicine25.stanford.edu/the25/ics.html

Teach Me Anatomy: The descending tracts. Available at: http://teachmeanatomy.info/neuro/pathways/descending-tracts-motor/

87. B. The left lateral superior cerebellar artery.

A. Left anterior inferior cerebellar artery (AICA) infarcts are rare. The classic AICA syndrome has ipsilateral involvement of the fifth, seventh, and the eighth clinical nerves with hearing loss, vertigo, vomiting, tinnitus, facial palsy, and facial sensory loss, Horner syndrome, contralateral temperature, and pain loss.

B. Correct answer: Left lateral superior cerebellar artery infarction is a part of superior cerebellar artery (SCA) infarction. The second division of the SCA is the medial artery. Lateral SCA infarcts are the most common type involving anterior rostral cerebellum. The features are described in the scenario described. Medial SCA infarct may cause ataxia and dysarthria, or present with an isolated tendency to fall to ipsilateral side (lateropulsion).

C. Left posterior inferior cerebellar artery (PICA) infarctions are common. If the medulla is not involved, patients may present with headache, vertigo, nystagmus, ipsilateral axial lateropulsion, gait, and appendicular ataxia. It may have laterobulbar extension producing dorsal lateral medullary syndrome (Wallenberg syndrome). The clinical features are ipsilateral vestibular (vertigo, vomiting, nystagmus, lateropulsion), fifth, ninth, tenth cranial nerve palsies, Horner syndrome, appendicular ataxia with contralateral loss of pain and temperature sensation. Hiccups may be frequent and prolonged.

D. Right AICA infarctions are similar to answer A: the symptoms would be present on the right side.

E. The right lateral SCA is similar to that described in answer B, but the features would be on the right side.

Ferro JM, Fonseca AC (2014). Clinical features of acute stroke. In: Norrving, B. (Ed.), *Oxford: Textbook of Stroke and Cerebrovascular Disease*. Oxford, UK: Oxford University Press.

88. E. Thalamus.

A. Infarction of basal ganglia may occur due to occlusion of the lenticulostriate branches of the middle cerebral artery (MCA). The clinical features may consist of motor or sensorimotor hemiparesis or hemiplegia with or without dysarthria.

B. Clinical features from involvement of internal capsule depend on the area involved. The patient may have purely motor hemiparesis, motor-sensory deficit, ataxic hemiparesis, and dysarthria and clumsy hands.

C. Precentral gyrus involvement occurs in occlusion of the very distal Rolandic artery, resulting in acute ischaemic distal arm paresis.

D. The temporal lobe may be affected on its lateral surface by occlusion of inferior trunk of MCA. The patients usually have no motor or sensory deficit, but they often have visual field defect (contralateral homonymous hemianopia or upper quadrant anopsia of the contralateral visual field). Dominant hemisphere involvement may lead to Wernicke-type aphasia.

E. Correct answer: Small infarctions (<15 mm) are limited to single lenticulostriate arteries, and are called lacular strokes. A pure sensory stroke affecting the face, arm, and leg is due to the impairment of blood supply of thalamus (called thalamic sensory loss).

Hennerici MG, Binder J, Szabo K, Kern R (2012). Clinical diagnosis. In: *Stroke*. Oxford, UK: Oxford University Press.

89. B. Neurohypophysis is an extension of the nervous system.

A. The anterior pituitary gland is derived from the ectoderm and is full of cellular tissue. It is connected to the hypothalamus via the circulatory system.

B. Correct answer: The posterior pituitary gland is connected to the hypothalamus by the pituitary stalk, which is sometimes referred to as neurohypothesis, as it acts as an extension of the nervous system.

C. The pituitary stalk is hollow and contains nerve fibres, which extend directly from the axonal terminals of hypothalamic neurons.

D. See answer B.

E. The hormone vasopressin (and oxytocin) is synthesized in the supraoptic and paraventricular nuclei of hypothalamus. They then migrate as secretory granules along the axons to the posterior pituitary before release into the circulation.

The most common cause of diabetes insipidus is trauma and tumours. Damage to posterior pituitary gland may cause a temporary DI lasing for six weeks to six months, but destruction at the level of upper pituitary stalk or hypothalamic nuclei may result in to permanent DI.

Pal A, Karavitake N, Wass JAH (2014). Disorder of posterior pituitary gland. In: Warrell DA, Cox TM, Firth JD (Eds.), *Oxford Textbook of Medicine*, 5th edition. Oxford, UK: Oxford University Press.

90. A. Brain stem.

The structure, which is responsible for the arousal and cortical activation, is the ascending reticular activating system (ARAS), located in the paramedian tegmental zone in the dorsal part of the brain stem. The ARAS controls the input of sensory and somatic stimuli to the cerebral cortex.

The pathological processes in the cerebral cortex or brain stem each can independently cause depressed consciousness or coma. To induce coma, both the cerebral hemispheres need to be affected depending on the speed and the extent of development of the pathology in the cortex. Unilateral involvement of cerebral cortex generally does not cause coma. However, a small focal lesion in the brain stem can affect the ARAS, resulting in coma. If the ARAS is affected, the cerebral cortex is unable to remain aroused. Other options are random. Psychogenic coma should not be associated with eye signs.

The eye signs are suggestive of brain stem lesion.

Gassin BS, Cooke JL (2014). Depressed consciousness and coma. In: Marx J, Hockberger RS, Walls RM (Eds.), *Rosen's Emergency Medicine*, 8th edition (Chapter 16; pp. 142–52). Philadelphia, PA: Elsevier.

91. D. Parietal.

In dementia, the predominant change is cortical atrophy most pronounced in the temporal and hippocampal regions of the brain. There is progressive loss of neurons and synapses in the cerebral grey matter. The grey matter loss is followed by loss of white matter, which is called subcortical atrophy. The cell loss is more significant in dementia than as part of the normal degenerative process.

The frontotemporal dementias are less prevalent than Alzheimer's disease (AD) and are characterized by frontal and temporal lobe atrophy. Multiinfarct dementia results from multiple vascular lesions in the cerebral hemispheres and the basal ganglia. The onset is at an earlier age than AD and occurs in men who are prone to atherosclerosis.

Smith JP, Seirafi J (2014). Delirium and dementia. In: Marx J, Hockberger RS, Walls RM (Eds.), *Rosen's Emergency Medicine*, 8th edition (Chapter 104; pp. 1398–408). Philadelphia, PA: Elsevier.

92. A. Both the cerebral cortex and subcortical structures are affected in delirium.

A. Correct answer: There is widespread alteration of cerebral metabolic activity. Because of involvement of cerebral cortex and subcortical structures, there are disturbances in arousal, attention, and the normal sleep-wake cycle.

B. The word delirium is derived from the Latin *delirare*, which means 'to go out of furrow'. Patients can experience disturbances of consciousness (inability to focus attention), memory, cognition (disorientation), and perception (delusions/hallucination). The hallmark of delirium is the fluctuating course of symptoms and inattention, developing during a short time over hours to days.

C. It may have an underlying cause, which could be treated. It is not an irreversible dysfunction.

D. See answer B.

E. Multiple neurotransmitters have been implicated in causing delirium. One of the theories is increased serum anticholinergic activity. The serotonin level is increased in delirium associated with sepsis, hepatic encephalopathy, serotonin syndrome, and so on.

Smith JP, Seirafi J (2014). Delirium and dementia. In: Marx J, Hockberger RS, Walls RM (Eds.), *Rosen's Emergency Medicine*. 8th edition (Chapter 104; pp. 1398–408). Philadelphia, PA: Elsevier.

93. E. Posterior communicating artery.

A. Majority of aneurysm is in the anterior cerebral and anterior communicating arteries. The clinical features may be of sudden increase in intracranial pressure (ICP) (headache, vomiting, reduced GCS, sixth nerve palsy, papilloedema, and so on).

B. As discussed in answer A.

C. Around 20% of aneurysms occur in the middle cerebral artery, rupture of which may cause the clinical features mentioned in answer A.

D. About 7% aneurysms arise in the basilar and 3% in the PICA.

E. Correct answer: The discussed patient has features of right-sided third nerve palsy with severe headache, which is associated with expanding aneurysm in the posterior communicating artery. About 25% of aneurysms occur in the posterior communicating artery.

Kwiatkowski T, Friedman BW (2014). Headache disorders. In: Marx J, Hockberger RS, Walls RM (Eds.), *Rosen's Emergency Medicine*, 8th edition (Chapter 103; pp. 1386–97. Philadelphia, PA: Elsevier Ltd.

94. D. Loss of postural reflex.

A. Bradykinesia is slowness of movements including fatiguing and decrement in size of repetitive movement. This does not cause directly into multiple falls in such patients.

B. Disturbances of higher mental functions as, for example, personality change, dementia, hallucinations, depression, and so on may be present, but do not directly contribute to the falls.

C. The loss of dopaminergic (pigmented) neurons in substantia nigra and the presence of Lewy bodies are the hallmarks of PD. The damage to substantial nigra is the major cause of motor symptoms.

D. Correct answer: The loss of postural reflex is the cause of unsteadiness or fall on turning. PD patients typically have 'festinant' gait. They walk with small shuffling steps with reduced swinging of the arms. Postural instability may occur, resulting in falls.

E. In PD, the rigidity is often of 'lead pipe' type: the rigidity is present to the same extent when flexing or extending the limb.

Edwards MJ, Stamelou M, Quinn N, et al. (2016). *Parkinson's Disease and other Movement Disorders*, 2nd edition. Oxford, UK: Oxford University Press.

Fuller G, Manford M (2014). *Neurology* (pp. 88–9. Edinburgh, UK: Churchill Livingstone.

UpToDate (2017). Diagnosis and differential diagnosis of Parkinson disease. Available at: https://www.uptodate.com/contents/diagnosis-and-differential-diagnosis-of-parkinson-disease

95. C. The aqueduct of Sylvius may be blocked.

A. The hypothalamus is situated at the lateral wall and floor of the third ventricle. There are two lateral ventricles projecting in to the cerebral hemispheres. Each has an anterior horn, a body (above and medial to the body of the caudate nucleus), a posterior horn (projecting into the occipital lobe), and an inferior horn (extending into the temporal lobe). The choroid plexus in the lateral ventricles produces most of the CSF.

B. In acute bacterial meningitis (as in this case), the hydrocephalus can occur because of thickened meninges obstructing CSF flow or adherence of the inflamed lining of the aqueduct of Sylvius or fourth ventricular outflow.

C. Correct answer, but see also answer B: The narrow cerebral aqueduct of Sylvius connects the third ventricle to the fourth ventricle through the midbrain.

D. The CSF is formed by the covering epithelium of the choroid plexus in the lateral, third, and fourth ventricles. After circulating through the ventricular system, it drains into the subarachnoid space from the roof of the fourth ventricle before being reabsorbed into the dural venous system.

E. Anatomically there are four ventricles within the brain in total, a pair of lateral ventricles, the third and the fourth ventricles. The subarachnoid space is enlarged to form cisterns in certain areas. The cisterna magna lies between the cerebellum and the dorsum of the medulla. The cisterna pontis lies over the ventral surface of the pons, while between the two cerebral peduncles lay the interpeduncular cistern, the cisterna ambiens between the splenium of the corpus callosum and the superior surface of the cerebellum, the chiasmatic cistern around the optic disc.

Ellis H, Mahadevan V (2006). The nervous system. In: *Clinical Anatomy: Applied Anatomy for Students and Junior Doctors*, 11th edition (pp. 386–7). Oxford, UK: John Wiley & Sons Ltd.

96. C. Bone and dura.

A. The CT scan shows the blood in a white well demarcated by a sharp border. The blood is collecting in-between the dura and skull bone after injury to an artery. The source of the bleeding is from a branch of middle meningeal artery. There is significant midline shift pushing the right cerebral hemisphere to the left. There is also escape of air into the brain tissue just anterior to the haematoma, showing the open fracture in the skull or the sinuses. The space between the arachnoid and pia is called the subarachnoid space, where blood collection often occurs after rupture of intracranial aneurysms.

B. Three meninges surround the brain and the spinal cord. From the outside in, they are called dura, arachnoid, and pia matter. The dura is a dense fibrous structure with two layers. The outer layer is adherent to the inner surface of the skull, and the inner layer is the true dura which covers the neural tissues. It is separated from arachnoid matter by a thin space called the subdural space.

C. Correct answer: The endosteal layer of the dura is adherent to the bone and fixed to the sutures, hence when the blood is collected in-between the bone and the dura, it is limited by the dural adherence to the skull sutures, giving the appearance of biconvexity.

D. Blood collection in the subdural space would not be biconvex in character, rather crescentic. Such collection in-between the dura and arachnoid is called acute subdural haemorrhage. It is typically caused by venous bleeding.

E. Pia is the inner most membrane which is in close contact with the brain surface. The interval between arachnoid and pia is called subarachnoid space. The space contains CSF and is traversed by trabeculae of fine fibrous strands running from arachnoid to pia.

Ellis H, Mahadevan V (2006). The nervous system. In: *Clinical Anatomy: Applied Anatomy for Students and Junior Doctors*, 11th edition (pp. 385–6). Oxford, UK: John Wiley & Sons Ltd.

97. D. Tongue biting is because of repeated jaw muscle contractions.

A. GABA neurotransmitters are inhibitory in action. Drugs, which block GABA receptors, are very potent convulsants. Acetylcholine is an excitatory neurotransmitter to cortical neurons, subtle changes in the local concentrations of which may also result in excitation of ictogenic focus.

B. In generalized seizures, the focus is often subcortical and midline, which results in prompt loss of consciousness and bilateral involvement. The alteration of consciousness may occur because of extension of ictal discharges to the reticular activating system in the brain stem.

C. During generalized seizures, hypertension, tachycardia, tachypnoea, and hyperglycaemia may occur because of sympathetic stimulation. Prolonged convulsions may result in muscle damage and lactic acidosis.

D. Correct answer: Repeated contractions of the jaw muscles may result in injury to the buccal mucosa and/or tongue.

E. Autonomic discharge and bulbar involvement may result in urinary or faecal incontinence, vomiting, tongue biting, and airway impairment.

Bear MF, Connors BW, Paradiso MA (2006). *Neuroscience: Exploring the Brain*, 3rd edition (pp. 592–4). Baltimore, MD: Lippincott Williams & Wilkins.

McMullan JT, Duvivier EH, Pollack CV (2014). Seizure disorders. In: Marx J, Hockberger RS, Walls RM (Eds.), *Rosen's Emergency Medicine*, 8th edition (pp. 1375–85). Philadelphia, PA: Saunders.

98. D. The patient is in spinal shock.

A. Return of bulbocavernosus reflex signifies the cessation of spinal shock from less than 24 hours to more than two weeks. Persistence of perianal sensation or rectal sphincter action (sacral sparing) in complete spinal cord injury indicates a partial lesion (usually central cord lesion), and therefore may have a significant functional recovery.

B. A complete spinal cord injury is defined as when there is total loss of motor and sensory input distal to the site of the injury.

C. The associated injuries (chest, cardiac, or other) must be excluded before ascertaining the reason of hypotension as spinal shock. The systolic BP in spinal shock is usually above 90 mmHg. Absence of tachycardia and peripheral vasoconstriction in association of hypotension, flaccidity, and areflexia should signpost towards spinal shock.

D. Correct answer: Spinal shock is a condition when there is total but temporary loss of neurologic and autonomic function distal of the injury site, due to concussion to the spinal cord. This condition may persist from a few days to a few weeks. During a spinal shock situation, prognosis cannot be ascertained.

E. Hypotension, whatever the origin might be, may lead to organ hypoperfusion resulting in secondary spinal cord injury adversely affecting prognosis. Therefore, try to avoid prolonged hypotension, which generally, if of spinal shock origin, will respond to fluids. But fluid overload may occur if pursued aggressively. So, in addition to cautious fluid administration, Trendelenburg positioning (if no contraindication), vasopressors and so on may be initiated under monitoring after excluding the traumatic hypovolumic shock.

Kaji AH, Newton EJ, Hockberger RS (2014). Spinal injuries. In: Marx J, Hockberger RS, Walls RM (Eds.), *Rosen's Emergency Medicine*, 8th edition (pp. 382–420). Philadelphia, PA: Saunders.

99. D. The proprioception is carried by the left posterior column.

A. Cranial nerve involvement is common in MS. Optic neuritis is the commonest cranial nerve abnormality in MS. Diplopia or nystagmus may occur as a result of lesions in vestibulo-ocular connections, including the occulomotor nerve. Abnormality of facial sensation is common. Unilateral facial paresis or TN may also occur in MS.

B. Corticospinal tract dysfunction may result in paraparesis or paraplegia because of motor involvement. Pins and needles or other sensory abnormalities are carried through the spinothalamic tract of the opposite side.

C. In MS, the paraplegia is usually associated with spasticity, increased reflexes, and extensor planter responses.

D. Correct answer: The vibration and joint position senses are carried by the ipsilateral posterior column.

E. See answer D.

Fuller G, Manford M (2006). *Neurology* (pp. 84–7). London, UK: Churchill Livingstone.

Stettler BA (2014). Brain and cranial nerve disorders. In: Marx J, Hockberger RS, Walls RM (Eds.), *Rosen's Emergency Medicine*, 8th edition (Chapter 205; pp. 1409–18). Philadelphia, PA: Saunders.

100. E. The vascular headache is mediated through the fifth nerve.

A. Most headaches occurring in patients over the age of 50 years have a secondary cause, temporal arteritis is the commonest.

B. The patients are poor in specifically localizing the headaches because of its diffuse nature. Origin of pain from specific structures (tooth, sinuses, and so on) may be localized, but not the diffuse pain in tension headaches.

C. The meninges and blood vessels within the skull are pain sensitive.

D. The brain parenchyma is insensitive to pain.

E. Correct answer: The headaches (particularly vascular headaches and migraines) are mediated through the fifth cranial nerve. The pain sensation is carried to the nucleus and then relayed through various branches to other areas which are not directly pathological.

Kernick D, Goadsby P (2012). Getting to grips with the basics. In: *Headache: A Practical Manual*. Oxford, UK: Oxford University Press.

Russi CS (2014). Headache. In: Marx J, Hockberger RS, Walls RM (Eds.), *Rosen's Emergency Medicine* (Chapter 20; pp. 170–5). Philadelphia, PA: Saunders.

101. D. Linked to Ramsey Hunt syndrome.

Bell's palsy is a condition affecting the facial (seventh) cranial nerve. It affects both sides of the face in less than 1% of cases. The facial nerve has a purely motor function and it is the trigeminal nerve that provides sensation to the face in three divisions.

A lower motor neurone palsy (Bell's palsy) is differentiated from an upper motor lesion by the inability to raise the eyebrow on the affected side. The orbicularis muscle has bicortical innervation. This means that with an upper motor neurone lesion the muscle is still under voluntary control from the other cortex, whereas with a lower motor neurone lesion there is no innervation and the muscle will not contract.

Ramsey Hunt syndrome is commonly linked to facial nerve palsies. It is a reactivation of the herpes zoster virus, which tracks along the nerve causing severe pain, dermatomal rash, and deafness.

UpToDate (2017). Bell's palsy: Pathogenesis, clinical features, and diagnosis in adults. Available at: https://www.uptodate.com/contents/bells-palsy-pathogenesis-clinical-features-and-diagnosis-in-adults

102. E. Posterior cranial fossa.

A. In cerebellar ischaemia (the commonest artery involved is PICA), patients have severe vertigo and prominent nystagmus. These may be associated with minor limb hypotonia and incoordination.

B. Labyrinth: If there is involvement of the cochlea and/or semicircular canal, the central signs may be absent.

C. Middle ear: The infection may spread to the inner ear causing vertigo or peripheral nystagmus.

D. Pons: Patients with pontine ischaemia (basilar artery occlusive disease) may have paresis and corticospinal tract abnormalities. The patients may have motor or reflex abnormalities in the non-affected side (e.g. hyperreflexia, extensor planter, twitching, shaking, and so on). The bulbar symptoms include dysphonia, dysarthria, and dysphagia. The pattern of motor weakness may be crossed, meaning thereby involvement of face with the contralateral side of the body.

E. Correct answer: Posterior cranial fossa. This patient may have acoustic neuroma. Some 95% of patients may have cochlear involvement resulting in deafness and tinnitus. The vestibular component may be affected and presented as unsteadiness on walking. If a large tumour presses on the cerebellum or brainstem, the patients may have ataxia.

UpToDate (2017). Vestibular schwannoma (acoustic neuroma). Available at: https://www.uptodate.com/contents/vestibular-schwannoma-acoustic-neuroma

103. D. Medial rectus.

Medial rectus paralysis causes the eye to lie in an abducted position at rest and causes limited adduction.

Inferior oblique paralysis causes elevation when the eye is adducted.

Inferior rectus paralysis causes limited depression, particularly when the eye is abducted.

Lateral rectus paralysis causes the eye to be adducted at rest and results in limited abduction.

Superior rectus paralysis causes limited elevation, particularly when the eye is abducted.

Superior oblique paralysis causes limited depression when the eye is adducted.

Sinnatamby CS (2011). Head and neck and spine. In: *Last's Anatomy Regional and Applied Anatomy*, 12th edition (pp. 329–454). London, UK: Elsevier Ltd.

104. B. Bitemporal hemianopia.

A lesion in the body of the optic chiasm is likely to affect the crossing nasal retinal fibres, leading to a loss of lateral vision fields bilaterally. At this point the optic nerves cross and form the optic tracts. This means that information from both eyes is now split and processed on the side of the brain according to the side of the visual field, rather than which eye it came from.

Binasal hemianopia can occur with middle lesions of optic chiasm when the uncrossed temporal fibres are affected, but are rare.

If the optic nerve is cut, then loss of vision from one eye occurs.

A homonymous hemianopia is caused by a lesion to the optic tract.

Complete loss of vision is rarely caused by a lesion of this kind.

Dean C, Pegington J (1995). *Core Anatomy for Students* (Vols. 1–3). Amsterdam, the Netherlands: Bailliere Tindall.

105. A. New olfactory receptors are formed repeatedly during adulthood.

A. Correct answer.

B. The mammalian olfactory epithelium can replace the olfactory neurons lost by injury.

C. The neuroepithelial cells are located on the superior and middle turbinates in the nasal cavity.

D. The neuroepithelial cells are also located in the upper part of the nasal septum. There are about 6–10 million chemoreceptor cells in each nasal cavity. The axons of these cells traverse the cribriform plate of the ethmoid bone to terminate in the olfactory bulb. The fine cilia project into the mucus lining of the surface epithelium. These cilia originate from the knob-like endings of dendrites in the chemoreceptor cells.

E. The submucosal glands (Bowman's glands) secret mucosa forms a layer on the epithelium. It contains immunoglobulins (IgA and IgM), lactoferricin, and lysozymes, which create a barrier to the entry of the organisms into the brain via the nose.

UpToDate (2017). Anatomy and etiology of taste and smell disorders. Available at: https://www. uptodate.com/contents/anatomy-and-etiology-of-taste-and-smell-disorders

106. A.   The alar part of the nose is painful when the maxillary division is affected.

The trigeminal nerve (V) supplies sensation to the face and the motor supply is to the muscle of mastication. It has three major divisions: ophthalmic (V1), maxillary (V2), and mandibular (V3). The ophthalmic division supplies the skin over the forehead, upper eyelid, much of the external surface of the nose and the conjunctiva.

A. Correct answer: The alar part of the nose is affected when the maxillary division is involved. The maxillary division supplies sensation to skin of the upper lip, the alar part of the nose, the prominence of the cheek, the lower eyelid, and the part of the temple.

B. The infraorbital nerve is a branch from maxillary nerve. It has three branches namely, palpebral, nasal, and superior labial, which supplies the skin as described in answer A.

C. See answers A and B.

D. The lower lip area is supplied by the mandibular division. In addition to this, it also innervates the skin over the mandible, the fleshy part of the cheek, a part of the auricle of the ear, and a part of the temple.

E. Please see answers A to D.

TN is described clinically by occurrence of paroxysmal intense sharp stabbing pain in the distribution of one or more branches of the trigeminal nerve. It is typically unilateral, but may affect bilaterally. The most common divisions affected are maxillary and/or mandibular.

UpToDate (2017). Trigeminal neuralgia. Available at: https://www.uptodate.com/contents/trigeminal-neuralgia

Standring S (2016). Head and neck. In: *Gray's Anatomy*, 41st edition (Chapter 26; pp. 399–415). London, UK: Elsevier Ltd.

107. B.   Perforation in the superior quadrant of the eardrum may cause significant hearing loss.

A. In conductive deafness (as in this case) the bone conduction is heard longer than the air conduction in Rinne's test. Conductive deafness may be caused by trauma to the external or middle ear cavity, acute or chronic infection of the middle ear, or disruption of the ossicles.

B. Correct answer: Perforations in superior or posterior part of the tympanic membrane tend to cause significant deafness, rather than the anterior or inferior quadrant of the eardrum.

C. Small perforations cause the least amount of deafness. The deafness following tympanic perforation is dependent on the size and the location of the perforation.

D. Such trauma may be confined to the external auditory canal or injury to tympanic membrane. Damage to the sensory hair cells results in sensorineural deafness. The hair cells are sensitive to barotraumas, infection or hypoxia, or drugs such as aminoglycoside antibiotics.

E. If a 512 Hz tuning fork is vibrated and placed in the centre of the forehead, the sound localizes to the deaf ear. In sensorineural deafness, the sound localizes to the good ear.

Standring S (2016). Inner ear. In: *Gray's Anatomy*, 41st edition (Chapter 38; pp. 641–57). London, UK: Elsevier Ltd.

UpToDate (2017). Etiology of hearing loss in adults. Available at: https://www.uptodate.com/contents/etiology-of-hearing-loss-in-adults

108. B. Glossopharyngeal nerve.

  A. The facial nerve carries taste fibres from the anterior two-thirds of the tongue (special visceral afferent). It also supplies the secretomotor fibres to the sublingual and submandibular glands in addition to the motor supply to the muscle of facial expression (special visceral efferent).

  B. Correct answer: The glossopharyngeal nerve provides parasympathetic secretomotor fibres to the parotid gland in addition to receiving taste fibres from the posterior third of the tongue. It also supplies motor fibres to the stylopharyngeus muscle (special visceral efferent), which if affected may cause some pharyngeal weakness. It also receives visceral input from carotid sinus (baroreceptor) and carotid body (chemoreceptor). The lesion mentioned in the scenario is difficult to detect, as these are often associated with vagus nerve involvement.

  C. Hypoglossal: The twelfth cranial nerve is entirely motor and supplies the extrinsic and intrinsic muscles of the tongue.

  D. Lingual: This is a branch from the mandibular division of the fifth nerve (trigeminal), which supplies the mucus membrane of the floor of the mouth, the anterior two-thirds of the tongue including the taste buds (carrying the fibres from chorda tympani), and the submandibular and sublingual salivary glands.

  E. Vagus: This is a mixed sensory and motor nerve.

  Sensory: Taste sensation comes from the epiglottis and posterior pharynx, while visceral sensation comes from the aortic baroreceptors and visceral receptors. Tactile sensation comes from the larynx, pharynx, and upper oesophagus.

  Motor: Pharyngeal and palatal muscles, laryngeal muscles, the cricothyroid and inferior constrictor muscles. It also provides parasympathetic input to the visceral organs. Isolated lesions are uncommon. In unilateral paralysis, the uvula deviates to the normal side when patient is asked to say 'Ah'.

Ellis H, Mahadevan V (2013). *Clinical Anatomy: Applied Anatomy for Students and Junior Doctors*, 13th edition (pp. 397–419). Oxford, UK: Wiley Blackwell.

Flemming KD (2015). Disorders of cranial nerves and brainstem. In: *Mayo Clinic Neurology Board Review: Clinical Neurology for Initial Certification and MOC*. Oxford, UK: Oxford University Press.

109. D. Posterior triangle of neck.

  A. Anterior triangle of neck: The nerve does not cross this area, so this is not the likely area where the nerve could be injured.

  B. The cranial nerve XI emerges through the jugular foramen with the vagus and glossopharyngeal nerves. The accessory nerve passes backwards over the internal jugular vein to the sternocleidomastoid muscle, which it supplies and pierces. It then crosses the posterior triangle of the neck to supply the deep surface of the trapezius muscle. Injury to this nerve at the base of the cranium may result in the paralysis of both the sternomastoid and trapezius muscles.

  C. Nuclear: This arises from the anterior horn cells of the upper five cervical segments. A nuclear lesion is usually caused by a vascular compromise or mass lesion or inflammatory, degenerative origin.

D. Correct answer: See answer B. Paralysis of the trapezius muscle only occurs when the nerve is injured in the posterior triangle surgery or trauma.

E. Injury in this area would also involve the sternocleidomastoid muscle.

Ellis H, Mahadevan V (2013). *Clinical Anatomy: Applied Anatomy for Students and Junior Doctors*, 13th edition (pp. 397–419). Oxford, UK: Wiley Blackwell.

Flemming KD (2015). Disorders of cranial nerves and brainstem. In: *Mayo Clinic Neurology Board Review: Clinical Neurology for Initial Certification and MOC.* Oxford, UK: Oxford University Press.

110. B. The left hypoglossal nerve.

The picture shows the atrophy of the left side of the tongue due to peripheral lesion of the left hypoglossal nerve.

A. The glossopharyngeal nerve is a mixed sensory and motor nerve. It carries sensation from the taste buds on the posterior third of the tongue. It has somatic sensation from pharynx, soft palate, middle ear, palatine tonsils, carotid sinus, Eustachian tube, and auditory canal. The motor supply is to the stylopharyngeus muscle. There is no motor supply to the tongue.

B. Correct answer: The left hypoglossal nerve. Lesion to this one-sided nerve or its nucleus causes atrophy and paralysis of the ipsilateral tongue. When the patient is asked to protrude his tongue, it deviates to the side of the lesion, which is due to the unopposed action of the genioglossus muscle pushing the tongue. The hypoglossal nerve is a purely motor nerve.

C. Left lingual nerve: This carries general sensation from the anterior two-thirds of the tongue and oral mucosa on the floor of the mouth. The chorda tympani branch of the facial nerve, which joins the lingual nerve, carries taste sensation from anterior two-thirds of the tongue and parasympathetic fibres to the sublingual and submandibular salivary glands. It is a major sensory nerve.

D. Left mandibular nerve; the mandibular division of the trigeminal nerve. The motor portion supplies the muscle of mastication and the tensor tympani and tensor veli palatini. It supplies the sensation to skin on the chin, lower jaw, TM joint, the dura of anterior and middle cranial fossa, the lower teeth and gums, and the oral mucosa. Lesion in the mandibular nerve may cause weakness in muscles of mastication.

E. The right lingual nerve is normal. The lesion is on the left hypoglossal nerve as explained in the answer B above.

Ellis H, Mahadevan V (2013). *Clinical Anatomy: Applied Anatomy for Students and Junior Doctors*, 13th edition (pp. 397–419). Oxford, UK: Wiley Blackwell.

Marcus EM, Jacobson S, Sabin TD (2014). The cranial nerves. In: *Integrated Neuroscience and Neurology: A Clinical Case History Problem Solving Approach* (Chapter 12). Oxford, UK: Oxford University Press.

111. C. Occulomotor.

The patient has left occulomotor nerve palsy. The left eye has ptosis, papillary dilatation, and abduction of the left eye. The cranial nerve III supplies the superior, medial, inferior rectus, and the inferior oblique muscles. The dilation of the pupil is because of unopposed action of sympathetic supply to the ciliary muscles.

A. The abducent (VI) supplies the lateral rectus muscles of the eye. When affected, it causes diplopia and convergent squint.

B. Facial—the cranial nerve VII has motor supply to the facial muscles of expression and secretory fibres to the salivary and lacrimal glands.

C. Correct answer: Occulomotor.

D. Ophthalmic division—the smallest branch from the trigeminal nerve is wholly sensory. It innervates the skin of the forehead, upper eyelid, cornea, and most of the nose.

E. Trochlear: The trochlear nerve innervates to the superior oblique muscle. It is unique as it arises from the dorsal surface of the brain, is the most slender, and has the longest intracranial course.

Ellis H, Mahadevan V (2013). *Clinical Anatomy: Applied Anatomy for Students and Junior Doctors*, 13th edition (pp. 397–419). Oxford, UK: Wiley Blackwell.

Kennard C (2011). Oculo motor disorders. In: *Brain's Diseases of the Nervous System*, 12th edition. Oxford, UK: Oxford University Press.

112. B.   The loss of the accommodation-convergence reflex is due to paralysis of constrictor pupillae.

A. The divergent squint is because of unopposed action of superior oblique muscle (innervated by the trochlear nerve) and lateral rectus (innervated by the abducent nerve).

B. Correct answer. Also see answer C.

C. Light reflex—the pupils constrict when light is shone in the eyes. The neural transmission travels through optic nerves to pretectal nuclei in the midbrain, then to the Edinger–Westphal nucleus, and back through the parasympathetic fibres to the constrictor pupillae. Paralysis to the constrictor pupillae causes the loss of right reflex and the accommodation-convergence reflex.

D. The pupil is dilated because of dilator action of the sympathetic fibres. The parasympathetic efferent fibres, while travelling from the midbrain, lie to the periphery of the occulomotor nerve which makes them susceptible to compression by the aneurysms or at the edge of the tentorium in trauma.

E. The ptosis is because of the paralysis of the levator palpebrae superioris supplied by the occulomotor nerve.

Ellis H, Mahadevan V (2013). *Clinical Anatomy: Applied Anatomy for Students and Junior Doctors*, 13th edition (pp. 397–419). Oxford, UK: Wiley Blackwell.

Kennard C (2011). Oculo motor disorders. In: *Brain's Diseases of the Nervous System*, 12th edition. Oxford, UK: Oxford University Press.

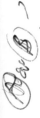

113. A.   Buccal.

A. The buccal branch supplies the zygomaticus major and levator labii superioris, levator anguli oris, levator labii superioris alaeque nasi, and the small nasal branches. They communicate with filaments of the buccal branch of the mandibular nerve.

B. Correct answer: The cervical branch of the facial nerve runs anteroinferiorly under platysma to the front of the neck. It supplies platysma.

C. A couple of the mandibular branches supply the risorius and muscles of the lower lip and chin, which communicate with the mental nerve.

D. The temporal branches supply intrinsic muscles on the lateral surface of the auricle, anterior, and superior auricular muscles. More anterior branches supply the frontal belly of the occipitofrontalis, orbicularis oculi, and corrugator.

E. The zygomatic branches supply the orbicularis oculi.

All the discussed branches form connections with the branches from ophthalmic, mandibular, and maxillary nerves and form plexuses supplying the various muscles of the face.

Standring S (2016). Face and scalp. In: *Gray's Anatomy*, 41st edition (pp. 475–506). London, UK: Elsevier Ltd.

114. E.   Posterior cranial fossa.

A. In cerebellar ischaemia (the commonest artery involved is the PICA), patients have severe vertigo and prominent nystagmus. These may be associated with minor limb hypotonia and incoordination.

B. Labyrinth: If there is involvement of the cochlea and/or semicircular canal, the central signs may be absent.

C. Middle ear: The infection may spread to the inner ear, causing vertigo or peripheral nystagmus.

D. Pons: Patients with pontine ischaemia (basilar artery occlusive disease) may have paresis and corticospinal tract abnormalities. The patients may have motor or reflex abnormalities in the non-affected side (e.g. hyperreflexia, extensor planter, twitching, shaking, and so on). The bulbar symptoms include dysphonia, dysarthria, and dysphagia. The pattern of motor weakness may be crossed, meaning thereby, involvement of face with contralateral side of the body.

E. Correct answer: Posterior cranial fossa. This patient may have acoustic neuroma. Some 95% of patients may have cochlear involvement resulting in deafness and tinnitus. The vestibular component may be affected and present as unsteadiness on walking. If a large tumour presses on the cerebellum or brainstem, the patients may have ataxia.

UpToDate (2017). Vestibular schwannoma (acoustic neuroma). Available at: https://www.uptodate.com/contents/vestibular-schwannoma-acoustic-neuroma

115. C.   Otorrhea may occur after temporal bone fractures.

A. Haemotympanum (blood behind the tympanic membrane) develops within hours of the occurrence of the petrous part of the temporal bone.

B. Bruising behind the ear (Battle sign) takes one to three days to develop.

C. Correct answer: Within hours or days of the occurrence of injury, clear rhinorrhoea or otorrhea may be found in up to 20% of the temporal bone fractures.

D. 'Raccoon eyes' (periorbital bruising) takes one to three days to develop after the anterior or middle cranial fossa fracture.

E. It is a rare but important complication following basal skull fracture. Incidence is 3.8% and mostly associated with middle cranial fossa fracture.

UpToDate (2017). Skull fractures in adults. Available at: https://www.uptodate.com/contents/skull-fractures-in-adults

1. **A 26-year-old woman and a 27-year-old man attended the emergency department (ED) with oral paraesthesia, generalized weakness, and dyspnoea after consuming dried pufferfish bought in London. Two friends who also ate the fish have similar but less severe symptoms and did not seek care. Which one of the following regarding action potentials is true?**
   A. Action potentials in skeletal muscle follow the same curve as in cardiac muscle
   B. Na+,K+-ATPase is electrogenic
   C. Only excitable cells have a resting membrane potential
   D. Relative refractory period describes the hyperpolarization of the membrane during which no other action potential can occur
   E. Voltage-dependent sodium channel activation generates the repolarization phase of the action potential

2. **A previously fit and well 28-year-old man is brought to the ED complaining of palpitations. On examination, his pulse is rapid and irregularly irregular. An electrocardiogram (ECG) demonstrates atrial fibrillation with rapid ventricular response. Vagal manoeuvres have been unsuccessful, and adenosine has been prescribed. Which of the following is responsible for the rapid upstroke of the cardiac action potential?**
   A. Funny current channels
   B. L-type calcium channels
   C. Na+,K+-ATPase channels
   D. Voltage-gated potassium channels
   E. Voltage-gated sodium channels

3. **A 92-year-old gentleman is brought to the ED following a fall while shopping with his wife. He is taking warfarin for a previous stroke. The computed tomography (CT) head scan demonstrates a subdural haemorrhage. His international normalized ratio (INR) is 2.7. Which of the statements regarding the coagulation screen is correct?**
   A. APTT is a measure of coagulation via the tissue factor pathway
   B. INR is calculated using the APTT
   C. Lithium heparin bottles are used to collect the blood sample
   D. Prothrombin time is a measure of coagulation via the tissue factor pathway
   E. The platelet count is not relevant

4. **A 92-year old woman has been brought in to the ED from her nursing home generally unwell. She has had very poor oral intake for several days and has not passed urine all day. On examination, her oral mucosae are dry, her eyes are sunken, and her capillary refill time (CRT) is 5 seconds. Initial observations are as follows: BP 81/46 mmHg, HR 112 bpm, RR 14 breaths per minute, T 36.7°C. Which statement regarding compartments and fluid spaces is true?**

A. Glucose and urea are effective osmoles

B. Higher proportions of adipose tissue indicate higher total body water

C. In a 70 kg adult, total body water is about 28 L

D. Of the extracellular fluid, approximately one-quarter makes up the plasma

E. The concentration of sodium is higher in the intracellular fluid than the extracellular fluid

5. **An 80-year-old woman has severe abdominal pain that is worsened by food. On examination, she is exquisitely tender in the epigastric region. Her BP is 112/72 mmHg, HR 104 bpm, RR 18 breaths per minute, T 36.90°C. Which statement regarding gastric acid secretion is false?**

A. Acetylcholine, histamine, and gastrin are agonists for gastric acid secretion

B. G proteins can be active or inactive

C. Gastric acid is secreted from parietal cells

D. Prolonged exposure to an agonist increases intracellular response by up-regulation and sensitization

E. Signal-transduction pathways link receptors to effectors by using a second messenger substance such as cAMP

6. **A 34-year-old otherwise fit and well gentleman attends the ED following a marathon. On examination, he is clinically dehydrated and drowsy. His blood glucose level is 2.4 mmol/L and his creatine kinase is 758, suggesting rhabdomyolysis. Which GLUT transporter is found predominantly in skeletal muscle?**

A. GLUT1

B. GLUT2

C. GLUT3

D. GLUT4

E. GLUT5

7. **A 57-year-old roofer has suffered from a 2 cm laceration across his nailbed. He has applied pressure with a cloth and appears to have achieved haemostasis. Which of the following mechanisms might have helped in haemostasis in this case?**

A. Fibrin converts prothrombin into thrombin, which is vital for coagulation

B. Haemostasis is achieved by vasodilatation, white cell aggregation, and coagulation of the blood

C. Serotonin is released by platelets to enhance vasoconstriction

D. Thromboxane A2 is released by normal endothelial cells to prevent platelet aggregation beyond the injury

E. Virchow's triad includes hypovolaemia, epithelial damage, and hypercoagulable state

8. **A 42-year old gentleman is found unconscious on the street. He smells of alcohol. Initial observations are as follows: BP 152/93 mmHg, HR 91 bpm, RR 14 breath per minute, T 36.7°C. A blood glucose reading is 6.1 mmol/L. Which of the following statements regarding blood glucose control is true?**

A. Blood glucose control is under positive feedback

B. Feedback mechanisms remain constant throughout the day

C. Negative feedback is an amplification process

D. Oscillation around a physiological 'set point' is due to lag time in the feedback loop

E. Positive feedback operates around a physiological 'set point'

9. **A 12-year-old boy is brought to paediatric ED with a cough and fever. He has a past medical history of Duchenne muscular dystrophy. On examination, he is wheelchair-bound with poor inspiratory effect and coarse right basal crepitations. His arms and legs are visibly wasted. Which of the following answers regarding muscle is true?**

A. Calcium is released from the sarcoplasmic reticulum of skeletal muscle

B. Cardiac muscle can increase force of contraction by recruitment

C. Myosin 'thin' filaments push actin 'thick' filaments away from the centre of the sarcomere

D. Strength training increases muscle mass by hyperplasia

E. Tetany increases the force of skeletal muscle contraction by activating more α neurons

10. **A 42-year-old woman has fallen at home and attends ED with leg weakness. She has a history of well-managed multiple sclerosis and is concerned about relapse. On examination, she has Medical Research Council (MRC) muscle power grading of 0/5 in extension of the knee and dorsiflexion of the foot. Which one of the following answers regarding nerve conduction is false?**

A. Cell diameter has a positive relationship with conduction velocity

B. Ion channels are concentrated at the nodes of Ranvier

C. Membrane resistance is increased by Schwann cells

D. Myelination increases the length constant

E. Saltatory conduction requires more energy than standard conduction in a cell of the same diameter.

11. **A 28-year-old man is brought to the ED following a seizure at home. He was given buccal midazolam by the paramedics and his seizure activity ceased en route. Which one of the following neurotransmitters has a predominantly inhibitory action within the central nervous system (CNS)?**

A. γ-aminobutyric acid

B. Acetylcholine

C. Dopamine

D. Glutamate

E. Substance P

12. **A 64-year-old gentleman is in resus with suspected non-ST-elevation myocardial infarction (NSTEMI), confirmed by changes in his inferolateral leads on ECG. You have commenced acute coronary syndrome (ACS) protocol, and after sublingual glyceryl trinitrate (GTN) spray, the patient's pain is alleviated. Which one of the following statements is true with regards to endothelial nitric oxide?**

A. NO acts exclusively in the venous system

B. NO is a neurotransmitter released in vesicles from post-synaptic membranes

C. NO is a paracrine mediator of vasodilatation

D. NO is an endocrine mediator of vasoconstriction

E. NO stimulates an increase intracellular cAMP levels in target cells

13. **A 72-year-old man tripped and fell while getting out of bed in the early hours of the morning. He has urinary frequency, dysuria, and feels sweaty and confused. On examination, he is tender in the suprapubic region and febrile. A diagnosis of urinary tract infection (UTI) is made and intravenous fluids are commenced. Which one of the following statements regarding osmosis is true?**

A. A 0.9% sodium chloride solution is isotonic and will not alter the osmotic gradient between the intra and extracellular compartments

B. Hypertonic saline alters the osmotic gradient such that water enters the intracellular compartment

C. Red cells swell and can lyse in hypertonic saline *~solute*

D. The more permeable a membrane is to a solid, the greater the osmotic pressure it exerts

E. Water moves from areas of high to low osmotic pressure

14. **A 92-year old gentleman is brought to the ED with severe abdominal discomfort. He has not passed urine in 48 hours and has a history of benign prostatic hypertrophy. On examination, he has a palpable bladder and suprapubic tenderness. A urinary catheter is inserted, and he immediately passes 2.5 L of urine. According to Poiseuille's Law regarding flow of liquids through tubes, which one of the following statements is correct?**

A. Doubling catheter length will double flow

B. Doubling catheter radius will quadruple flow

C. Flow is directly proportional to resistance

D. Flow is independent of the pressure gradient across the catheter

E. Flow is inversely proportional to fluid viscosity

15. **A 36-year-old body builder attends the ED with sudden-onset, right shoulder pain following a session at the gym. On examination, there is a suspicion of biceps rupture. You recall studying the components of striated muscle fibres as a student. Which of the following most accurately describes the area containing the myosin thick filaments?**

    A. A band

    B. I band

    C. Sarcomere

    D. T tubule

    E. Z line

16. **A 10-month-old is brought to the ED with difficulty breathing. On examination, he is coryzal with subcostal recessions and head bobbing with widespread crepitations and expiratory wheeze bilaterally. Rapid analysis of the nasopharyngeal aspirate suggests respiratory syncytial virus (RSV) infection. Your colleague recommends a α-adrenergic agonist, but you question the benefit of this treatment. Which of the following mechanisms best describes the aim of treatment with beta-agonists?**

    A. Activation of α1-adrenergic receptors to stimulate smooth muscle relaxation

    B. cGMP-mediated increase in cytosolic [Ca2+], causing widening of the smaller airways

    C. Hormonal stimulation of InsP3 production to increase pharmacomechanical coupling

    D. Inhibition of troponin phosphorylation to generate bronchodilatation

    E. Myosin phosphorylation is inhibited by an increase in cAMP, leading to improved ventilation

17. **A 37-year-old gentleman attends ED with generalized weakness, particularly after prolonged exertion. On examination, there is bilateral ptosis and his mouth hangs open. The remainder of the neurological examination is normal, but the patient complains of fatigue. Given the likely diagnosis, which one of the following regarding neuromuscular synaptic transmission in this patient is true?**

    A. Action potentials arriving in the presynaptic neuron trigger influx of Mg2+ ions

    B. Neurotransmitter release occurs via voltage-gated channels

    C. Post-synaptic receptors for acetylcholine are inhibitory

    D. Recycling of choline occurs by endocytosis of coated vesicles

    E. Transmission at chemical synapses is bi-directional

18. **A 24-year-old is in resus following an intentional overdose. You suspect that she may have taken a non-lethal dose of cyanide, and you remember that cyanide irreversibly binds to cytochrome oxidase and prevents the production of adenosine triphosphate (ATP) via oxidative phosphorylation. Which one of the following membrane transport proteins requires ATP?**

    A. Aquaporin 1
    B. Desmoglein-1
    C. GLUT2 transporter
    D. Nicotinic acetylcholine receptor
    E. Voltage-gated Na+ channel

19. **A 47-year-old woman is brought in to the ED as a trauma call following a road traffic accident. She has sustained significant injuries to her head and abdomen and is unresponsive. What are the components of the triad of death?**

    A. Hypertension, bradycardia, and irregular breathing
    B. Hypothermia, coagulopathy, and acidosis
    C. Muffled heart sounds, distended neck veins, and hypotension
    D. Right upper quadrant abdominal pain, jaundice, and fever
    E. Tachycardia, tachypnoea, and tender hepatomegaly

20. **A 26-year-old woman attends ED with shortness of breath and haemoptysis. She recently started taking an oestrogen-containing oral contraceptive pill and has a family history of venous thromboembolism. Her Aa gradient is elevated in arterial blood gas (ABG) sample. Which of the following best describes the Aa gradient?**

    A. Difference between ideal PAO_2 and measured PaO_2
    B. Difference between ideal $PACO_2$ and measured $PaCO_2$
    C. Ratio of ideal PAO_2 and measured PaO_2
    D. Ratio of ideal $PACO_2$ and measured $PaCO_2$
    E. Relationship between PAO_2 and $PACO_2$

21. **A 17-year-old boy is brought to the ED with a two-hour history of severe dyspnoea. He has a past medical history of asthma. In the previous few days he has been using his salbutamol inhaler up to ten times a day. On examination, he is pale, clammy, and has increased work of breathing with quiet breath sounds. Which one of the following answers regarding airway resistance is true?**

    A. Airway resistance is reduced by turbulent flow
    B. Bronchial smooth muscle receives a sympathetic bronchoconstrictor nerve supply
    C. Doubling airway radius increases the airway resistance 16-fold
    D. Peak expiratory flow rate is increased at higher lung volumes
    E. Wheeze is an indication of severe bronchoconstriction

22. **A 32-year-old pregnant woman attends the ED with acute dyspnoea, chest pain, and haemoptysis. She is at 32 weeks gestation and reports having a deep vein thrombosis (DVT) during her previous pregnancy. Which one of the following answers best explains the mechanism of hypoxaemia in this case?**

    A. Anatomical shunt
    B. Hypoventilation
    C. Increase in dead space
    D. Physiological shunt
    E. V/Q mismatch

23. **A 66-year-old man attends the ED with shortness of breath. He has a 100-pack year smoking history and a persistent cough productive of pale grey sputum. The cough has persisted for more than three months on several occasions in the last five years. On examination, he has nicotine-stained fingers and a smoker's cough, but his chest is clear. Which of the following statements regarding ventilation and perfusion in this case is most likely?**

    A. Both mucus production and perfusion are reduced
    B. Both ventilation and perfusion are unaffected
    C. Mucus production and ventilation are reduced
    D. Perfusion is reduced due to smoking, while ventilation is increased due to emphysema
    E. Ventilation is reduced to a greater extent than perfusion

24. **A 79-year-old gentleman is brought to ED from his nursing home with dyspnoea and a productive cough. He has a past medical history of chronic obstructive pulmonary disease (COPD) and is taking a steroid inhaler. His ABG result shows the following: pH 7.37, $PaCO_2$ 8.2, base excess 6.2, HCO_3- 29.7. Which statement regarding carbon dioxide transport is true?**

    A. ABG analysis in this gentleman is most likely to indicate a metabolic alkalosis with respiratory compensation
    B. Carbonic anhydrase catalyses the reaction of CO_2 with H_2O to form H_2CO_3 within the red blood cells
    C. Chloride shift maintains red blood cells homeostasis and involves the diffusion of chloride out of red blood cells in exchange for bicarbonate
    D. Haemoglobin buffers the production of H+ ions within the bloodstream, preventing synthesis of bicarbonate
    E. The Haldane effect describes the relationship between oxyhaemoglobin saturation and the CO_2 dissociation curve, which is S-shaped

25. **A 72-year-old gentleman attends ED with dyspnoea and a productive cough. On examination, he has a barrel chest, widespread crackles throughout his lung fields, and tar staining on his fingers. His initial observations are as follows: BP 134/78 mmHg, HR 91 bpm, RR 21 breaths per min, SaO$_2$ 89% (room air), and T 36.7°C. What is the single best answer regarding lung function and compliance in this gentleman?**

    A. Compliance is a measure of the elastic properties of the lung and is measured in mL/cm H$_2$O
    B. Functional residual capacity is decreased in emphysema
    C. Lung compliance is a static variable
    D. Lung compliance will be increased in COPD
    E. Surface area for gas exchange increases in emphysema

26. **A 67-year-old man is brought to the ED with double pneumonia. His respiratory effort is worsening, and the anaesthetist has intubated and sedated him. Once he is ventilated, the tidal volume is set to 1,200 mL, the end inspiratory pressure is 20 cmH$_2$O and the end expiratory pressure is 5 cmH$_2$O. What is the value for lung compliance in this gentleman?**

    A. 60 mL/cmH$_2$O
    B. 80 mL/cmH$_2$O
    C. 300 mL/cmH$_2$O
    D. 6,000 mL/cmH$_2$O
    E. 24,000 mL/cmH$_2$O

27. **A 24-year-old student is brought to the ED following a quad-bike accident. He had not been wearing a helmet when he turned sharply, overturning the vehicle, and launching himself headfirst into a tree. During the initial assessment, you note that he is breathing independently, but that his breaths have a long inspiratory phase lasting several seconds followed by a brief expiration. This pattern is consistently repeated. Which one of the following answers best explains this example of respiratory control?**

    A. Agonal breathing, secondary to damage to the forebrain
    B. Apneustic breathing, secondary to damage to the pons and vagus nerve
    C. Central sleep apnoea, secondary to damage to the phrenic nerve
    D. Cheyne–Stokes breathing, secondary to damage to the medulla oblongata
    E. Kussmaul breathing, secondary to damage to the nucleus tractus solitarius

28. **A 34-year-old man with Down's syndrome and a known atrioventricular septal defect attends with a productive cough and fever. He is centrally cyanosed at rest despite oxygen therapy. Which one of the following best explains the cyanosis?**

    A. Anaemia of chronic disease
    B. Decreased alveolo-arteriolar gas exchange
    C. Eisenmenger syndrome
    D. Left-to-right shunt
    E. Polycythaemia

29. **A 22-year-old gentleman attends ED with severe foot pain. He has a past medical history of sickle cell anaemia and multiple attendances in crisis. On examination, his right foot is exquisitely tender to palpation and movement, with red, swollen, sausage-like toes. You recall that haemoglobinopathies such as sickle cell anaemia can shift the oxyhaemoglobin dissociation curve to the right. Which one of the following does not shift the oxyhaemoglobin dissociation curve to the right?**

    A. Acidosis
    B. Concentration of 2,3-diphosphoglycerate
    C. Foetal haemoglobin
    D. Living at altitude
    E. Partial pressure of CO_2

30. **A 55-year-old man attends the ED with shortness of breath. His recent pulmonary function tests demonstrate reduced full vital capacity (FVC), FEV1, and FEV1/FVC. The residual volume (RV) is elevated and the diffusion capacity of the lungs for CO_2 ($DLCO_2$) is reduced. Based on this information alone, what is the likely diagnosis?**

    A. Asthma
    B. Bronchiectasis
    C. Emphysema
    D. Pneumonia
    E. Pulmonary fibrosis

31. **An 84-year-old man is brought to the ED with infective exacerbation of COPD. On examination, he has a barrel chest and appears confused. He has generalized inspiratory crackles on auscultation. His BP is 125/82 mmHg, HR 112 bpm, RR 32 breaths per minute, T 38.1 C. Which of the following mechanisms leads to premature airway closure in expiration?**

    A. Airway hypersensitivity
    B. Degradation of airway cartilage
    C. Increased lung compliance
    D. Shifting of the equal pressure point towards the alveoli
    E. Widening of the small airways and bulla formation

32. **A 79-year-old gentleman is brought to ED from his nursing home with dyspnoea and a productive cough. He has a past medical history of COPD and is taking a steroid inhaler. Prior to examination, you inspect his recent lung function testing results. Which one of the following sets of results indicates COPD?**

 A. FEV_1 = 2.47 L; FVC = 2.50 L
 B. FEV_1 = 2.47 L; FVC = 3.50 L
 C. FEV_1 = 1.43 L; FVC = 2.00 L
 D. FEV_1 = 1.43 L; FVC = 2.50 L
 E. FEV_1 = 2.47 L; FVC = 3.00 L

33. **A 47-year-old woman is brought in by her neighbour after being found unconscious in her vintage car. She had been running the exhaust fumes into the car via a hose, presumably in an attempt to end her life. Which one of the following answers regarding gas transfer is true?**

 A. Carbon monoxide has an affinity for haemoglobin approximately 200 times greater than oxygen
 B. Diffusion of a gas across a membrane is inversely related to surface area
 C. Gas transfer occurs more readily from the alveoli to the pulmonary capillaries in interstitial fibrosis
 D. Oxygen is a diffusion-limited gas
 E. Under normal conditions, there is no methaemoglobin in the blood

34. **A 21-year-old professional basketball player attends ED with sudden-onset shortness of breath. On general inspection, the patient is tall and slim. There is reduced air entry on the right-hand side and increased resonance on percussion. The chest radiograph reveals a right-sided pneumothorax of greater than 2 cm. The ABG indicates a reduced PaO_2. Which of the following is the physiological cause of this patient's hypoxaemia?**

 A. Anatomical shunt
 B. Hypoventilation
 C. Increase dead space
 D. Reduced cardiac output
 E. V/Q mismatch

35. **A 41-year-old woman attends the ED with facial pain, foul nasal discharge, and fever. She has a history of recurrent ear and chest infections, and fertility problems. On examination, her skin has a greasy appearance and her breath sounds are coarse at the right lung base. You are unable to hear the apex beat on the left. Given the likely diagnosis, which physiological change underlies the recurrent infections?**

 A. Deficiency of vitamin C
 B. IgG subclass deficiency
 C. Immotile cilia
 D. Mutation of a chloride transporter
 E. Severe combined immunodeficiency

36. **A 28-year-old woman attends ED with difficulty breathing, cough productive of thick green sputum, and fever. She has a past medical history of cystic fibrosis with double lung transplant. On examination, her breath sounds are generally quiet with coarse crepitations at the right base. Which one of the following answers regarding the lung epithelium is true?**

   A. Ciliated squamous epithelium lines the respiratory tract from the nose to the bronchi
   B. Goblet cells produce periciliary fluid
   C. Mucus composes the sol phase of the mucociliary transport system
   D. Three fluids line the respiratory epithelium: periciliary fluid, mucus, and surfactant
   E. Type I pneumocytes produce surfactant

37. **A 41-year-old man attends the ED with an hour history of sudden-onset shortness of breath. He has a history of Factor V Leiden thrombophilia and previous DVT. On examination, his breath sounds are normal, but his respiratory rate is 36. Which of the following is most responsible for causing tachypnoea?**

   A. Central and peripheral chemoreceptors responding to change in PCO_2
   B. Central chemoreceptors responding to change in PO_2
   C. Irritant receptors in the lower respiratory tract
   D. Peripheral chemoreceptors responding to change in pH
   E. Pulmonary mechanoreceptors

38. **A 65-year-old man with a 100-pack year smoking history attends the ED with cough and shortness of breath. On examination, he has nicotine-stained fingers and a barrel chest. He has inspiratory crackles throughout his lung fields. He has had recent pulmonary function tests. Which single pulmonary function test can distinguish between chronic bronchitis and emphysema?**

   A. $DLCO_2$
   B. FEV_1
   C. FEV_1/FVC
   D. FVC
   E. Tidal volume

39. **A 26-year-old woman attends ED with a cough and fever. She has a history of asthma and started a new job in a nursery recently. On examination, her tonsils are bilaterally red and enlarged. Which epithelial cells line the respiratory tract from the nose to the larynx?**

   A. Ciliated columnar
   B. Ciliated cuboidal
   C. Cuboidal with glandular cells
   D. Stratified columnar
   E. Stratified squamous

40. A 60-year-old woman is brought to the ED in cardiac arrest. Ventricular fibrillation is confirmed, and you proceed along the shockable rhythm side of the cardiac arrest algorithm by delivering DC cardioversion. Spontaneous return of circulation is achieved with which sinus rhythm on the monitor?

A. Phase 0

B. Phase 1

C. Phase 2

D. Phase 3

E. Phase 4

41. A 92-year-old man is brought to the ED with shortness of breath. He has a history of hypertension and congestive cardiac failure. On examination, he is grossly oedematous in peripheral areas with bilateral basal crepitations on auscultation. His wife brings in a list of his medications. Which of the following is afterload-reducing to the heart?

A. Digoxin

B. Gelofusine 4%

C. Rabeprazole

D. Ramipril

E. Terlipressin

42. A 67-year-old man attends the ED with palpitations, who has a history of three previous failed DC cardioversions and is due for ablation next month. His ECG demonstrates atrial fibrillation with a fast ventricular response. What is the site at which ablation therapy should largely be targeted?

A. Atrioventricular node

B. Base of the pulmonary arteries

C. Base of the pulmonary veins

D. Bundle of His

E. Bundle of Kent

43. A four-year old boy is brought to the ED with difficulty in breathing and cyanosis. He has been noted to squat when he becomes breathless. An ECG is requested that shows an abnormal cardiac axis. Cardiac axis is a key component of ECG interpretation. Which one of the following statements is correct?

A. Cardiac axis is perpendicular to any given lead with a positive QRS

B. Extreme axis deviation occurs between -90 and 180 degrees

C. Normal cardiac axis occurs between 30 and -90 degrees

D. Positive QRS in lead I and negative QRS in lead aVF indicate right axis deviation

E. Right axis deviation is always demonstrated by a positive QRS in lead aVF

44. **A 28-year-old gentleman is brought to the ED following sudden collapse while playing football this afternoon. On examination, he has a harsh crescendo-decrescendo systolic murmur heard throughout the praecordium, but loudest at the left sternal edge in the second intercostal space. Which one of the following answers regarding the cardiac cycle is true?**

    A. During isovolumetric contraction, the mitral valve and the aortic valve are both open
    B. During isovolumetric contraction, the ventricular pressure reaches the maximal value, approximately 120 mmHg
    C. The second heart sound coincides with the closure of the mitral valve
    D. The T wave on the ECG occurs at the same time as ventricular filling begins
    E. Ventricular volume remains constant at the points during which the heart sounds are heard

45. **A 48-year-old gentleman is brought to the ED with chest pain and reduced exercise tolerance. He was playing football with his children this afternoon when the symptoms came on and he needed to stop. The pain resolved with rest. On examination, he has normal heart sounds, nicotine-stained fingers, and enlarged body habitus. Which one of the following answers regarding cardiac cycle is true?**

    A. Aortic blood flow is greater than 1 L/min after aortic valve closure
    B. Atrial systole coincides with the third heart sound
    C. Mitral valve closure occurs simultaneously to the P wave on the ECG
    D. Perfusion of the coronary arteries occurs mainly during diastole
    E. Ventricular pressure is approximately 60 mmHg during ventricular filling

46. **An 82-year-old gentleman is brought to the ED with dyspnoea and reduced exercise tolerance. He was unable to get out of bed this morning and has been sleeping on five pillows recently. On examination, he has fine basal crepitations bilaterally and significant pitting oedema in dependent areas. Which one of the following answers regarding cardiac output is true?**

    A. Catastrophic haemorrhage results in increased preload
    B. Dilated cardiomyopathy increases preload
    C. Hypertension causes increased preload
    D. Pulmonary oedema predisposes right heart strain by increasing the preload
    E. Tachycardia leads to increased preload

47. **A 54-year-old schoolteacher is brought to the ED with palpitations and chest pain. She also reports feeling tremulous in her hands and needing to dress more lightly in the past two weeks. She has a moderate-sized goitre, pulsatile nailbeds, and a degree of exophthalmos. Which one of the following answers best explains why this patient has pulsatile nailbeds?**

A. Autoantibodies effect changes in the capillary wall to increase elasticity

B. Capillary blood flow increases secondary to tachycardia

C. Dilatation of small arteries and arterioles decreases systemic vascular resistance and reduces the damping effect on cardiac contraction

D. Muscular contraction of the venules and small veins generates back-pressure in the capillary beds

E. Viscosity of the blood increases in this condition

48. **A 14-year-old boy with cerebral palsy is brought to ED by his mother as he has been 'out of sorts' for the last couple of days and vomited twice today. He was discharged from a tertiary hospital seven days ago following the insertion of a ventriculo-peritoneal shunt. On examination, he has papilloedema and fixed, mid-position pupils. Which one of the following does not alter cerebral perfusion pressure?**

A. Blood glucose concentration

B. Intracranial pressure

C. Jugular venous pressure

D. Mean arterial pressure

E. Partial pressure of carbon dioxide in the blood

49. **A 79-year-old is brought to the ED following a collapse at home. He has a history of ischaemic heart disease. On examination, he is diaphoretic and tachycardic. His ECG is shown in Figure 2.1. Given the likely diagnosis, what is the most common site of disease?**

A. Left circumflex artery

B. Left main stem

C. Normal variant left anterior descending artery

D. Right coronary artery

E. Type III left anterior descending artery

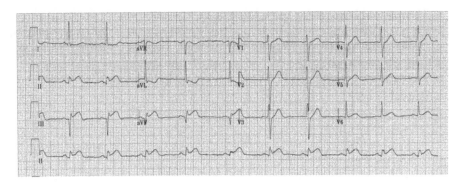

Figure 2.1 Electrocardiogram (ECG).

Courtesy of lifeinthefastlane.com. Copyright © 2007–2017.

50. **A 22-year-old man is brought to the ED following a collapse while running for a bus. He has a history of syncopal episodes and is deaf. On examination, he is well with a regular pulse. His ECG is shown in Figure 2.2. Given the likely diagnosis, what is the physiological change underlying this condition?**

   A. Accessory pathway
   B. Ectopic pacemaker function
   C. Impaired conduction through the His-Purkinje system
   D. Mutation in cardiac sodium ion channels
   E. Slowing of potassium ion channels

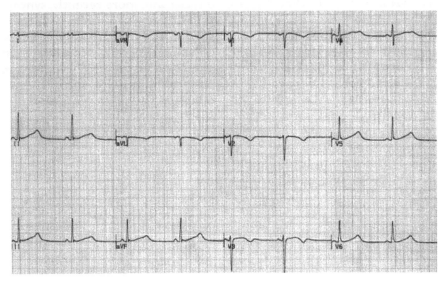

Figure 2.2 ECG.

Courtesy of lifeinthefastlane.com. Copyright © 2007–2017.

51. **A 21-year-old man walks in to Minors ED complaining of palpitations. He has a history of psychosis and is taking olanzapine. On examination, his heart sounds are normal with a regularly regular rhythm. His ECG demonstrates a prolonged QT interval. What one of the following answers shows the upper limit for a normal QT interval?**

    A. 250 milliseconds
    B. 350 milliseconds
    C. 440 milliseconds
    D. 460 milliseconds
    E. 500 milliseconds

52. **A 27-year-old manual labourer attends the ED with a painful right arm. He was carrying bricks in a hod when he slipped and fell, dropping the load onto his upper arm. He was unable to get up until help arrived, by which time his right arm was numb and pale. On examination however, the arm is now flushed red, warm to touch with reduced CRT. Which one of the following metabolites does not cause metabolic hyperaemia?**

    A. Adenosine
    B. Adrenaline
    C. Carbon dioxide
    D. Lactic acid
    E. Nitric acid

53. **A 62-year-old man is brought to the ED following a collapse at home. He has a history of ischaemic heart disease and, more recently, syncopal episodes. On examination, his pulse is rate is approximately 40 beats per minute. His ECG demonstrates total dissociation between P waves and QRS complexes. You recall that the physiological process preventing ventricular rhythms during sinus rhythm is called overdrive suppression. Which membrane transport protein is responsible for overdrive suppression?**

    A. Funny current channels
    B. L-type Ca2+ channels
    C. Na+,K+-ATPase transporters
    D. Voltage-gated K+ channels
    E. Voltage-gated Na+ channels

54. **A 57-year-old man attends the ED referred from his GP with severe hypertension. He has no significant medical history and was attending the GP for a Well Man check. On examination, he has enlarged body habitus. Initial observations in the ED are as follows: BP 194/98 mmHg, HR 92 bpm, RR 24 breaths per minute, and T 37.2°C. What is the physiological reason for the high pulse pressure in this case?**

   A. Increased total cross-sectional area of the capillary beds
   B. Reduced arterial compliance secondary to hypertension and ageing
   C. Reduced systemic vascular resistance
   D. Shorter duration of the reduced ejection phase
   E. White coat hypertension

55. **A 44-year-old woman attends the ED with palpitations and feeling faint. The episodes are intermittent, and she starts to experience the symptoms during your history. On examination, her pulse is rapid but regular, and she is otherwise well. Initial observations are as follows: BP 94/58 mmHg, HR 142 bpm, RR 28 breaths/min, and T 37.2°C. The symptoms stop quickly while you are examining for cervical lymph nodes. Repeat observations are as follows: BP 126/77 mmHg, HR 91 bpm, RR 22 breaths/min. Given the likely diagnosis, which physiological change would you expect to occur during the episode?**

   A. Decreased noradrenaline release
   B. Decreased Ca_2+ concentration in the cardiac myocyte cytoplasm
   C. Increased myocardial contractility
   D. Increased vagal tone
   E. Metabolic alkalosis

56. **A 30-year-old woman is brought to the ED by her boyfriend after she collapsed while they were walking on the beach. While they were descending from the promenade she struck her knee on a protruding rock and cried out in pain. Seconds later she turned white and her legs gave way beneath her. She recovered almost instantaneously with good orientation and no other symptoms. On examination, she has bruising over the left tibial tuberosity and her pulse is regular. Initial observations are as follows: BP 122/83, HR 81, RR 16, T 36.7°C. Which one of the following mechanisms best explains the physiology of this collapse?**

   A. Increased parasympathetic activity, increased acetylcholine release, reduced rate of diastolic depolarization in pacemaker cells
   B. Increased parasympathetic activity, increased noradrenaline release, reduced threshold for pacemaker cell action potential firing
   C. Increased sympathetic nervous activity, increased acetylcholine release, hyperpolarization of pacemaker cell membranes
   D. Increased sympathetic nervous activity, increased noradrenaline release, increased rate of diastolic depolarization in pacemaker cell
   E. Induction of a 'funny' current during repolarization of pacemaker cells

57. A 79-year-old is brought to the ED following a fainting episode at home. He has a history of ischaemic heart disease. On examination, he is warm and well-perfused, and his pulse is regularly irregular. His ECG is shown in Figure 2.3. Given the likely diagnosis, what is the most common site of disease?

A. Atrioventricular node

B. Distal His-Purkinje system

C. Infranodal block

D. Proximal His-Purkinje system

E. Sinoatrial node

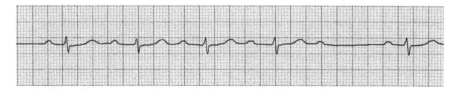

Figure 2.3 ECG.

Courtesy of lifeinthefastlane.com. Copyright © 2007–2017.

58. A 22-year-old man attends the ED with intermittent palpitations. He reports having similar episodes as a child, but these are becoming more frequent and preventing him from working as a manual labourer. He can usually terminate the episodes by pinching his nose, closing his mouth, and exhaling forcefully. On examination, he is sweaty and pale with a rapid pulse rate. Initial observations are as follows: BP 102/63, HR 131, RR 22, T 36.7°C. His ECG demonstrates a small up-sloping prior to the QRS complex. Which one of the following answers regarding the atrioventricular node is true?

A. Absence of fast Na+ channels decreases the duration of the action potential in the atrioventricular (AV) node

B. Conduction through the AV node is rapid compared to the bundle of His

C. Diltiazem is indicated for hypertension in patients with first degree heart block

D. Post-repolarization refractoriness is one of the mechanisms by which impulses are blocked in the AV node

E. Presence of an accessory pathway causes syncope by ventricular pre-excitation

59. **A 50-year-old Caucasian woman is brought to the ED by her children with abdominal pain and steatorrhoea. On examination, she has enlarged body habitus and is slightly jaundiced. When exerting pressure in the right upper quadrant, she is unable to take a complete breath without suddenly crying out in pain. Which one of the following regarding biliary secretion is true?**

    A. Bile consists of bicarbonate, bile salts, lecithin, and cholesterol
    B. Bile salts in the portal circulation inhibit further bile salt secretion by the hepatocytes
    C. Cholecystokinin directly stimulates bicarbonate secretion from the bile ducts
    D. Functions of the gallbladder include storage and dilution of bile
    E. Secretin stimulates secretion from the hepatocytes

60. **An 80-year-old woman attends the ED with abdominal pain, nausea, and reduced oral intake. She has a history of transient ischaemic attack (TIA) and takes clopidogrel. On examination, she is exquisitely tender in the epigastric region. Initial observations are as follows: BP 92/53, HR 112, RR 26, T 36.7°C. Which of the following statements regarding gastric emptying is true?**

    A. Cholecystokinin is secreted from G cells
    B. Gastrin promotes gastric emptying
    C. Increased duodenal pH decreases gastric emptying
    D. Parasympathetic stimulation to the pylorus is always inhibitory
    E. Secretin decreases gastric emptying

61. **A 27-year-old male nurse attends the ED with abdominal pain and vomiting. He has not opened his bowels in seven days. One week ago he had a Hartmann's procedure for perforated bowel, but is otherwise well. On examination, his abdomen is slightly distended with absent bowel sounds. Initial observations are as follows: BP 122/83, HR 106, RR 22, T 36.7°C. An abdominal film indicates significant faecal loading. Which one of the following is responsible for propulsion of intestinal contents along the gastrointestinal (GI) tract?**

    A. Adventitia
    B. Epithelium
    C. Muscularis externa
    D. Muscularis mucosae
    E. Submucosa

62. **A 27-year-old male nurse attends the ED with abdominal pain and vomiting. He has passed some dark blood per rectum today. As a child he suffered several episodes of volvulus. On examination, his abdomen is grossly distended with tinkling bowel sounds. Initial observations are as follows: BP 122/83, HR 126, RR 32, T 38.7°C. An abdominal film indicates a coffee bean pattern. Which one of the following transmits large nerves trunks and blood vessels within the gut wall?**

   A. Lamina propria
   B. Mucosa
   C. Muscularis externa
   D. Serosa
   E. Submucosa

63. **A 27-year-old nurse attends the ED with weight loss and diarrhoea. One month ago, he had a bowel resection for Crohn's disease. On examination, he is cachectic with multiple abdominal scars from previous surgery. Initial observations are as follows: BP 102/63, HR 116, RR 28, T 36.7°C. An abdominal film demonstrates a sparse-looking abdomen. Which one of the following is most responsible for increasing the surface area of the gut?**

   A. Lamina propria
   B. Muscularis mucosae
   C. Myenteric plexus
   D. Serosa
   E. Submucosal plexus

64. **A 25-year-old woman attends the ED with dehydration and diarrhoea. She has a history of ulcerative colitis and total colectomy. On examination, she has sunken eyes and prolonged CRT peripherally. Initial observations are as follows: BP 102/53, HR 92, RR 20, T 36.7°C. Which one of the following answers regarding the large intestine is true?**

   A. Mass movements occur one to three times a minute
   B. Segmental contractions of the caecum are responsible for propulsion of chyme
   C. The defaecation reflex is controlled by the enteric plexus
   D. The internal anal sphincter is under voluntary control
   E. The longitudinal smooth muscle layer around the large intestine is divided into bands

65. **A 40-year-old policewoman attends the ED with severe abdominal pain. She has a history of biliary colic and recent endoscopic retrograde cholangio-pancreatography (ERCP). On examination, she is slightly jaundiced and tender in the epigastric region. Initial observations are as follows: BP 132/93, HR 112, RR 26, T 38.3°C. Which one of the following functions of pancreatic exocrine juice is false?**
   A. Digestion of RNA
   B. Digestion of triglycerides
   C. Emulsification of fats
   D. Neutralization of gastric acid
   E. Prevention of premature proteolysis

66. **A 62-year-old semi-retired teacher attends the ED with difficulty swallowing. He was recently commenced on an antidepressant and describes dry mouth and worsening oral hygiene since that time. On examination, his tongue is dry, and you note multiple dental caries and halitosis. Which one of the following answers regarding saliva production is false?**
   A. Innervation to salivary glands is parasympathetic
   B. Innervation to salivary glands is sympathetic
   C. Saliva is involved in the digestion of carbohydrate
   D. Saliva is primarily hypertonic
   E. Taste and smell receptors stimulate salivation

67. **A 19-year-old woman attends the ED with very heavy periods and fatigue. On examination, she has general and conjunctival pallor. Initial observations are as follows: HR 92 bpm, BP 112/73 mmHg, RR 20 breaths per in, T 36.9°C. Which one of the following answers regarding iron absorption is true?**
   A. 90% of ingested iron is absorbed in the gastrointestinal tract
   B. Ascorbic acid is an inhibitor of iron absorption
   C. Enterocytes absorb Fe^{2+} ions via the DCT1 co-transporter
   D. This patient will have reduced capacity to absorb iron
   E. Transferrin binds Fe^{2+} in the enterocytes

68. **An 86-year-old woman is brought to the ED by her husband with dehydration and weight loss. She is suffering from Parkinson's disease and recently began to have difficulty swallowing, often choking in the process. On examination, she is cachectic with dry oral mucosae and increased skin turgor. She demonstrates Parkinsonian tremor and rigidity and when given a sip of water begins to cough. Initial observations are as follows: BP 82/53, HR 112, RR 26, T 36.7°C. Which one of the following answers regarding swallowing is true?**

    A. Secondary peristalsis occurs if a food bolus does not completely pass down the oesophagus
    B. The oesophageal phase occurs in less than one second
    C. The oesophagus contains smooth muscle only
    D. The pharyngeal phase is under voluntary control
    E. The upper oesophageal sphincter opens during respiration

69. **An obese 34-year-old woman attends the ED complaining of chronic symptoms: a sore and red tongue, mouth ulcers, paraesthesiae in the hands and feet, feeling foggy with her memory, and generally fatigued. You elicit that she had a Roux-en-Y gastric bypass performed three months ago at a private clinic. Her blood tests reveal a macrocytic anaemia. What most accurately describes the reasons the patient may have her current symptoms?**

    A. B12 absorption is dependent on intrinsic factor which is produced by chief cells of the stomach
    B. B12 is a fat-soluble vitamin and her lipase deficiency prevents absorption at the jejunum
    C. Her dietary B12 has been drastically reduced since her bariatric surgery
    D. She has a deficiency in R-binder protein and therefore free B12 cannot bind to R-binder in the duodenum for transport and absorption
    E. Surgery has resulted in pernicious anaemia due to removal of parietal cells

70. **An 86-year-old gentleman is awaiting medical admission in the ED; however, the hospital is at 'black' status for beds, and he has been in the ED for eight hours now. You are aware that the patient is diabetic, and ask the nurse looking after him to get him a cup of tea and some biscuits. Which one of the following is an example of a monosaccharide produced as a result of carbohydrate digestion?**

    A. Fructose
    B. Lactose
    C. Maltose
    D. Sucrose
    E. Trehalose

71. **A 24-year-old beautician has been referred by her GP to the ED due to chronic diarrhoea and significant postural drop in the surgery. On examination, she looks clinically dehydrated and says she has been using milk and yoghurts to maintain her fluid and energy levels. Her observations are as follows: lying BP 140/88, standing BP 111/60, HR 120, RR 18, Sats 97% in room air, T 36.8°C. Which one of the following statements is true with regards to osmotic diarrhoea?**

    A. Chloride channels in the apical membrane are open and result in excessive chloride loss
    B. Excessive secretion of water by crypt cells leads to increased water in the lumen
    C. Non-absorbable solutes in the intestine cause retention of water in the lumen
    D. Osmotic diarrhoea is secondary to an overgrowth of enteropathic bacteria in the gut
    E. Shortened gut length is the principal cause of osmotic diarrhoea

72. **A 43-year-old overweight woman attends the ED complaining of severe right upper quadrant pain which she describes as 'worse than childbirth'. On careful questioning, she has had dark brown urine and pale stools for the last few days, and has been suffering with nausea and vomiting. On examination, she is Murphy's sign positive and is guarding her upper abdomen. Which one of the following statements accurately describes the process of gallstone formation?**

    A. Excessive absorption of bile salts and water results in cholesterol precipitating into crystals
    B. Not enough cholesterol is absorbed from plasma into the bile resulting in a higher circulating cholesterol concentration in the blood
    C. Not enough water is absorbed from bile in the gall bladder
    D. The condition of the gallbladder epithelium is not a contributing factor to stone formation
    E. Most gallstones are comprised of calcium

73. **A 12-year-old with learning difficulties and multiple previous attendances is seen in the ED complaining of severe abdominal pain and vomiting. His mother reveals he suffers with pica, and you suspect he may have acute bowel obstruction as he has had absolute constipation for three days. Which one of the following hormones is most likely to inhibit gastric secretions?**

    A. Acetylcholine
    B. Gastrin
    C. Ghrelin
    D. Histamine
    E. Secretin

74. **A 22-year-old arts student attends the ED with upper abdominal pain and diarrhoea. You are aware that he suffers with Crohn's disease and has an ileostomy following perforation two years ago. In this particular visit, he complains of greasy pale stool which is difficult to flush and wipe away. Which one of the following statements is true with regards to lipid metabolism?**
    A. Emulsification of fats begins in the duodenum
    B. Emulsification of fats in the intestine increases surface area by a factor of 10
    C. Fats are emulsified exclusively by bile salts
    D. Pancreatic lipases are fat-soluble compounds
    E. Triglycerides are broken down into free fatty acids and monoglycerides by lipase

75. **A 63-year-old man has represented to the ED shortly after surgical discharge. He had been admitted with gallstone pancreatitis three days ago, and in spite of medical advice, self-discharged prior to treatment. He has admitted to a diet rich in red meat and cheese since discharge. What best describes the role of the enzyme trypsin in protein digestion in the small intestine?**
    A. Cleaving of individual amino acids from the carboxyl terminus
    B. Collagen breakdown in an acidic environment
    C. Digestion of elastin fibres
    D. Splitting proteins into smaller polypeptides
    E. Stimulates pancreas to release more proteolytic pancreatic enzymes

76. **A 19-year-old girl is brought to the ED by her friends who are worried about her because she has a reduced conscious level, has been crying hysterically and vomited three times. On careful history taking, you unveil she had consumed a large quantity of different types of alcohol prior to being removed from the party she was at. Which one of the following neurotransmitters is least likely to be a cause of vomiting?**
    A. Acetylcholine
    B. Dopamine
    C. Histamine
    D. Noradrenaline
    E. Serotonin

77. **A young man is brought to the ED after being found unconscious in his own home. Neighbours became concerned for his well-being and the police were called. Blood gas analysis demonstrates the following: pH 6.95, PCO_2 2.8, BE -19.4, anion gap 29. Which of the following causes is most likely to generate these results?**
    A. Addison's disease
    B. Administration of chloride
    C. Cyanide intoxication
    D. Diarrhoeal illness
    E. Renal tubular acidosis

78. **A medical student has taken an ABG sample for a 60-year-old gentleman who has attended with a febrile illness. They present you with the following results for interpretation: pH 7.28, PaCO$_2$ 7.4, HCO$_3$⁻ 22.6, BE -1.4. Which one of the following answers regarding the interpretation of this result is most likely to be true?**

A. Fully compensated respiratory acidosis

B. Metabolic acidosis

C. Partially compensated respiratory acidosis

D. Respiratory acidosis

E. Venous sample

79. **The FY2 doctor has taken an ABG sample for a 60-year-old woman who has attended with a febrile illness. They present you with the following results for interpretation: pH 7.49, PaCO$_2$ 6.9, HCO$_3$⁻ 27.6, BE 9.4. Which one of the following answers regarding the interpretation of this result is most likely to be true?**

A. Fully compensated metabolic alkalosis

B. Metabolic alkalosis

C. Normal sample

D. Partially compensated metabolic alkalosis

E. Respiratory alkalosis

80. **A 72-year-old woman is brought to the ED with slurred speech and right-sided weakness. She has a history of previous DVT, smoking, and hypertension. She has no allergies but is treated with ramipril. The circulating level of which one of the following is reduced by angiotensin converting enzyme (ACE) inhibitors?**

A. Aldosterone

B. Angiotensin I

C. Bradykinin

D. Renin

E. Serum albumin

81. **A 48-year-old pub landlady attends the ED with vomiting, cramps, and very dark urine. She has a history of central diabetes insipidus, treated with terlipressin. While inspecting her medication, you realize she has been taking a 10-fold overdose. On examination, she appears well hydrated with moist mucosae and normal capillary refill. Blood tests demonstrate the following: Na 118, K 2.9, Ur 1.4, Cre 22. Which of the following transport proteins is only active in the presence of antidiuretic hormone (ADH)?**

A. 1Na+,1K+,2Cl- symporter

B. Apical aquaporin 2

C. Basolateral aquaporin 3

D. Na+,K+ ATPase pump

E. Na+,Cl- symporter

82. **A 48-year-old pub landlord attends the ED with vomiting, cramps, and very dark urine. He was diagnosed with small-cell carcinoma of the lung one year ago and is receiving chemotherapy. On examination, he appears well hydrated with moist mucosae and normal capillary refill. Blood tests demonstrate the following: Na 118, K 2.9, Ur 1.4, Cre 22. Which one of the following answers regarding regulation of plasma osmolality is true?**

    A. ADH binds to V2 receptors in cells lining the loop of Henle
    B. ADH is produced in the hypothalamus and secreted by the anterior pituitary gland
    C. ADH is released in response to a decrease in plasma osmolality
    D. Thirst is more responsive to changes in plasma osmolality than blood volume
    E. This gentleman has central diabetes insipidus

83. **A 96-year-old woman is brought to the ED from her nursing home with confusion and reduced oral intake. On examination, she is clinically dehydrated and has a pan-systolic murmur in the mitral area. While checking her list of medications, you note she is taking spironolactone, an aldosterone antagonist. Which one of the following functions of aldosterone is correct?**

    A. Conversion of angiotensin I to angiotensin II
    B. Inhibition of Na^+ reabsorption by the collecting duct via second messenger compounds
    C. Insertion of aquaporin 2 into the membranes of cells lining the collecting duct
    D. Stimulation of Na^+ entry across the apical membranes of the cells of the distal convoluted tubule
    E. Vasoconstriction of the afferent arterioles and enhancement of Na^+ reabsorption by the proximal convoluted tubule

84. **A 17-year-old male is brought to the ED following a motorcycle collision with an oncoming vehicle. There is evidence of catastrophic haemorrhage from a compound fracture of the left femur and a tense, distended abdomen. Initial observations are as follows: BP 82/53, HR 152, RR 42, T 34.7°C. Which one of the following answers regarding renal autoregulation is true?**

    A. Angiotensin II acts to increase renal blood flow
    B. Autoregulation is absent at this blood pressure
    C. Haemorrhage decreases renin secretion
    D. Nitric oxide is a vasoconstrictor
    E. Sympathetic stimulation acts to increase glomerular filtration rate

85. **A 19-year-old patient attends the ED with diarrhoea and vomiting for several days. He recently attended a pop-up street food festival in East London and thinks he may have food poisoning. On examination, he is tachycardic with sunken eyes, cool peripheries, and dry mucosae. Blood tests demonstrate the following: WCC 15.7, CRP 29, Na 149, K 3.5. In which part of the nephron does aldosterone stimulate sodium ion reabsorption?**

   A. Collecting duct
   B. Descending limb of the loop of Henle
   C. Juxtaglomerular apparatus
   D. Proximal convoluted tubule
   E. Thin ascending limb of the loop of Henle

86. **A 47-year-old woman attends the ED with debilitating diarrhoea. She recently returned from a business trip to India and has been passing watery stools over 10 times a day since. On examination, she appears clinically dehydrated and has active bowel sounds. Initial observations are as follows: BP 102/53, HR 102, RR 19, T 37.7°C. An ABG is taken, which demonstrates the following: pH 7.32. Which one of the following is a variable in the Henderson–Hasselbalch equation?**

   A. Cl^-
   B. O_2
   C. H^+
   D. HCO_3^-
   E. Na^+

87. **A 32-year-old woman is brought to the ED with a displaced percutaneous endoscopic gastrostomy (PEG) tube. She has a history of cerebral palsy with swallowing difficulties and previous aspiration pneumonia. On examination, she appears dehydrated. There is no one on site who is competent to replace the PEG tube and after discussion with your consultant, who knows the patient well, you decide that nasogastric (NG) tube insertion is unlikely to be tolerated. You therefore cannulate and commence IV fluids. Which of the following responses to hypovolaemia is likely to occur?**

   A. Decrease in sympathetic outflow to the kidneys
   B. Glomerular filtration rate is enhanced
   C. Na+ reabsorption increases
   D. Release of natriuretic peptides from the heart and kidneys
   E. Suppression of the renin-angiotensin-aldosterone system

88. **A 92-year-old gentleman is brought to the ED with abdominal pain. He has not passed urine in over 24 hours. On examination, there is a large, palpable mass in the suprapubic area. Initial observations in the ED are as follows: BP 172/91, HR 118, RR 28, T 36.8. Which of the following statements about micturition is correct?**

A. Detrusor muscle is composed of skeletal muscle
B. External sphincter relaxation is under autonomic control
C. Loss of sympathetic innervation results in bladder dysfunction
D. Pudendal nerve forms the afferent arm of the micturition reflex
E. Stimulation of parasympathetic fibres causes detrusor contraction

89. **A 77-year-old woman is brought to the ED following a collapse at home. She reports she stood up to make herself a cup of tea, but felt light-headed by the time she reached the kitchen and her legs gave way beneath her. She takes ramipril and bendroflumethiazide. On examination, she has normal, regular heart sounds, and a small laceration on her forehead. Initial observations are as follows: BP 152/63, HR 62, RR 14, T 36.7°C. Which one of the following components of the nephron responds to pressure changes in the afferent arteriole to release renin?**

A. Bowman's capsule
B. Descending loop of Henle
C. Juxtaglomerular apparatus
D. Podocytes
E. Vasa recta

90. **A 29-year-old woman attends the ED with facial swelling. This started a couple of days ago and is accompanied by a 'butterfly' rash across her cheeks that has been present for several weeks. On examination, she is oedematous in her dependent areas and her urine sample appears milky. Which of the following features supports the diagnosis of a nephrotic syndrome rather than a nephritic syndrome?**

A. Haematuria
B. History of recent upper respiratory tract infection
C. Hypertension
D. Oliguria <300 mL/day
E. Proteinuria >3.5 g/day/1.73 m^2

91. A 91-year-old gentleman is brought to the ED from his home after an unresponsive episode. He has recently been experiencing dysuria and confusion. He has a past medical history of stage 4 chronic kidney disease. On examination, he is disorientated and appears clinically dehydrated. Initial observations are as follows: BP 104/68, HR 92, RR 20, T 38.7°C. His initial blood results demonstrate his potassium level to be 6.8. Which one of the following answers regarding potassium excretion is true?

A. Potassium is secreted by principal cells in the distal tubule and collecting duct

B. Reabsorption of potassium from the tubular lumen occurs via the Na+,K+-ATPase pump

C. Renal failure causes hyperkalaemia due to increased reabsorption of K+

D. The main route of potassium excretion is in the stool

E. Treatment with insulin-dextrose increases potassium excretion

92. A 57-year-old roofer attends the ED with a red, swollen, hot, and painful thumb. He injured himself at work while cutting tiles three days before. He reports no allergies but takes ibuprofen regularly for joint pain. On examination, there is purulent discharge from the wound with surrounding erythema that has spread to the first metacarpophalangeal (MCP) joint on the affected side. Blood tests demonstrate the following: WCC 17.8, CRP 46, Ur 8.2, Cre 157. Which of the following increase GFR?

A. Angiotensin II

B. Endothelin

C. Noradrenaline

D. Prostaglandins

E. Sympathetic stimulation

93. A 19-year-old patient attends the ED with diarrhoea and vomiting. He has a history of maple syrup urine disease (MSUD) and liver transplant. You recall that MSUD is an organic acidaemia, the result of an inborn error of metabolism. Which part of the nephron is primarily responsible for reabsorption of organic acids?

A. Ascending limb of the loop of Henle

B. Collecting duct

C. Descending limb of the loop of Henle

D. Distal convoluted tubule

E. Proximal convoluted tubule

94. **A 60-year-old woman is brought to the ED following a seizure at home. She is a nutritionist and her family report that she eats healthily and drinks plenty of water. Once recovered, she states that she regularly drinks in excess of 12 L water a day. Which one of the following answers regarding urine production is true?**

A. ADH will be present at high levels in this patient
B. Dilution occurs in the thick ascending limb
C. The descending limb of the loop of Henle is impermeable to H_2O
D. Urea is an ineffective osmole in the medulla of the kidney
E. Urine osmolality will be approximately 290 mOsm/kg H_2O in this patient

95. **A 72-year-old woman attends the ED with vomiting and abdominal pain. She has not opened her bowels for three days. On further questioning, she has been feeling lethargic and low in mood for several months. She has a history of hypertension and renal stones. On examination, her abdomen is soft, but you can palpate faecal loading on the left side. Comprehensive blood tests taken in triage have just come back. Which of the following results is consistent with a diagnosis of hyperparathyroidism?**

A. Decreased Ca^{2+}; decreased PO_{4-}
B. Decreased Ca^{2+}; increased PO_{4-}
C. Increased Ca^{2+}; decreased PO_{4-}
D. Increased Ca^{2+}; increased PO_{4-}
E. Unchanged Ca^{2+}; unchanged PO_{4-}

96. **A 72-year-old woman was brought in to the ED following a fall at home. She tripped over a plant pot while gardening and landed onto the turf on her left side. On examination, she has a shortened, externally rotated left leg, and is in a lot of pain. A plain radiograph confirms the presence of an intracapsular neck of femur fracture on the left-hand side, while initial blood tests demonstrate elevated calcium and low phosphate levels. You suspect hyperparathyroidism. Which one of the following answers regarding renal absorption of calcium and phosphate in hyperparathyroidism is true?**

A. Activation of vitamin D increases excretion of calcium and phosphate
B. Calcium reabsorption is decreased in the collecting duct AND phosphate reabsorption is decreased in the thick ascending loop of Henle
C. Calcium reabsorption is decreased in the distal tubule AND phosphate reabsorption is increased in the thick ascending loop of Henle
D. Calcium reabsorption is increased in the distal tubule AND phosphate reabsorption is decreased in the proximal tubule
E. Phosphate secretion is increased throughout the nephron AND calcium reabsorption is increased in the distal tubule

97) **A 29-year-old gentleman is brought to the ED after being found unresponsive in his own home by a neighbour. On examination, he is cachectic and appears to have a darkening of the skin around his mouth that his neighbour states is new. Initial observations in the ED are as follows: BP 72/48, HR 121, RR 40, T 39.1°C, SaO$_2$ 99% (on 15 L O$_2$). His capillary blood glucose is measured at 2.3. Which one of the following mechanisms best explains why this gentleman has darkening of his skin?**

A. Catalysis of tyrosine into dihydroxyphenylalanine (DOPA) is the first step of melanogenesis and results from direct exposure to ultraviolet (UV) light

B. Hypersecretion of insulin leading to activation of keratinocyte insulin-like growth factor (ILGF) receptors

C. Increased levels of DCT1 in the luminal membrane of enterocytes leading to levels of Fe^{3+} in the body

D. Mutation of the *STK11* gene leading to development of melanotic macules on the lips and oral mucosa

E. Removal of negative feedback to adrenocorticotropic hormone (ACTH) secretion

98. **A 62-year-old woman attends the ED with headaches, palpitations, and a sense of impending doom. These symptoms have been occurring intermittently over the preceding few months. On examination, she is diaphoretic and tremulous. Initial observations in the ED are as follows: BP 202/128, HR 151, RR 22, T 37.1°C, SaO$_2$ 100% (on room air). Which one of the following answers regarding layers of the adrenal gland is true?**

A. Capsule produces no hormones

B. Medulla produces cortisol

C. Zona fasciculata produces aldosterone

D. Zona glomerulosa produces adrenaline and noradrenaline

E. Zona reticularis produces mineralocorticoids

99. **A 79-year-old woman attends the ED following a fall at home. She describes falling forward onto her outstretched right hand. Since the injury, her right wrist has been very painful, and she has been unable to move it. On examination, there is a 'dinner fork' deformity of the right wrist. Which one of the following answers regarding bone turnover is correct?**

A. Formation precedes resorption in bone remodelling

B. Hydroxyapatite forms the organic matrix of bone

C. Hydroxyproline and hydroxylysine concentrations in the urine reflect bone turnover rate

D. Osteoblasts comprise 90% of all bone cells

E. Osteoclasts arise from pluripotential mesenchymal cells

100. A 59-year-old woman attends the ED with abdominal pain. On examination, she has left-sided abdominal tenderness with a palpable mass. Initial observations in the ED are as follows: BP 172/108, HR 114, RR 28, T 37.1°C. A CT scan of the abdomen and pelvis is requested, which demonstrated a 5 × 7 cm mass associated with the left adrenal gland. Which of the following is a common feature of Conn syndrome?

A. Dehydration
B. Hyperchloraemic acidosis
C. Hypokalaemia
D. Natriuresis
E. Peripheral oedema

101. A 38-year-old woman attends the ED with headaches, weakness, and irregular menstruation. She has noticed that she has put on weight around her abdomen but that her arms and legs are much thinner. On examination, she has striae and bruising over her abdomen and hirsutism. Initial observations in the ED are as follows: BP 152/98, HR 81, RR 20, T 37.1°C. Her blood glucose is 15.8. Which one of the following answers regarding the effects of cortisol is true? Cortisol ...

A. ... directly stimulates vasoconstriction
B. ... increases bone density
C. ... increases proteolysis
D. ... inhibits glycogen formation
E. ... promotes the immune response

102. A 54-year-old man is brought to the ED with generalized weakness and inability to get out of his armchair. He reports recent low mood and weight gain. On examination, he has a dorsocervical fat pad with abdominal obesity and striae. His limbs appear wasted. Initial observations in the ED are as follows: BP 174/116, HR 98, RR 29, and T 37.2°C. Which of the following factors suggests Cushing's disease rather than Cushing's syndrome?

A. Circulating level of ACTH is reduced
B. Galactorrhoea
C. Male gender
D. Positive low-dose dexamethasone suppression test
E. Use of exogenous glucocorticoids

103. **A 21-year-old medical student is brought to the ED with reduced level of consciousness, vomiting, and abdominal pain. His friends tell you that he has type 1 diabetes mellitus and has been participating in 'Freshers Week' events for the past couple of days and may have forgotten to take his insulin. On examination, the patient appears clinically dehydrated and demonstrates Kussmaul breathing. He opens his eyes to voice and localizes pain, but his speech is confused. Initial observations in the ED are as follows: BP 92/48, HR 121, RR 32, T 37.1°C and SaO$_2$ 100% (on 10 L O$_2$). Which one of the following will be elevated?**

A. Arterial partial pressure of CO_2
B. Glucokinase activity
C. Lipoprotein lipase activity
D. Serum C-peptide level
E. Serum triglyceride level

104. **An 18-year-old male is brought into the ED by the police following a violent altercation at a football match. Before he was apprehended, he tried to escape arrest on foot and ran for over an hour. Once caught, a short fist-fight ensued, and the patient was knocked unconscious. He was brought immediately to the ED. On examination, the patient is now alert but is breathing heavily and bleeding from a laceration to his left cheekbone. Initial observations in the ED are as follows: BP 112/78, HR 121, RR 28, T 37.1°C, SaO$_2$ 99% (on room air). Which one of the following will be reduced in this patient?**

A. Basal metabolic rate
B. Serum cortisol level
C. Serum C-peptide level
D. Serum glucagon level
E. Sympathetic tone

105. **A 62-year-old man attends the ED with a minor hand laceration while sawing timber in his garage. On further questioning, he reluctantly states the accident occurred because his hands seem to be getting bigger. He has no significant past medical history. On examination, he has thick, spade-like digits, and a large tongue. Blood glucose is measured at 11.2. Given the probable diagnosis, which of the following would most likely be effective treatment?**

A. Dopamine analogues
B. Insulin therapy
C. Insulin growth factor 1 supplementation
D. Ketogenic diet
E. Somatostatin analogues

106. A 32-year-old man attends the ED with a flare of Crohn's disease. He is on long-term steroids and confides in you that he is concerned about the risk this poses to his normal hormonal function. Which one of the following answers regarding the hypothalamic-pituitary-adrenal axis is true?

A. Adrenal medulla is ACTH-dependent and atrophies during periods of prolonged exogenous steroid administration

B. Cortisol is the only product of the adrenal cortex that participates in negative feedback to corticotropin-releasing hormone (CRH) and ACTH

C. CRH is produced in the anterior pituitary gland from proopiomelanocortin

D. Exogenous steroids do not suppress CRH or ACTH release

E. Serotonin inhibits CRH release

107. A 62-year-old woman attends the ED with abdominal pain and vomiting. On questioning, she also reports a longer history of back pain and low mood since she had a gallstone removed. On examination, her abdomen is soft and non-tender. Initial observations in the ED are as follows: BP 114/76, HR 81, RR 18, T 37.1°C. Initial blood tests demonstrate her albumin-corrected calcium level is 2.98. Which one of the following answers regarding calcium metabolism is true?

A. Calcitonin is synthesized in the parathyroid glands in response to hypocalcaemia

B. Extracellular (Ca^{2+}) undergoes wide, transient swings in order to maintain intracellular (Ca^{2+}) within tight limits

C. Osteoporosis is characterized by a disproportionate decrease in bone mineral content compared to bone matrix

D. Parathyroid hormone (PTH) synthesis will be suppressed in this patient

E. Vitamin D3 binds to membrane receptors on the enterocytes to decrease intestinal absorption of calcium

108. A 57-year-old woman attends the ED with palpitations. She gives a history of recent unintentional weight loss of 3 kg, tremulous hands, and feeling hot most of the time. On examination, she has a visible goitre. Initial observations in the ED are as follows: BP 142/98, HR 121, RR 20, T 37.1°C. In this patient, which one of the following would you expect to be reduced?

A. Calorie intake

B. Cardiac output

C. Minute ventilation

D. Serum rT3 level

E. Thyroid peroxidase activity

109. A 57-year-old woman attends the ED with her partner having expressed suicidal ideas. She gives a history of recent weight gain, cold intolerance, and feeling low in mood. On examination, she has coarse features, thin hair, dry skin, and a visible goitre. Initial observations in the ED are as follows: BP 102/68, HR 51, RR 20, T 36.1°C. In this patient, which one of the following physiological changes would you expect?

A. Increased cardiac output

B. Increased gluconeogenesis

C. Reduced number of cardiac α adrenergic receptors

D. Reduced thyrotropin levels

E. Reduced colloid production

110. A 62-year-old man is brought to the ED after being found unconscious while shopping. He is unaccompanied but carries a patient information card stating that he has type 2 diabetes mellitus on insulin therapy. He has been cannulated by the paramedics. On examination, he opens his eyes to pain and withdraws from painful stimuli. His speech is sparse but unintelligible. Initial observations in the ED are as follows: BP 159/98, HR 113, RR 22, T 37.1°C. His capillary blood glucose is measured at 2.1. Which one of the following processes is stimulated by insulin?

A. Catabolysis

B. Hepatic glycogenolysis

C. Ketogenesis

D. Lipolysis of adipose tissue

E. Muscle glucose uptake

111. A 62-year-old gentleman is brought to the ED following an unresponsive episode at home. He was doing the laundry when his wife noticed his speech was confused and he was supporting himself against the counter. He has known type 2 diabetes mellitus and had just taken his evening insulin, but appeared unconscious when offered a sugary drink. He has been given oral glucose gel by the paramedics. On examination, he is disorientated and has abdominal bruising. Initial observations in the ED are as follows: BP 159/98, HR 113, RR 22, T 37.1°C. His capillary blood glucose is measured at 2.1. Which one of the following answers regarding insulin is true?

A. Destruction of the pancreatic islet α cells underlies this gentleman's condition

B. Insulin secretion occurs independently from α cell function

C. Serum insulin levels are an inaccurate proxy of α cell function in diabetic patients

D. This gentleman will have an elevated serum C-peptide level

E. Zinc joins insulin molecules into dimers within secretory granules

112. **A 49-year-old woman attends the ED with a painful rash on her abdomen that has not responded to the medication her GP has prescribed. On examination, her body mass index (BMI) is 49 and there is a red, tender rash with skin sloughing and a foul odour in the skin fold underlying her abdominal fat. What is the site of leptin secretion?**

A. Adipose tissue

B. Duodenum

C. Endocrine pancreas

D. Exocrine pancreas

E. Hypothalamus

113. **A 47-year-old woman attends the ED with headache, blurred vision, and extreme anxiety. These symptoms have been occurring in bursts for the last month and she has lost 3 kg in weight. She is feeling better at present. On examination, she has a left-sided palpable mass. Initial observations in the ED are as follows: BP 122/78, HR 84, RR 28, T 37.3°C. She then complains of sudden chest pain and profuse sweating. Repeat observations are taken: BP 208/149, HR 162. A CT scan of the abdomen and pelvis is requested, which demonstrates a 5 × 7 cm mass associated with the left adrenal gland. Which of the following statements regarding the adrenal medulla is correct?**

A. Adrenaline is synthesized from cholesterol

B. Cholinergic preganglionic fibres stimulate catecholamine release

C. Hyperglycaemia is a trigger for adrenaline release

D. Phaeochromocytoma is a tumour of the parietal cells

E. Noradrenaline release is independent of CRH

114. **A 27-year-old woman is brought to the ED after collapsing spontaneously at home. She had been complaining of difficulty breast-feeding but was otherwise well. She lost 2.5 L of blood at the delivery of her first child six months ago. On examination, there is no evidence of bleeding. Initial observations in the ED are as follows: BP 52/28, HR 121, RR 40, T 37.1°C, SaO$_2$ 99% (on 15 L O$_2$). Her ECG shows sinus tachycardia. Which single answer best explains the physiology of this case?**

A. Adrenal crisis secondary to pituitary ischaemic necrosis

B. Bilateral adrenal haemorrhage secondary to sepsis

C. Hypotensive crisis secondary to hypothalamic ischaemic necrosis

D. Tachycardia-induced cardiomyopathy

E. Thyrotoxic crisis secondary to pituitary ischaemic necrosis

115. A 58-year-old gentleman attends the ED with a painful rash across his shoulders. He has a history of dermatomyositis and takes long-term steroids. Which one of the statements regarding steroid hormones is MOST correct?

A. Specific plasma membrane receptors are the target of steroid hormones
B. Steroid hormones are produced from cholesterol
C. Steroid hormones are released by exocytosis
D. Steroid hormones are stored in secretory granules
E. Tyrosine is vital to production of steroid hormones

116. A 58-year-old man attends the ED with abdominal pain and steatorrhoea. The pain resolves slightly after eating. He has been treated with ranitidine for several months with no significant improvement in symptoms. On examination, he is exquisitely tender in the epigastric region. Which of the following is characteristic for Zollinger–Ellison syndrome?

A. G-cell activity is reduced compared to normal state
B. Gastrin levels increase significantly following a test meal
C. Parietal cell numbers are reduced due to negative feedback
D. Proton pump inhibitors are less effective than H_2-receptor antagonists
E. Somatostatin levels are reduced compared to normal state

1. B. Na⁺,K⁺-ATPase is electrogenic

A. Excitable tissues produce action potentials of different shapes and durations because they have different types of voltage-dependent ion channels. In cardiac muscle after the rapid depolarization, slow L-type calcium channels cause a plateau phase that is not seen in skeletal muscle. This is why the action potential lasts 5 msec in skeletal muscle and 200 msec in cardiac muscle.

B. Correct answer: The Na^+-K^+ pump moves three sodium ions out of the cell for every two potassium ions it brings in. This causes a net transfer of positive charge out of the cell and means the cytoplasm is negatively charged compared to the interstitial fluid. It is this process that generates the resting membrane potential and makes the Na^+-K^+ pump electrogenic.

C. All cells have a resting membrane potential, but not all cells are excitable. Excitable tissues have the capacity to produce action potentials and include neurons, skeletal, smooth, and cardiac muscle.

D. During the absolute refractory period, the cell is unresponsive, and an action potential cannot occur, no matter how strongly the cell is stimulated. During the relative refractory period, some voltage-dependent sodium channels are inactivated but if enough are recruited by a stronger-than-usual stimulus then a further action potential could be fired.

E. The voltage-dependent sodium channel is activated at the start of the action potential and the resulting influx of sodium ions correlates with the rapid depolarization of the action potential. The sodium gradient approaches electrochemical equilibrium but is counterbalanced by inactivation of sodium channels and activation of potassium channels. Further efflux of potassium generates repolarization of the membrane potential.

Cole JB, Heegaard WG, Deeds JR, et al. (2015). Tetrodotoxin poisoning outbreak from imported dried puffer fish—Minneapolis, Minnesota, 2014. *Morbidity and Mortality Weekly Report,* **63**(51), 1222–5.

Kutchai HC (2006). Generation and conduction of action potentials. In: Levy MN, Stanton BA, Koeppen BM (Eds.), *Berne & Levy Principles of Physiology,* 4th edition (Chapter 3). Maryland Heights, MO: Elsevier Mosby.

2. E. Voltage-gated sodium channels.

A. The channels responsible for the so-called 'funny' current are also known as pacemaker channels. They predominantly reside in the sino-atrial node and Purkinje fibres and transmit sodium ions inwards and more slowly at a more negative electrical potential than other sodium channels. This results in a shorter refractory period potentiating slow depolarization immediately at the end of the previous cardiac action potential.

B. These slow channels are responsible for calcium influx during the plateau (phase 2) of the cardiac action potential.

C. This electrogenic channel is partly responsible for achieving the resting membrane potential (phase 4) of excitable cells.

D. These channels open slowly as L-type calcium channels start to close. This results in repolarization of the myocyte membrane (phase 3).

E. Correct answer: Voltage-gated sodium channels are opened at approximately −80 mV, resulting in a rapid influx of sodium ions that have been concentrated in the extracellular fluid by the Na^+,K^+-ATPase pump. Phase 0 of the cardiac action potential is seen as a rapid upstroke.

Levy MN, Pappano A (2006). Electrical activity of the heart. In: Levy MN, Stanton BA, Koeppen BM (Eds.), *Berne & Levy Principles of Physiology*, 4th edition (Chapter 16). Maryland Heights, MO: Elsevier Mosby.

3. D. Prothrombin time is a measure of coagulation via the tissue factor pathway.

A. APTT is reflective of the contact activation pathway (previously known as the intrinsic pathway).

B. This is incorrect, as INR is calculated using the prothrombin time.

C. Sodium citrate (commonly the blue bottle in most UK hospital trusts) are used to collect coagulation samples. Sodium citrate binds calcium ions in the sample and acts as a reversible anticoagulant. Lithium heparin (green bottles) contain both anticoagulant and gel separate to separate the serum. It is usually used in biochemistry.

D. Correct answer: The tissue factor pathway (previously known as the extrinsic pathway), alongside the intrinsic or contact activation pathway, is responsible for the activation of Factor X and indirectly responsible for the conversion of prothrombin to thrombin.

E. Platelets are integral to the effective clotting and are responsible for providing us with the bleeding time. Absolute platelet counts are performed in a full blood count.

Levy MN, Pappano A (2006). Overview of the circulation, blood, and hemostasis. In: Levy MN, Stanton BA, Koeppen BM (Eds.), *Berne & Levy Principles of Physiology*, 4th edition (Chapter 15). Maryland Heights, MO: Elsevier Mosby.

4. D. Of the extracellular fluid, approximately one-quarter makes up the plasma.

A. Effective osmoles are those ions and molecules that are less permeable across the plasma membrane and so exert a greater osmotic pressure. Of these, the major determinant of extracellular fluid osmolality is sodium. One can roughly estimate the osmolality of extracellular fluid (ECF) by doubling the concentration of sodium.

B. Adipose tissue is hydrophobic and carries less water. Therefore, individual with greater amounts of adipose tissue have proportionally lower total body water.

C. The human body is at least 60% water. In this way, we estimate that a 70 kg adult has approximately 42 L (70 x 0.6 = 42) of total body water. This is then subdivided into one-third of ECF (14 L) and two-thirds of intracellular fluid (28 L).

D. Correct answer: ECF can be further subdivided into the interstitial fluid that surrounds cells and the intravascular fluid or plasma. The plasma constitutes one-quarter of the ECF, which in a 70 kg adult amounts to approximately 3.5 L.

E. The concentration of sodium in the ECF is about 145 mEq/L, while the intracellular concentration is about 12 mEq/L. This chemical gradient is the result of the Na^+,K^+-ATPase, or sodium pump.

Koeppen BM, Stanton BA (2006). Control of body fluid osmolality and extracellular fluid volume. In: Levy MN, Stanton BA, Koeppen BM (Eds.), *Berne & Levy Principles of Physiology*, 4th edition (Chapter 38). Maryland Heights, MO: Elsevier Mosby.

5. D. Prolonged exposure to an agonist increases intracellular response by up-regulation and sensitization.

  A. These are all secretagogues for gastric acid and each of them binds to a different G-protein coupled receptor. Histamine is the most potent of these and binds to H_2 receptors linked to stimulatory or Gs proteins. Receptor activation stimulates adenylyl cyclase to produce cAMP.

  B. G proteins are activated when the receptor they are linked to is bound to the correct agonist or ligand.

  C. Parietal, or oxyntic, cells secrete gastric acid and intrinsic factor.

  D. Correct answer: Prolonged exposure to an agonist often decreases the intracellular response by down-regulation and de-sensitization. This can occur by endocytosis and lysosomal degradation of receptors or by phosphorylation of the G protein.

  E. These are the components of a generalized signal-transduction pathway.

Kutchai HC (2006). Membrane receptors, second messengers, and signal-transduction pathways. In: Levy MN, Stanton BA, Koeppen BM (Eds.), *Berne & Levy Principles of Physiology*, 4th edition (Chapter 5). Maryland Heights, MO: Elsevier Mosby.

6. D. GLUT4.

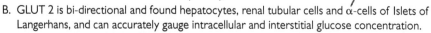

  A. GLUT 1 is found in foetal cells and erythrocytes.

  B. GLUT 2 is bi-directional and found hepatocytes, renal tubular cells and α-cells of Islets of Langerhans, and can accurately gauge intracellular and interstitial glucose concentration.

  C. GLUT3 is found in neurons and the placenta.

  D. Correct answer: GLUT4 is predominantly found in adipose tissue and striated muscle which includes skeletal and cardiac muscle. It is stored in cytoplasmic vesicles and recruited to the plasma membrane as a result of activation of insulin receptors.

  E. GLUT5 is responsible for fructose transport in enterocytes.

Genuth SM (2006). Hormones of the pancreatic islets. In: Levy MN, Stanton BA, Koeppen BM (Eds.), *Berne & Levy Principles of Physiology*, 4th edition (Chapter 43). Maryland Heights, MO: Elsevier Mosby.

7. C. Serotonin is released by platelets to enhance vasoconstriction.

  A. Thrombin converts fibrinogen into fibrin, which is the key step in coagulation.

  B. The three major factors involved in haemostasis are vasoconstriction, platelet aggregation, and coagulation of the blood. Vasoconstriction occurs as the direct result of mechanical stimulation to an injured vessel, causing smooth muscle constriction.

  C. Correct answer: Serotonin also contributes to vasoconstriction and is released by platelets during aggregation.

  D. Thromboxane A2 is released by platelets that have started to adhere to form a clot. This promotes further platelet aggregation and is an example of a positive feedback mechanism. Prostacyclin is released by normal endothelial cells and is part of the mechanism that prevents clot forming along the entirety of a vessel.

  E. Virchow's triad describes the key conditions that promote clot formation. It includes disturbance of blood flow, which may include stasis or turbulent flow such as occurs in the atria of the heart during atrial fibrillation. It also includes a hypercoagulable state, such as occurs in various forms of thrombophilia. The last component is endothelial damage, which provides a negatively charged surface that initiates the intrinsic pathway of the clotting cascade. Exposure of collagen also stimulates this process.

Levy MN, Pappano A (2006). Overview of the circulation, blood, and hemostasis. In: Levy MN, Stanton BA, Koeppen BM (Eds.), *Berne & Levy Principles of Physiology*, 4th edition (Chapter 15). Maryland Heights, MO: Elsevier Mosby.

8. D. Oscillation around a physiological 'set point' is due to lag time in the feedback loop.

A. Blood glucose control is under negative feedback, as are most homeostatic mechanisms.

B. Feedback loops are dictated by several factors, including emotion, pain, and sexual arousal. Additionally, patterns of hormone release vary through the day and may follow diurnal, ultradian (within a day) or seasonal patterns.

C. Positive feedback is an amplification process and therefore more unstable than negative feedback. An example is platelet aggregation during clot formation.

D. Correct answer: Since negative feedback requires the combined function of target cells, transport in the bloodstream, receptors, comparators and effectors (usually glands) there is an inevitable lag period between stimulus and response. As such, a value may continue to deviate away from the physiological set point until the homeostatic response counteracts the change and effects a return to the set point.

E. As discussed, negative feedback loops operate around a set point, while positive feedback loops are amplification processes in which response increases exponentially with time.

Genuth SM (2006). General principles of endocrine physiology. In: Levy MN, Stanton BA, Koeppen BM (Eds.), *Berne & Levy Principles of Physiology*, 4th edition (Chapter 41). Maryland Heights, MO: Elsevier Mosby.

9. A. Calcium is released from the sarcoplasmic reticulum of skeletal muscle.

A. Correct answer: Skeletal muscle is under voluntary control, innervated by α motor neurons. When the action potential reaches the motor end plate, acetylcholine is released and binds to nicotinic receptors. This generates an action potential that leads release of calcium ions from the sarcoplasmic reticulum, causing contraction of the entire muscle fibre. The motor unit is the term given to all the muscle innervated by a single neuron. In cardiac muscle, the influx of calcium ions is from the ECF.

B. Skeletal muscle differs from cardiac muscle in that it can increase the force of contraction by recruitment of other muscle fibres. In cardiac muscle, sympathetic innervation and stretch increase force.

C. Quite the opposite: myosin filaments ('thick') pull actin filaments ('thin') towards the centre of the sarcomere, which is bounded by Z lines.

D. Muscle mass increase secondary to strength training is due to hypertrophy of muscle fibres, which increase in diameter. No new muscle fibres are developed, as occurs in hyperplasia.

E. Tetany increases the frequency of action potentials in the muscle fibre, while recruitment is the process by which activating more α neurons increases force of skeletal muscle contraction.

Watras J (2006). Skeletal muscle. In: Levy MN, Stanton BA, Koeppen BM (Eds.), *Berne & Levy Principles of Physiology*, 4th edition (Chapter 12). Maryland Heights, MO: Elsevier Mosby.

10. E. Saltatory conduction requires more energy than standard conduction in a cell of the same diameter.

A. Larger diameter cells transmit action potentials at higher velocity due to the decreased longitudinal resistance of the cell.

B. Since action potentials 'jump' from one node to the next, up-regulation of voltage-gated ion channels occurs at these sites.

C. Schwann cells may consist of over 100 layers around a nerve cell, which greatly increases the membrane resistance at these points.

D. Since the length constant is calculated using the membrane resistance divided by the longitudinal resistance, myelination increases the length constant by dramatically increasing the membrane resistance. This increases conduction velocity and maintains amplification of the action potential.

E. Correct answer: Myelination improves metabolic efficiency of conduction pathways. The major expenditure of energy in electrical conduction is the Na^+,K^+-ATPase pump, which regenerates the electrochemical gradients of sodium and potassium after an action potential. Since the influx and efflux of ions occurs only at the nodes of Ranvier, the total energy required to achieve the resting membrane potential for the cell decreases significantly.

Kutchai HC (2006). Generation and conduction of action potentials. In: Levy MN, Stanton BA, Koeppen BM (Eds.), *Berne & Levy Principles of Physiology*, 4th edition (Chapter 3). Maryland Heights, MO: Elsevier Mosby.

11. A. γ-aminobutyric acid.

A. Correct answer: γ-aminobutyric acid (GABA) is an inhibitory neurotransmitter in the CNS. It is derived from glutamate and receptors are subdivided into the two major subclasses, $GABA_A$ and $GABA_B$. $GABA_A$ is a ligand-gated chloride channel, the activation of which hyperpolarizes the post-synaptic neuron. $GABA_B$ receptors act via protein kinase C to decrease calcium conductance.

B. Acetylcholine is responsible for stimulating nicotinic and muscarinic receptors, most prevalent at the neuromuscular junction and in the parasympathetic nervous system. Acetylcholine pathway degeneration has been implicated in Alzheimer's disease.

C. Dopamine is a catecholamine derived from tyrosine. Dopaminergic transmission is prevalent in the midbrain and disease of these pathways is implicated in Parkinson's disease and psychotic conditions.

D. Glutamate is the major excitatory neurotransmitter in the CNS. Glutamate receptors are also known as excitatory amino acid receptors.

E. Substance P pathways are present in the central and enteric nervous systems and are involved in the transmission of pain signals.

Kutchai HC (2006). Synaptic transmission. In: Levy MN, Stanton BA, Koeppen BM (Eds.), *Berne & Levy Principles of Physiology*, 4th edition (Chapter 4). Maryland Heights, MO: Elsevier Mosby.

12. C. NO is a paracrine mediator of vasodilatation.

A. This is incorrect because NO acts on both arterial and venous smooth muscle. In this way, both preload and afterload are reduced, alleviating ischaemic cardiac pain.

B. NO is released as a gas, and a well-established neurotransmitter in the enteric and CNS. Due to its high solubility, it is not released in vesicles, but instead diffuses from the presynaptic membrane.

C. Correct answer: Since endothelial NO is released by endothelial cells and acts upon neighbouring smooth muscle cells, its mode of action is paracrine. Its production is catalysed by endothelial NO synthase which is largely calcium-dependent.

D. NO is a potent vasodilator, and as stated here, acts in a paracrine rather than endocrine fashion.

E. The receptor for NO is guanylyl cyclase on smooth muscle cells. Activation of this receptor increases intracellular levels of cGMP and subsequently stimulating protein kinase to relax the cell.

Levy MN, Pappano A (2006). Overview of the circulation, blood, and hemostasis. In: Levy MN, Stanton BA, Koeppen BM (Eds.), *Berne & Levy Principles of Physiology*, 4th edition (Chapter 15). Maryland Heights, MO: Elsevier Mosby.

13. A.   A 0.9% sodium chloride solution is isotonic and will not alter the osmotic gradient between the intra and extracellular compartments.

A. Correct answer: The osmolarity of normal saline is approximately equal to the osmolarity of the body fluid, which is 286 milliosmolar. As such, administration of this isotonic solution should not alter the osmotic pressure gradient between the intra- and extracellular compartments.

B. This is incorrect because hypertonic saline increases net water movement out of the intracellular compartment, which is why it is used to treat cerebral oedema.

C. This is false because red cells shrink in hypertonic solutions and can lyse in hypotonic solutions.

D. If a membrane is more permeable to a solute, then movement of the solute down the concentration gradient will decrease the osmotic pressure gradient between the compartments and decrease water movement. The ideal semi-permeable membrane is permeable to water but impermeable to all solutes.

E. This is incorrect because water moves from areas of low to high osmotic pressure across a semi-permeable membrane.

Kutchai HC (2006). Cellular membranes and transmembrane transport of solutes and water. In: Levy MN, Stanton BA, Koeppen BM (Eds.), *Berne & Levy Principles of Physiology*, 4th edition (Chapter 1). Maryland Heights, MO: Elsevier Mosby.

14. E.   Flow is inversely proportional to fluid viscosity.

A. This will halve flow according to the equation shown in Box 2.1.

B. This will lead to a 16-fold increase in flow.

C. Flow is inversely proportional to resistance.

D. Flow is proportional to the pressure difference.

E. Correct answer: Poiseuille described the flow of fluids through a tube, such as an intravenous catheter. Flow (Q) is related to four variables: pressure gradient across the tubing (P), fluid viscosity (n), tubing length (L) and tubing diameter (r). Resistance to flow (R) can also be derived from these variables.

Levy MN, Pappano A (2006). Haemodynamics. In: Levy MN, Stanton BA, Koeppen BM (Eds.), *Berne & Levy Principles of Physiology*, 4th edition (Chapter 20). Maryland Heights, MO: Elsevier Mosby.

Box 2.1 Equation

$$\text{Volume Flowrate} = \mathcal{F} = \frac{P_1 - P_2}{\Re} = \frac{\pi(\text{Pressure difference})(\text{radius})^4}{8(\text{viscosity})(\text{length})}$$

$$\text{Resistance to Flow } \Re = \frac{8\eta L}{\pi r^4}$$

15. A. A band.

A. Correct answer: Striated muscle is so-called because of the striped appearance it demonstrates under the microscope. The dark bands of the myofibril are due to myosin thick filaments and are constant in length during muscle contraction.

B. The light band, or I band, describes the area containing only actin thin filaments. In contrast to the A band, this band shortens during muscle contraction, as more actin overlaps with myosin filaments.

C. The sarcomere is the basic contractile unit of the myofibril, and describes the space between two Z lines.

D. The T tubules are invaginations of the muscle plasma membrane, the sarcolemma. They extend into the muscle fibre and stimulate Ca^{2+} release from the sarcoplasmic reticulum.

E. The Z line is a plate of connective tissue from which the actin filaments extend towards the midline of the sarcomere.

Watras J (2006). Skeletal muscle. In: Levy MN, Stanton BA, Koeppen BM (Eds.), *Berne & Levy Principles of Physiology*, 4th edition (Chapter 12). Maryland Heights, MO: Elsevier Mosby.

 16. E. Myosin phosphorylation is inhibited by an increase in cAMP, leading to improved ventilation.

A. Smooth muscle contraction and narrowing the smaller airways is a major part of the pathophysiology of bronchiolitis. Nevertheless, smooth muscle in the bronchiolar walls contains α_2- rather than α_1-receptors.

B. While not increasing cytosolic Ca^{2+} concentration—which would increase smooth muscle contraction—cGMP does stimulate myosin dephosphorylation leading to smooth muscle relaxation. However, α_2-adrenergic agonists do not cause increased cGMP levels in smooth muscle.

C. Hormones can stimulate smooth muscle contraction, as seen in asthma attacks triggered by fear or emotion. Hormones, such as adrenaline, bind to receptors on the smooth muscle cell membrane, activating phospholipase C and increasing inositol 1,4,5-triphosphate (InsP3) levels.

D. Smooth muscle differs from striated muscle, in that it lacks sarcomeres, T tubules, and troponin.

E. Correct answer: α_2-adrenergic agonists, such as salbutamol, activate adenylyl cyclase to increase cytosolic cAMP levels in smooth muscle. This inhibits myosin light-chain kinase, which decreases myosin phosphorylation and so relaxes the smooth muscle. As bronchiolar diameter increases, air flow increases to the fourth power, improving ventilation significantly. Unfortunately, while it has been demonstrated that humans develop α_2-adrenergic receptors from the sixteenth week of gestation, there is no good evidence to support the use of α_2-adrenergic agonists for wheeze in under-2's.

Chavasse R, Seddon P, Bara A, McKean M (2002). Short acting beta agonists for recurrent wheeze in children under 2 years of age. *The Cochrane Database of Systematic Reviews*, (2), CD002873.

Watras J (2006). Smooth muscle. In: Levy MN, Stanton BA, Koeppen BM (Eds.), *Berne & Levy Principles of Physiology*, 4th edition (Chapter 14). Maryland Heights, MO: Elsevier Mosby.

17. D. Recycling of choline occurs by endocytosis of coated vesicles.

A. When the action potential reaches the presynaptic neuron, voltage-gated calcium channels open triggering an increase in intracellular calcium concentration.

B. Influx of calcium ions stimulates release of acetylcholine, which occurs by exocytosis into the synaptic cleft.

C. Acetylcholine binds to nicotinic receptors on the post-synaptic membrane, which are excitatory. These are ligand-gated channels that increase conductance of sodium and potassium, generating an end-plate potential.

D. Correct answer: Acetylcholinesterase is abundant on the post-synaptic membrane, cleaving acetylcholine into acetate and choline. This action terminates the conductance of sodium and potassium, so terminating the end-plate potential. In myasthenia gravis, anticholinesterase medications such as pyridostigmine prolong and amplify the end-plate potential. Choline is not produced in neurons and is recycled.

E. Transmission at electrical synapses, such as those in cardiac muscle, can be bi-directional. However, due to the nature of neurotransmitter release and receptors, chemical synapses are only ever one-way.

Kutchai HC (2006). Synaptic transmission. In: Levy MN, Stanton BA, Koeppen BM (Eds.), *Berne & Levy Principles of Physiology*, 4th edition (Chapter 4). Maryland Heights, MO: Elsevier Mosby.

18. C. GLUT2 transporter.

A. Aquaporin 1 is an example of a pore, a channel that transports small molecules such as water along the concentration gradient. They remain constantly open.

B. Desmoglein-1 is not a membrane transport protein, but an adhesion protein that forms part of the desmosome, a structure that joins adjacent epithelial cells.

C. Correct answer: GLUT2 is a transporter protein. Transporters, or carriers, bind a substrate and undergo conformational change to allow the substrate to traverse the membrane. They can transport molecules against the concentration gradient. Due to this, they are ATP-dependent.

D. These post-synaptic receptors are an example of a ligand-gated channel.

E. Channels resemble pores in that they facilitate substrates in a bi-directional manner. Channels have open or closed states: an open channel allows rapid diffusion of substrate along the electrochemical gradient, whereas a closed channel results in a much slower rate of transport.

Kutchai HC (2006). Cellular membranes and transmembrane transport of solutes and water. In: Levy MN, Stanton BA, Koeppen BM (Eds.), *Berne & Levy Principles of Physiology*, 4th edition (Chapter 1). Maryland Heights, MO: Elsevier Mosby.

19. B. Hypothermia, coagulopathy, and acidosis.

A. Cushing's triad describes the physiological changes observed in the late stages of raised intracranial pressure.

B. Correct answer: The trauma triad of death, also known as the lethal triad, describes the signs that may be observed following significant traumatic injury, particularly involving massive haemorrhage. The loss of blood reduces body temperature and reduces tissue perfusion, increasing lactate production and reducing renal excretion of H^+. The resulting hypothermia and metabolic acidosis both impair the clotting cascade, worsening haemorrhage, and decreasing cardiac output. This positive feedback loop is associated with significantly increased mortality rates.

C. Beck's triad describes the examination findings in cardiac tamponade.

D. Charcot's triad describes the clinical picture commonly observed in ascending cholangitis.

E. This triad is suggestive of congestive heart failure.

Levy MN, Pappano A (2006). Interplay of central and peripheral factors in control of the circulation. In: Levy MN, Stanton BA, Koeppen BM (Eds.), *Berne & Levy Principles of Physiology*, 4th edition (Chapter 26). Maryland Heights, MO: Elsevier Mosby.

20. A. Difference between ideal P_AO_2 and measured PaO_2.

A. Correct answer: This patient has symptoms, risk factors, and clinical evidence of pulmonary embolism. The Aa gradient is used to detect impaired gas transfer by comparing the alveolar partial pressure of oxygen (P_AO_2), calculated using the alveolar air equation, with the arterial partial pressure of oxygen in the ABG (PaO_2).

B. The Aa gradient is not a comparison of CO_2 gas transfer, as the diffusion properties of CO_2 mean that P_ACO_2 and measured $PaCO_2$ are equivalent.

C. The Aa gradient is calculated as P_AO_2—PaO_2.

D. The Aa gradient is not a comparison of CO_2 gas transfer.

E. The relationship between P_AO_2 and P_ACO_2 is described by the alveolar air equation, a calculation that utilizes barometric pressure, water vapour pressure, inspired O_2 fraction (FiO_2) and the respiratory quotient (R).

Cloutier MM, Thrall RS (2006). Ventilation, perfusion and their relationship. In: Levy MN, Stanton BA, Koeppen BM (Eds.), *Berne & Levy Principles of Physiology*, 4th edition (Chapter 29). Maryland Heights, MO: Elsevier Mosby.

21. D. Peak expiratory flow rate is increased at higher lung volumes.

A. Laminar flow generates less airway resistance than turbulent flow. This is partly because the wave front in laminar flow is conical, with central particles moving faster than peripheral ones. The wave front in turbulent flow is square.

B. Airway irritant receptors stimulate a reflex loop, the efferent limb of which is a parasympathetic bronchoconstrictor nerve supply. Sympathetic innervation to the bronchial smooth muscle is sparse in humans.

C. According to Poiseuille's equation, resistance is inversely proportional to the fourth power of radius. Therefore, halving airway radius will increase airway resistance 16-fold.

D. Correct answer: Lung volume is a major factor in airway resistance, since the airways are higher calibre when lung volume is higher. As such, PEFR is much lower when the patient has not taken a full breath.

E. Wheeze requires turbulent flow between two closely opposed airway walls. However, reasonable airflow is required to generate the sound. As such, in severe bronchoconstriction when airflow is greatly reduced, the chest can be silent.

Cloutier MM, Thrall RS (2006). Mechanical properties of the lung and chest wall. In: Levy MN, Stanton BA, Koeppen BM (Eds.), *Berne & Levy Principles of Physiology*, 4th edition (Chapter 28). Maryland Heights, MO: Elsevier Mosby.

Ward JPT, Ward J, Leach RM, Wiener CM (Eds.) (2006). Lung mechanics: airway resistance. In: *The Respiratory System at a Glance*, 2nd edition (Chapter 7). Hoboken, NJ: Blackwell Publishing.

22. E. V/Q mismatch.

A. Anatomical shunts are most commonly caused by congenital heart disease, in which deoxygenated blood from right side of the heart bypasses the lungs and enters the systemic circulation, causing hypoxaemia.

B. Hypoventilation causes hypoxaemia by decreasing the partial pressure of oxygen in the alveoli (PAO_2). Since the airways and capillaries are morphologically normal, the PaO_2 (arterial) falls accordingly. As such, the alveolo-arterial (Aa) gradient is normal, which distinguishes hypoventilation from other causes of hypoxaemia. An example might be diaphragmatic paralysis.

C. Increase in dead space is the one answer that does not cause hypoxaemia. However, in diseases such as emphysema, increased dead space can cause hypercapnia.

D. Physiological shunts are those in which ventilation to an airway is completely blocked, leading to perfused blood passing through the lungs without oxygenation. This is a right-to-left shunt in the presence of normal anatomy and causes hypoxaemia. It is also an example of a ventilation-perfusion mismatch. Clinical examples include atelectasis.

E. Correct answer: This woman has a pulmonary embolism, unsurprisingly. Blood is not being perfused to areas of ventilated lung as the result of the thrombosis in the pulmonary vasculature, therefore, deoxygenated blood is returning to the left side of the heart. Ventilation-perfusion mismatching is the most common cause of hypoxaemia.

Cloutier MM & Thrall RS (2006). Ventilation, perfusion, and their relationship. In: Levy MN, Stanton BA, Koeppen BM (Eds.), *Berne & Levy Principles of Physiology*, 4th edition (Chapter 29). Maryland Heights, MO: Elsevier Mosby.

23. E. Ventilation is reduced to a greater extent than perfusion.

A. This gentleman meets the criteria for chronic bronchitis, a disease characterized by impaired ventilation and increased mucus production.

B. As a form of obstructive respiratory disease, chronic bronchitis is likely to impair ventilation due to both airway inflammation and narrowing and increased mucus production.

C. As described, mucus production will be increased.

D. Perfusion may be impaired secondary to arterial disease and smoking. However, emphysema reduces ventilation by destroying gas exchange surfaces and alveolar air spaces.

E. Correct answer: The pathology of obstructive pulmonary disease primarily affects ventilation.

Cloutier MM, Thrall RS (2006). Overview of the respiratory system. In: Levy MN, Stanton BA, Koeppen BM (Eds.), *Berne & Levy Principles of Physiology*, 4th edition (Chapter 27). Maryland Heights, MO: Elsevier Mosby.

24. B. Carbonic anhydrase catalyses the reaction of CO_2 with H_2O to form H_2CO_3 within the red blood cells.

A. This is a possible explanation for normal pH with high PaCO2 and high HCO_3^-. However, given the diagnosis of COPD and the history of likely exacerbation, the most plausible interpretation of the result is a respiratory acidosis in a chronic CO_2 retainer with full metabolic compensation over time.

B. Correct answer: $CO_2 + H_2O \leftrightarrow H_2CO_3 \leftrightarrow H^+ + HCO_3^-$
Bicarbonate synthesis is the main transport mechanism of CO_2 in the blood. This hydration reaction happens slowly in the plasma, but quickly in the red cells due to presence of carbonic anhydrase. Both stages are reversible, that is to say in equilibrium, and multiple factors shift the direction of the reaction, for instance pH.

C. Chloride shift also maintains the osmotic equilibrium of the red cell with the plasma, but involves the diffusion of bicarbonate produced by the hydration of CO_2 out of the red cell in exchange for chloride.

D. Haemoglobin does buffer the protons produced by the reaction, maintaining the blood pH within tight limits and potentiating further bicarbonate production, which would otherwise be inhibited by falling pH.

E. The Haldane effect does describe this relationship, however the O_2 dissociation curve is sigmoid (S-shaped) while the CO_2 dissociation curve is linear. In areas of low oxyhaemoglobin concentration (i.e. venous blood) the CO_2 dissociation curve shifts to the left—that is to say, the affinity of CO_2 for haemoglobin increases and more is bound for transport to the lungs and elimination.

Cloutier MM, Thrall RS (2006). Oxygen and carbon dioxide transport. In: Levy MN, Stanton BA, Koeppen BM (Eds.), *Berne & Levy Principles of Physiology*, 4th edition (Chapter 30). Maryland Heights, MO: Elsevier Mosby.

25. A. Compliance is a measure of the elastic properties of the lung and is measured in mL/cm H_2O.

A. Correct answer: This is the definition of lung compliance, defined as the change in lung volume produced by a transpulmonary pressure of 1 cm H_2O. Lung compliance is increased in emphysema and decreased in restrictive diseases, such as lung fibrosis. The same transpulmonary pressure increase would result in a greater increase lung volume in emphysema than in lung fibrosis.

B. Functional residual capacity is the volume of air in the lungs at the end of a normal expiration and is increased in emphysema. At this point, the inward elastic recoil of the lung is in equilibrium with the outward force exerted by the chest wall. Transpulmonary pressure is zero at both this point and the end of normal inspiration.

C. Lung compliance has static factors, such as age, gender, and body size. However, there is a dynamic component including airway resistance, which varies throughout inspiration and expiration and is inversely proportional to the fourth power of the airway radius (see Poiseuille's Law). Furthemore, compliance varies with lung volume: a partially-expanded lung is less compliant than an unexpanded lung.

D. Although we expect lung compliance to be increased in emphysema, COPD is the combination of two disease processes: chronic bronchitis and emphysema. In chronic bronchitis, factors such as airway resistance, RV, and total lung capacity are increased. However, lung compliance and surface area for gas exchange are normal. As such, not every patient with COPD is guaranteed to have increased lung compliance, though it is common.

E. Emphysema destroys the alveolar and capillary walls and so decreases the total surface area for gas exchange, measured as the DLCO.

Cloutier MM, Thrall RS (2006). Mechanical properties of the lung and chest wall. In: Levy MN, Stanton BA, Koeppen BM (Eds.), *Berne & Levy Principles of Physiology*, 4th edition (Chapter 28). Maryland Heights, MO: Elsevier Mosby.

26. B. 80 mL/cmH$_2$O.

Lung compliance is a measure of how elastic the lung tissue is. In this case, it takes a volume of 1,200 mL to inflate the lungs from end expiration to end inspiration, generating a pressure increase of 15 cmH$_2$O. Both are points of no air movement, as the forces of lung expansion and elastic recoil are in balance. This calculation requires that there be no physical effort from the subject.

A. This is incorrect; the calculation is as follows:
   Lung compliance = tidal volume / pressure difference

B. Correct answer: 1,200 mL/(20 cmH$_2$O—5 cmH$_2$O) = 80 mL/cmH$_2$O

C. This is incorrect.

D. This is incorrect.

E. This is incorrect.

Cloutier MM, Thrall RS (2006). Mechanical properties of the lung and chest wall. In: Levy MN, Stanton BA, Koeppen BM (Eds.), *Berne & Levy Principles of Physiology*, 4th edition (Chapter 28). Maryland Heights, MO: Elsevier Mosby.

27. B. Apneustic breathing, secondary to damage to the pons and vagus nerve.

A. Agonal gasps are seen in cardiac arrest situations as the result of generalized cerebral hypoxia or anoxia. They appear laboured, with a short inspiratory phase and longer expiratory phase.

B. Correct answer: Apneustic breathing follows this pattern and occurs as the result of damage to the pontine respiratory group with loss of sensory information from the vagus nerve. The dorsal respiratory group in the medulla oblongata provides continuous inspiratory drive that is 'turned off' by expiratory input from the cerebrum, pons, and cranial nerves. Without the pontine or vagal input, unopposed inspiration is only sporadically punctuated by inhibition from the ventral respiratory group in the medulla.

C. The patient is not apnoeic, although this pattern of breathing is seen in some individuals who lose respiratory drive when asleep due to defects in the autonomic system.

D. Cheyne–Stokes breathing describes an alternation between rapid, shallow breaths and slow, deep breaths. This is seen is brainstem disease, chronic heart failure, premature newborns, and during sleep at high altitude.

E. Kussmaul breathing is the laboured breathing seen in metabolic disorders such as diabetic ketoacedosis (DKA) and renal failure. Tidal volume is increased in an attempt to eliminate carbon dioxide and increase the pH of the blood.

Cloutier MM, Thrall RS (2006). Control of respiration. In: Levy MN, Stanton BA, Koeppen BM (Eds.), *Berne & Levy Principles of Physiology*, 4th edition (Chapter 31). Maryland Heights, MO: Elsevier Mosby.

28. C. Eisenmenger syndrome.

A. Although anaemia is common in Down's syndrome, it is highly unlikely to cause cyanosis. This is because approximately 50 g/L deoxygenated haemoglobin is required to give the bluish appearance. In addition, cyanosis from this cause would likely respond to oxygen therapy.

B. Although the patient presents with symptoms of lower respiratory tract infection, cyanosis from this cause would likely respond to oxygen therapy.

C. Correct answer Eisenmenger syndrome describes the conversion from a left-to-right cardiac shunt to a right-to-left shunt, occurring as the result of a chronic pulmonary hypertension and right heart overload. As the disease progresses, the pulmonary vascular resistance becomes so great that the direction of the shunt is reversed, and deoxygenated blood is pumped directly into the systemic circulation. Of the options, only this condition would be expected not to respond to oxygen therapy. The prognosis is poor as low oxygen saturations predispose end-organ damage.

D. Oxygenated blood returning to the pulmonary circulation is unlikely to cause cyanosis.

E. Although polycythaemia is common in Down's syndrome, it is unlikely to be the cause of cyanosis in this cause. However, cyanosis is common in this condition since due to the increased haemoglobin content of the blood, patients can tolerate quantities of deoxygenated haemoglobin over 50 g/L quite easily.

Inaba AS, Horeczko T (2010). Cardiac disorders. In: Marx JA, Hockberger RS, Wall RM, (Eds.), *Rosen's Emergency Medicine*, 7th edition. Philadelphia, PA: Mosby Elsevier.

Körten MA, Helm PC, Abdul-Khaliq H, et al. (2016). Eisenmenger syndrome and long-term survival in patients with Down syndrome and congenital heart disease, *Heart*, **102**(19), 1552–7.

29. C. Foetal haemoglobin.

A. This is known at the Bohr shift. Lower blood pH values occur when carbon dioxide and other metabolites are released into the bloodstream, generating increased H^+. This is an indicator of metabolic demand. It is beneficial that oxygen dissociates more readily from haemoglobin under these conditions.

B. 2,3-DPG is a product of the glycolysis pathway in red blood cells, another indicator of metabolic demand.

C. Correct answer: Foetal haemoglobin has a higher affinity for oxygen than adult haemoglobin and shifts the oxyhaemoglobin dissociation curve to the left. This ameliorates the right shift that occurs in sickle cell disease and is why babies with the disease have fewer crises than older children.

D. The chronic hypoxaemia resulting from living at altitude shifts the dissociation curve to the right, liberating O_2 for use by the tissues at higher partial pressures.

E. As with acidosis, the Bohr shift means that areas of high metabolic activity such as those with high partial pressure of CO_2 are supplied with O_2 more readily.

Cloutier MM & Thrall RS (2006). Oxygen and carbon dioxide transport. In: Levy MN, Stanton BA, Koeppen BM (Eds.), *Berne & Levy Principles of Physiology*, 4th edition (Chapter 30). Maryland Heights, MO: Elsevier Mosby.

30. C. Emphysema.

A. The reduced FEV_1/FVC ratio indicates obstructive disease, while air trapping and increased RV does occur in acute asthma. Reduced DLCO is not a feature of asthma.

B. There is no indication in the question that the gentleman has bronchiectasis.

C. Correct answer: Emphysema, a form of COPD, is characterized by degradation of elastin in airways, reducing lung compliance and leading to bulla formation. This increased RV and reduces the available surface for gas exchange, as measured by the diffusion capacity for carbon monoxide (DLCO).

D. Pneumonia does not affect the DLCO significantly.

E. Pulmonary fibrosis is a restrictive disease and should present an increased FEV_1/FVC ratio. A reduced DLCO is a feature of pulmonary fibrosis.

Cloutier MM & Thrall RS (2006). Mechanical properties of the lung and chest wall. In: Levy MN, Stanton BA, Koeppen BM (Eds.), *Berne & Levy Principles of Physiology*, 4th edition (Chapter 28). Maryland Heights, MO: Elsevier Mosby.

31. D. Shifting of the equal pressure point towards the alveoli.

A. This mechanism underlies allergic and atopic airway conditions such as asthma and extrinsic allergic alveolitis.

B. Elastic tissue may be degraded in emphysema, but the cartilage in the walls of larger airways is unaffected.

C. Lung compliance is reduced in obstructive airway diseases such as COPD.

D. Correct answer: Air trapping occurs in COPD due to collapse of the smaller airways during expiration. This occurs because the forces driving expiration, namely elastic recoil and positive pleural pressure, reduce throughout expiration as lung volume decreases and airway resistance increases. An equal pressure point is reached when pressure within the airway is equal to the forces driving expiration. In healthy individuals, this point occurs in the larger airways that contain cartilage to prevent collapse. In COPD, airway resistance is greater and the equal pressure point shifts towards the alveoli. In the smaller airways that do not contain cartilage, airway collapse, and air trapping occurs. This premature airway closure causes crackles as the airways re-open during inspiration.

E. This process may occur in emphysema, but does not contribute to expiratory airway collapse directly.

Cloutier MM, Thrall RS (2006). Mechanical properties of the lung and chest wall. In: Levy MN, Stanton BA, Koeppen BM (Eds.), *Berne & Levy Principles of Physiology*, 4th edition (Chapter 28). Maryland Heights, MO: Elsevier Mosby.

32. D. FEV_1 = 1.43 L; FVC = 2.50 L.

In obstructive respiratory diseases, the forced expiratory volume in one second (FEV_1) is reduced by a proportionally greater amount than the FVC of the lungs. The FEV_1/FVC ratio, with a normal value of approximately 0.8, is therefore reduced. The British Thoracic Society requires a FEV_1/FVC of <0.7 in order to diagnose COPD.

  A. 2.47/2.50 = 0.988
  B. 2.47/3.50 = 0.705
  C. 1.43/2.00 = 0.715
  D. Correct answer: 1.43/2.50 = 0.572
  E. 2.47/3.00 = 0.823

NICE (June 2010) Chronic obstructive pulmonary disease in over 16s: Diagnosis and management. Clinical guideline [CG101]. Available at: http://www.nice.org.uk/guidance/cg101

33. A. Carbon monoxide has an affinity for haemoglobin approximately 200 times greater than oxygen.

  A. Correct answer: Haemoglobin binds four oxygen molecules for every haem unit. Carbon monoxide binds to haemoglobin at the same site as oxygen and also increases oxygen affinity at the other sites, limiting oxygen delivery to tissues. Symptoms of carbon dioxide poisoning include headache, nausea, breathing difficulties, and neurological disturbances. Incidence has decreased since the advent of catalytic converters in car exhausts. Treatment is based around administration of high flow oxygen and barometric therapy in an attempt to displace the carbon monoxide.
  B. Fick's law states that diffusion of a gas across a sheet of tissue is directly related to surface area, permeability of the gas, and the partial pressure gradient across the tissue. Diffusion is inversely proportional to tissue thickness.
  C. As suggested by Fick's law, interstitial fibrosis, which thickens the alveolocapillary membrane by scar tissue formation, will impede diffusion and gas transfer. Diffusion is inversely proportional to membrane thickness.
  D. Oxygen and carbon dioxide are perfusion-limited, in that they readily equilibrate by diffusion between the alveolar gas and blood. This takes place while the red cell is in transit in the capillary bed and so the amount of diffusion depends on the amount of perfused blood. Carbon monoxide is less soluble in the alveolar-capillary membrane but highly soluble in blood because of its affinity with haemoglobin. As such, it is diffusion-limited.
  E. Methemoglobin accounts for 1–2% of total haemoglobin under normal conditions.

Cloutier MM & Thrall RS (2006). Oxygen and carbon dioxide transport. In: Levy MN, Stanton BA, Koeppen BM (Eds.), *Berne & Levy Principles of Physiology*, 4th edition (Chapter 30). Maryland Heights, MO: Elsevier Mosby.

34. E. V/Q mismatch.

  A. The four major physiological causes of hypoxaemia are: anatomical shunt, physiological shunt, hypoventilation, and ventilation-perfusion mismatching. The most common type of anatomical shunts are the cyanotic congenital heart diseases.
  B. Hypoventilation is a feature of musculoskeletal and neurological disorders.

C. Increased dead space is a feature of COPD and causes hypercapnia, rather than hypoxaemia.

D. Reduced cardiac output is the only non-respiratory factor to cause hypoxaemia.

E. Correct answer: Ventilation-perfusion mismatching is the most common cause of hypoxaemia. Examples include consolidation, pulmonary embolism, pneumothorax, mucous plugging, foreign bodies, and tumours.

Cloutier MM, Thrall RS (2006). Ventilation, perfusion and their relationship. In: Levy MN, Stanton BA, Koeppen BM (Eds.), *Berne & Levy Principles of Physiology*, 4th edition (Chapter 29). Maryland Heights, MO: Elsevier Mosby.

35. C. Immotile cilia.

A. Vitamin C deficiency is the cause of scurvy.

B. While this form of immunodeficiency may present with recurrent ear, sinus, and chest infections, the presence of dextrocardia and oily skin point to another diagnosis.

C. Correct answer: Kartagener syndrome, or primary ciliary dyskinesia, is an autosomal recessive condition in which the cilia beat ineffectively, in a disorganized manner or not at all. The importance of cilia in structures such as the respiratory tract, Eustachian and fallopian tubes is evident in the recurrent infections and fertility problems these patients experience. Embryological changes can range from dextrocardia to situs inversus.

D. Mutation of the *CFTR* chloride channel is seen in cystic fibrosis.

E. SCID causes recurrent infections, but the condition is so severe many patients die before one year of age without effective diagnosis and treatment.

Cloutier MM, Thrall RS (2006). Nonrespiratory functions of the lung. In: Levy MN, Stanton BA, Koeppen BM (Eds.), *Berne & Levy Principles of Physiology*, 4th edition (Chapter 32). Maryland Heights, MO: Elsevier Mosby.

36. D. Three fluids line the respiratory epithelium: periciliary fluid, mucus, and surfactant.

A. Respiratory epithelium is composed of pseudostratified ciliated columnar epithelial cells from the nose to the bronchi. From the bronchioles the cells are more cuboidal but remain ciliated.

B. Goblet cells are the histologically wine glass-shaped cells that produce mucus. In cystic fibrosis, this mucus is thicker and more viscous due to the impaired *CFTR* chloride channel. As such, particulate matter and pathogens are more likely to remain in the lungs and cause chronic infection.

C. The fluid in the mucociliary transport system is divided into the mucus (gel phase) and the periciliary fluid (sol phase). The cilia beat in one direction in the thin, watery sol phase which allows the viscous gel phase to carry particulate matter and pathogens out of the lungs to be swallowed.

D. Correct answer: Periciliary fluid and mucus line the respiratory tract from the nose to the bronchi. From the bronchioles there are virtually no goblet cells and therefore no mucus.

E. The type II pneumocytes produce surfactant, which is predominantly composed of phospholipids acting as detergents to reduce the surface tension and allow expansion of the alveoli.

Cloutier MM, Thrall RS (2006). Overview of the respiratory system. In: Levy MN, Stanton BA, Koeppen BM (Eds.), *Berne & Levy Principles of Physiology*, 4th edition (Chapter 27). Maryland Heights, MO: Elsevier Mosby.

37. A. Central and peripheral chemoreceptors responding to change in PCO_2.

A. Correct answer: The major physiological factor controlling ventilation is PCO_2. Both central and peripheral chemoreceptors respond to even small changes in the carbon dioxide concentration of arterial blood to maintain the PCO_2 within tight limits.

B. Only the peripheral chemoreceptors in the aortic and carotid bodies respond to changes in PO_2.

C. Irritant receptors prevent particulate matter and noxious gases from damaging the respiratory tract by inducing cough.

D. Peripheral chemoreceptors do respond to changes in arterial pH, but these changes occur slowly, as demonstrated by the time to respiratory compensation of chronic metabolic acidosis.

E. Pulmonary mechanoreceptors are responsible for breathing patterns and reflexes such as the Hering–Breuer inspiratory-inhibitory reflex.

Cloutier MM, Thrall RS (2006). Control of respiration. In: Levy MN, Stanton BA, Koeppen BM (Eds.), *Berne & Levy Principles of Physiology*, 4th edition (Chapter 31). Maryland Heights, MO: Elsevier Mosby.

38. A. $DLCO_2$.

A. Correct answer: Diffusion capacity for carbon dioxide ($DLCO_2$) is a measure of the functioning surface area for gas exchange. While lung compliance and DLCO may be unaffected in chronic bronchitis, emphysema is characterized by increased lung compliance and reduced DLCO.

B. Forced expiratory volume in one second (FEV_1) is likely to be reduced in both forms of COPD.

C. Reduction of the FEV_1/FVC ratio below 0.7 is diagnostic of obstructive lung disease, and will not distinguish between chronic bronchitis and emphysema.

D. Forced vital capacity is likely to be reduced in both conditions.

E. The volume of air inspired during a normal breath, this test is unlikely to differentiate between the disorders.

Cloutier MM, Thrall RS (2006). Mechanical properties of the lung and chest wall. In: Levy MN, Stanton BA, Koeppen BM (Eds.), *Berne & Levy Principles of Physiology*, 4th edition (Chapter 28). Maryland Heights, MO: Elsevier Mosby.

39. A. Ciliated columnar.

A. Correct answer: Respiratory epithelium is composed of pseudostratified ciliated columnar epithelial cells from the nose to the bronchi. Below this point, the epithelium becomes cuboidal in nature.

B. From the bronchioles the cells are more cuboidal but remain ciliated.

C. Simple cuboidal epithelium with glandular cells line the GI tract below the oesophagus.

D. Without cilia, these cells would not be able to remove particular matter and pathogens.

E. Stratified squamous epithelium line the oropharynx and oesophagus.

Cloutier MM, Thrall RS (2006). Overview of the respiratory system. In: Levy MN, Stanton BA, Koeppen BM (Eds.), *Berne & Levy Principles of Physiology*, 4th edition (Chapter 27). Maryland Heights, MO: Elsevier Mosby.

40. B. Phase 1.

A. When the threshold for a membrane action potential is reached, there is a rapid depolarization as fast sodium ion channels are activated. The sodium influx is seen as a rapid upstroke.

B. Correct answer: As efflux of potassium ions through several types of potassium channels begins, this causes an early repolarization, seen as a notch in the action potential trace.

C. An electrical equilibrium occurs as potassium ion efflux matches calcium ion influx, visualized as a plateau.

D. Eventually, potassium ion efflux exceeds calcium ion influx and the membrane starts to repolarize. A positive feedback loop occurs as partial repolarization opens further potassium ion channels.

E. The myocyte membrane is fully repolarized and achieves the resting membrane potential, prior to the threshold of the next action potential being reached.

Levy MN, Pappano A (2006). Electrical activity of the heart. In: Levy MN, Stanton BA, Koeppen BM (Eds.), *Berne & Levy Principles of Physiology*, 4th edition (Chapter 16). Maryland Heights, MO: Elsevier Mosby.

41. D. Ramipril.

A. Digoxin is a cardiac glycoside that slows AV nodal conduction and increases diastolic filling time. This improves cardiac output and gives symptomatic relief in heart failure, but does not reduce the afterload.

B. This colloid will increase the intravascular volume and increase both preload and afterload.

C. Rabeprazole is a proton pump inhibitor and does not affect afterload.

D. Correct answer: Ramipril is an ACE inhibitor, which reduces peripheral conversion of angiotensin 1 to the active form, angiotensin 2. In doing so, ramipril causes vasodilatation, decreases the systemic vascular resistance and reduces the afterload to the heart.

E. Terlipressin is an ADH analogue that increases reabsorption of water in the collecting ducts of the nephrons. This increases intravascular volume and also afterload to the heart.

Levy MN, Pappano A (2006). Electrical activity of the heart. In: Levy MN, Stanton BA, Koeppen BM (Eds.), *Berne & Levy Principles of Physiology*, 4th edition (Chapter 16). Maryland Heights, MO: Elsevier Mosby.

42. C. Base of the pulmonary veins.

A. This is incorrect, because the cause of atrial fibrillation is ectopic atrial foci causing disorganized contraction of the atria, rather than AV nodal disease causing block or re-entrant tachycardia. Ablation here would cause complete heart block, unless an accessory pathway existed.

B. This is a red herring, as the four pulmonary arteries branching from the pulmonary trunk are rarely implicated in atrial fibrillation.

C. Correct answer: Research from the early 1990s has provided substantial evidence to suggest that most cases of atrial fibrillation (AF) are triggered from the pulmonary veins entering the left atrium, the superior pair generating more rapid atrial firing than the inferior pair of veins. Catheter ablation therapy is therefore targeted largely to the base of the pulmonary vein which eradicates 75–80% of AF. Extrapulmonary vein sites of AF are rare, but can include areas near the superior vena cava or the coronary sinus.

D. The bundle of His describes the fibres conducting the cardiac impulse from the AV node and down the interventricular septum. Ablation here would cause complete heart block.

E. The bundle of Kent is an anatomical variant seen in Wolff-Parkinson-White syndrome. While ablation at this site can be beneficial to sufferers of this disease, it will not affect AF.

Mahida S, Sacher F, Derval N, et al. (2015). Science linking pulmonary veins and AF. *Arrhythmia & Electrophysiology Review*, **4**(1), 40–3.

Olshansky B, Arora R (2017). Mechanisms of atrial fibrillation. In: Knight BP, Calkins H (Eds.), UpToDate, Waltham, MA. Available at: https://www.uptodate.com/contents/mechanisms-of-atrial-fibrillation

43. B. Extreme axis deviation occurs between -90 and 180 degrees (Figure 2.4).

A. Cardiac axis (or QRS axis) is defined using the limb leads on an ECG, where the zero-degree point exists in the same direction as lead I. Positive deflection of the QRS complex in a lead suggests shared direction with the cardiac axis.

B. Correct answer: Extreme axis deviation is possible, for instance in ventricular rhythms or severe right ventricular hypertrophy, beyond 180 degrees to the right or beyond -90 degrees to the left. In this case, a cardiac anomaly such as Tetralogy of Fallot may be the cause. Some children present with 'tet spells', when deoxygenated blood is shunted right-to-left. Squatting increases systemic vascular resistance and can ameliorate the effects of the shunt.

C. Normal axis exists between -30 and 90 degrees.

D. This conformation suggests either normal or left axis deviation. Some methods of interpretation utilize leads I and aVF, while others utilize the isoelectric lead which will be perpendicular to the axis.

E. 'Always' is a dangerous word in multiple choice questions (MCQs). Positive QRS in aVF can represent either right or normal axis.

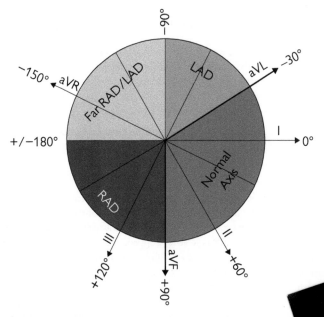

Figure 2.4 ECG axis interpretation.

Courtesy of lifeinthefastlane.com. Copyright © 2007–2017.

Levy MN, Pappano A (2006). Electrical activity of the heart. In: Levy MN, Stanton BA, Koeppen BM (Eds.), *Berne & Levy Principles of Physiology*, 4th edition (Chapter 16). Maryland Heights, MO: Elsevier Mosby.

44. E. Ventricular volume remains constant at the points during which the heart sounds are heard.

    A. During isovolumetric contraction, the mitral valve and the aortic valve are both closed.

    B. The maximal ventricular chamber pressure occurs during the ejection phase, demarcating the rapid and reduced ejection phases. During isovolumetric contraction, the ventricular pressure reaches 60–80 mmHg, roughly equal to the aortic pressure at that point. It is at this stage that the aortic valve opens, and ejection begins.

    C. The second heart sound coincides with the closure of the aortic valve.

    D. The T wave represents ventricular repolarization and occurs during the reduced ejection phase. This precedes isovolumetric relaxation and then ventricular filling begins.

    E. Correct answer: The heart sounds represent closure of the mitral and aortic valves, respectively. At these points, both valves are closed. During ventricular contraction, pressure increases but volume remains constant at approximately 100 mL (see variations for men and women). During relaxation, pressure falls but volume is approximately 20 mL.

Levy MN, Pappano A (2006). Cardiac pump. In: Levy MN, Stanton BA, Koeppen BM (Eds.), *Berne & Levy Principles of Physiology*, 4th edition (Chapter 18). Maryland Heights, MO: Elsevier Mosby.

45. D. Perfusion of the coronary arteries occurs mainly during diastole.

    A. Aortic flow falls to less than 0 L/min briefly before aortic valve closure, thereafter oscillating slightly above 0 L/min due to elastic recoil.

    B. Atrial systole coincides with the fourth heart sound and is often heard in healthy individuals with thin chest walls.

    C. The P wave signals the start of atrial systole, the end of which coincides with the closure of the mitral valve.

    D. Correct answer: This explains why patients with angina experience pain with increased heart rate. During tachycardia, the duration of systole is relatively maintained compared to the duration of diastole, which is significantly shorter. This reduces the amount of perfusion the coronary arteries receive and results in myocardial ischaemia, causing pain.

    E. During ventricular filling, ventricular chamber pressure is approximately 10 mmHg.

Levy MN, Pappano A (2006). Cardiac pump. In: Levy MN, Stanton BA, Koeppen BM (Eds.), *Berne & Levy Principles of Physiology*, 4th edition (Chapter 18). Maryland Heights, MO: Elsevier Mosby.

46. B. Dilated cardiomyopathy increases preload.

    A. Preload is often presented by the proxy value of the end diastolic filling pressure. In catastrophic haemorrhage, the circulating volume is significantly reduced beyond the scope of normal compensatory mechanisms. There is less ventricular filling during diastole and the preload at the start of ventricular systole is reduced.

    B. Correct answer: According to the Law of Laplace, for a chamber with a constant internal pressure the wall tension is directly proportional to the radius of the chamber. In dilated cardiomyopathy the chamber radius has increased, as must the wall tension generated during isovolumetric contraction. The increase in volume of blood to be pumped directly increases the preload. In addition, when the actin and myosin filaments of the sarcomere are stretched beyond their optimal degree of overlap, there are fewer cross-bridges formed to provide force to the contraction. This leads to further dilatation and over time, failure of the cardiac pump.

C. Systemic hypertension is the primary cause of increased afterload to the left ventricle.

D. Similarly to hypertension, pulmonary oedema is associated with increased pulmonary vascular pressures and therefore increased afterload to the right ventricle.

E. Diastole is shortened in tachycardia and leads to reduced ventricular filling, lower end diastolic pressures, and reduced preload.

Levy MN, Pappano A (2006). Cardiac pump. In: Levy MN, Stanton BA, Koeppen BM (Eds.), *Berne & Levy Principles of Physiology*, 4th edition (Chapter 18). Maryland Heights, MO: Elsevier Mosby.

47. C. Dilatation of small arteries and arterioles decreases systemic vascular resistance and reduces the damping effect on cardiac contraction.

A. While autoantibodies are a feature of Grave's disease, capillary walls do not contain significant quantities of elastic tissue in either healthy or disease states.

B. Cardiac output is a product of heart rate and stroke volume ($CO = HR \times SV$), and as such tachycardia does increase total blood flow. This in itself does not explain the nailbed pulsatility, which is not seen in healthy patients after exercise.

C. Correct answer: Blood pressure is a product of cardiac output and systemic vascular resistance ($BP = CO \times SVR$). This patient's low blood pressure is the result of vasodilatation and decreased vascular resistance. The small arteries and arterioles provide much of the systemic vascular resistance due to their low cross-sectional area, generating friction, and high elastin content, or distensibility. In Grave's disease the arteries and arterioles are generally dilated, which reduces the damping effect on the arterial blood and can lead to pulsatile capillary flow.

D. Small veins and venules do not contain smooth muscle in their walls, unlike veins over 4 mm diameter and arterial vessels.

E. Viscosity in the cardiovascular system is largely defined by frictional resistance, which will be reduced in this vase due to vasodilation.

Levy MN, Pappano A (2006). Overview of the circulation, blood, and hemostasis. In: Levy MN, Stanton BA, Koeppen BM (Eds.), *Berne & Levy Principles of Physiology*, 4th edition (Chapter 15). Maryland Heights, MO: Elsevier Mosby.

48. A. Blood glucose concentration.

A. Correct answer: This boy has Cushing's triad of raised intracranial pressure: bradycardia, bradypnoea, and hypertension. The likely pathophysiology is a blockage in the recently inserted venous pressure (VP) shunt. Many factors influence intracranial pressure. Hyperglycaemia worsens cerebral ischaemia and should be avoided in this case, but does not directly alter cerebral perfusion pressure (CPP). CPP needs to be maintained to ensure adequate oxygen transport to the brain cells and can be defined by the following equations:

$$CPP = MAP - ICP \; (\text{where } ICP > JVP)$$

Or

$$CPP = MAP - JVP \; (\text{where } JVP > ICP)$$

B. Raised intracranial pressure (ICP) leads to decreased CPP and thereby cerebral ischaemia.

C. Raised jugular venous pressure (JVP) leads to decreased CPP and thereby cerebral ischaemia.

D. Maintaining (mean arterial) blood pressure within normal limits is a major component of healthy CPP. In hypotensive patients, CPP will fall and lead to cerebral ischaemia. In hypertensive patients, excess fluid administration may cause cerebral oedema.

E. Hypocapnia reduces CPP and cerebral blood flow by increasing cerebral vascular resistance.

Posner JB, Saper CB, Schiff N, Plum F (2007). *Plum and Posner's Diagnosis of Stupor and Coma* (Contemporary Neurology 71). New York, NY: Oxford University Press.

Ramrakha PS, Moore K, Sam A (2010). Neurological emergencies. In: *Oxford Handbook of Acute Medicine* (Chapter 6). Oxford: UK: Oxford University Press

Grüne F, Kazmaier S, Stolker RJ, Visser GH, Weyland A (2015). Carbon dioxide induced changes in cerebral blood flow and flow velocity: role of cerebrovascular resistance and effective cerebral perfusion pressure. *Journal of Cerebral Blood Flow & Metabolism*, **35**(9), 1470–7.

49. D. Right coronary artery.

A. The diagnosis is inferior ST-elevation myocardial infarction, which is caused by disease of the left circumflex artery in approximately 15% of cases. This is because the left circumflex supplies the lateral edge of the inferior heart.

B. Occlusion of the left main stem causes anterolateral changes on the ECG, known euphemistically as 'the widow-maker'.

C. Occlusion of this artery causes anterior changes on the ECG.

D. Correct answer: The right coronary artery supplies most of the inferior heart. Approximately 80% of inferior ST-elevation myocardial infarction (STEMI)s are caused by disease of the right coronary artery, which account for almost half of all STEMIs. While prognosis is generally better than in anterior STEMI, inferior STEMI can be associated with right ventricular failure and second- to third-degree heart block. In-hospital survival rate is approximately 2–9%.

E. The type II variant left anterior descending (LAD) artery is also known as the 'wraparound' LAD, and causes less than 5% of all inferior STEMI's.

Levy MN, Pappano A (2006). Cardiac pump. In: Levy MN, Stanton BA, Koeppen BM (Eds.), *Berne & Levy Principles of Physiology*, 4th edition (Chapter 18). Maryland Heights, MO: Elsevier Mosby.

50. E. Slowing of potassium ion channels.

A. Accessory pathway is the anatomical variant in atrioventricular nodal re-entry tachycardia (AVNRT) and Wolff-Parkinson-White syndrome.

B. Ectopic pacemaker function is the physiological change in atrial flutter.

C. Disease of the distal conduction system is the pathology described in some cases of second- and third-degree heart block.

D. While this might be correct, the fact that the patient is deaf differentiates this form of long QT syndrome from other forms. In LQT3, mutation of sodium channel SCN5A speeds up sodium transport, prolonging ventricular repolarization. This condition is known as Romano-Ward syndrome.

E. Correct answer: This patient has a QT interval of 550 milliseconds, and their history is consistent with Lange-Nielsen syndrome, or LQT1. In this condition, mutation of the KCNQ1 potassium channels slows potassium ion transport and prolongs ventricular repolarization. Syncope can be provoked by physical exertion. These channels are also found in the inner ear, which is why the condition is associated with congenital deafness.

Levy MN, Pappano A (2006). Electrical activity of the heart. In: Levy MN, Stanton BA, Koeppen BM (Eds.), *Berne & Levy Principles of Physiology*, 4th edition (Chapter 18). Maryland Heights, MO: Elsevier Mosby.

51. C. 440 milliseconds.

    A. This is incorrect and represents a short QT interval. Short QT syndrome can present with palpitations, syncope or ventricular fibrillation (VF) cardiac arrest.

    B. This is the lower limit for a normal QT interval.

    C. Correct answer: Normal QT interval falls between 350–440 milliseconds. Several formulae exist to calculate corrected QT interval (QTc), which allows comparison of QT interval at different heart rates.

    D. Studies have shown that in women QTc can be greater than in men, up to 460 milliseconds.

    E. Above 500 milliseconds, the risk of fatal arrhythmias such as torsades de pointes increases significantly.

Chauhan VS, Krahn AD, Walker BD, et al. (2002). Sex differences in QTc interval and QT dispersion: dynamics during exercise and recovery in healthy subjects. *American Heart Journal*, **144**(5), 858–64.

Trinkley KE, Page RL 2nd, Lien H, Yamanouye K, Tisdale JE (2013). QT interval prolongation and the risk of torsades de pointes: essentials for clinicians. *Current Medical Research and Opinion*, **29**(12), 1719–26.

52. B. Adrenaline.

    A. Adenosine is a component of energy-carrying molecules and exists in higher concentrations at areas of high metabolic activity. ATP acts as an inhibitor to smooth muscle contraction.

    B. Correct answer: In reactive hyperaemia, where the blood supply is occluded temporarily followed by a period of increased blood flow, metabolites build up in the area to promote vasodilatation until metabolic activity returns to normal (metabolic washout). Adrenaline is a potent vasoconstrictor and does not result in metabolic hyperaemia.

    C. Carbon dioxide is a product of respiration and exists at higher partial pressures in areas of higher metabolic activity or vascular occlusion.

    D. Lactic acid, and the build-up of H^+, signifies increased metabolic activity, particularly anaerobic respiration.

    E. Nitric acid is a potent vasodilator, acting on the smooth muscle to promote increased perfusion in metabolically active areas.

Levy MN, Pappano A (2006). Peripheral circulation and its control. In: Levy MN, Stanton BA, Koeppen BM (Eds.), *Berne & Levy Principles of Physiology*, 4th edition (Chapter 23). Maryland Heights, MO: Elsevier Mosby.

53. C. Na^+,K^+-ATPase transporters.

    A. This woman has sick sinus syndrome, sometimes referred to as tachy-brady syndrome. So-called funny channels are actually sodium channels, which decrease the refractory period between action potentials in pacemaker cells.

    B. These calcium channels are open during the plateau phase of the action potential.

    C. Correct answer: Cardiac pacemaker cells that depolarize at a lower frequency do not trigger cardiac impulses while a faster pacemaker is doing so. This is due to overdrive suppression, which increases the refractory period in slower pacemaker cells. These electrogenic channels have increased activity in more frequently depolarizing cells. When the faster pacemaker signal is withdrawn, the active Na^+,K^+-ATPase pumps hyperpolarize the myocyte membrane, increasing the refractory period.

    D. These potassium channels are responsible for repolarization of the myocyte membrane during phases 1–3 of the action potential.

E. The rapid influx of sodium ions when the cardiac action potential is triggered occurs via these channels.

Levy MN, Pappano A (2006). Natural excitation of the heart. In: Levy MN, Stanton BA, Koeppen BM (Eds.), *Berne & Levy Principles of Physiology*, 4th edition (Chapter 17). Maryland Heights, MO: Elsevier Mosby.

54. B. Reduced arterial compliance secondary to hypertension and ageing.

A. Neither hypertension nor ageing have significant effects on the cross-sectional area of the capillary beds.

B. Correct answer: Both hypertension and ageing reduce arterial compliance. The elastic nature of arterial walls allows buffering of the cardiac systolic impulse, giving a smaller pulse pressure. At higher blood pressures, the arteries are less able to expand further and so the buffering effect is reduced. Similarly, breakdown of the elastic components of arterial walls occurs with age. As such, the cardiac systolic impulse generates higher systolic pressures and relatively lower diastolic pressures in elderly patients.

C. Systemic vascular resistance is likely to be the same or increased in this patient, who may have arteriosclerotic changes.

D. The duration of the reduced ejection phase of cardiac systole is most reduced during tachycardia, but this will have only a negligible effect on pulse pressure.

E. Patients with white coat hypertension have both elevated systolic and diastolic pressures.

Levy MN, Pappano A (2006). Arterial system. In: Levy MN, Stanton BA, Koeppen BM (Eds.), *Berne & Levy Principles of Physiology*, 4th edition (Chapter 21). Maryland Heights, MO: Elsevier Mosby.

55. C. Increased myocardial contractility.

A. This woman has a paroxysmal supraventricular tachycardia, responding to carotid sinus massage. During the episode she has tachycardia and reduced blood pressure due to reduced cardiac output. Carotid baroreceptors, among others, will detect the hypotension and stimulate a reflex sympathetic response, increasing noradrenaline release.

B. Noradrenaline will increase the conductance of Ca^{2+} channels in the myocyte membrane, increasing cytoplasmic Ca^{2+} concentration.

C. Correct answer: Increased cytoplasmic Ca^{2+} concentration will increase myocardial contractility.

D. While vagal tone is increased by carotid sinus massage, parasympathetic tone is not raised during paroxysmal tachycardia.

E. The patient is breathing more rapidly during the episode, however, this would be more likely to cause a respiratory alkalosis than a metabolic alkalosis.

Levy MN, Pappano A (2006). Regulation of the heartbeat. In: Levy MN, Stanton BA, Koeppen BM (Eds.), *Berne & Levy Principles of Physiology*, 4th edition (Chapter 19). Maryland Heights, MO: Elsevier Mosby.

56. A. Increased parasympathetic activity, increased acetylcholine release, reduced rate of diastolic depolarization in pacemaker cells.

A. Correct answer: This woman has had a vasovagal syncopal episode. This can be provoked by stimuli such as pain or strong emotion and results in increased vagal discharge. This slows the depolarization that occurs in the pacemaker cells of the sinoatrial node during atrial diastole, reducing the rate at which the next heart beat can be initiated. As the heart rates drops, this combines with other cardiovascular consequences of increased vagal tone such as vasodilatation to drop systemic blood pressure and momentarily reduce cerebral blood flow. The result is light-headedness or syncope.

B. Parasympathetic activity is not mediated by noradrenaline and reducing the threshold of pacemaker cell firing would result in increased heart rate.

C. Sympathetic activity is not increased in vasovagal syncope and is not mediated by acetylcholine. Although hyperpolarization of pacemaker cell membranes would result in reduced heart rate.

D. While sympathetic activity is mediated by noradrenaline, increasing the rate of diastolic depolarization of pacemaker cells would result in more rapid firing of the sinoatrial node and increased heart rate, not seen in vasovagal syncope.

E. The 'funny' current describes an influx of sodium ions into the pacemaker cells that occurs during late repolarization and is characteristic of pacemaker cells. This is a normal process that occurs during health.

Levy MN, Pappano A (2006). Natural excitation of the heart. In: Levy MN, Stanton BA, Koeppen BM (Eds.), *Berne & Levy Principles of Physiology*, 4th edition (Chapter 17). Maryland Heights, MO: Elsevier Mosby.

57. A. Atrioventricular node.

A. Correct answer: The ECG confirms a diagnosis of second degree heart block, subclassified as Mobitz type I or Wenckebach periodicity. In this condition, the PR interval gradually increases until a P wave is not conducted through the AV node. The PR interval then resets and the pattern repeats. Although usually asymptomatic, patients can present with dizziness or syncope. Disease is usually at the AV node and the condition is generally considered benign and does not merit further intervention.

B. Second degree heart block of the Mobitz type II pattern is considered more dangerous. Seen as 2.1 or 3.1 conduction of P waves to the ventricles, disease is normally in the distal conduction system.

C. Sometimes referred to as infranodal block, disease in the distal conduction system is more typical of Mobitz type II disease.

D. This is incorrect, as the His-Purkinje system is generally intact in Mobitz type I disease and the QRS will be of normal duration.

E. It is important to check that the sinus rhythm is regular when making a diagnosis of Wenckebach periodicity. If the P waves are irregular, it can give a false impression of increasing PR interval.

Levy MN, Pappano A (2006. Electrical activity of the heart. In: Levy MN, Stanton BA, Koeppen BM (Eds.), *Berne & Levy Principles of Physiology*, 4th edition (Chapter 16). Maryland Heights, MO: Elsevier Mosby.

58. D. Post-repolarization refractoriness is one of the mechanisms by which impulses are blocked in the AV node.

A. AV nodal action potentials have increased duration due to the relative absence of fast Na^+ channels, which are responsible for the rapid upstroke of the depolarization.

B. AV nodal conduction is slow compared to other parts of the conduction system, due in part to the small size of the cells in the AV node.

C. Since the depolarization of AV nodal cells relies on L-type Ca^{2+} channels, rather than Na^+ channels, calcium channel blockers such as nifedipine and diltiazem have a greater effect on AV node conduction. As such, they are contra-indicated in AV nodal block.

D. Correct answer: This is seen in patients with atrial flutter. While the sinoatrial (SA) node and atrial myocytes are contracting at a rate of 300 beats per minute, the rate of conduction through the AV node is limited to approximately 150 bpm by factors such as post-repolarization refractoriness.

E. Wolff-Parkinson-White syndrome is characterized by the presence of a congenital accessory pathway from the atrial to ventricular myocytes. While this does not generally cause any functional disturbance, it can be seen on the ECG as an up-slope to the QRS complex caused by pre-excitation of a portion of the ventricular myocytes. When a re-entrant rhythm forms through retrograde conduction of the impulse via either the AV node or the accessory pathway, a supraventricular tachycardia ensues. Vagal manoeuvres such as carotid body massage or the Valsalva manoeuvre can terminate re-entrant rhythms by increasing vagal tone. If this fails, adenosine is used for transient AV nodal block to restore sinus rhythm.

Levy MN, Pappano A (2006). Natural excitation of the heart. In: Levy MN, Stanton BA, Koeppen BM (Eds.), *Berne & Levy Principles of Physiology*, 4th edition (Chapter 17). Maryland Heights, MO: Elsevier Mosby.

59. A. Bile consists of bicarbonate, bile salts, lecithin, and cholesterol.

A. Correct answer: These are some of the major components of bile and serve to neutralize gastric contents in the duodenum and to emulsify fats and form micelles for enzymatic digestion. Biliary secretion is the only route of cholesterol excretion.

B. On the contrary, bile salts pass through the enterohepatic circulation and are reabsorbed in the terminal ileum before returning to the liver via the portal vein. Here, they are rapidly absorbed by the hepatocytes to be secreted again. However, their presence stimulates further bile salt production, as approximately 30% of bile salts are lost in the faeces.

C. Cholecystokinin (CCK) stimulates the primary secretion of hepatic bile from the hepatocytes, as it stimulates the primary secretion of pancreatic exocrine juice from the acinar cells of the pancreas. Indirectly, CCK does enhance the action of secretion. Furthermore, as the name suggests, CCK is also the major stimulant to gallbladder emptying.

D. The gallbladder stores and concentrates the bile by water absorption using the standing osmotic gradient mechanism. In this way, bile can be concentrated up to 20 times the original concentration.

E. Secretin stimulates the secretion of a bicarbonate rich fluid from the bile ducts, as it stimulates a similar secretion from the pancreatic ducts.

Dawson PA (2012). Bile formation and the enterohepatic circulation. In: Johnson LR (Ed.), *Physiology of the Gastrointestinal Tract*. 5th edition (Chapter 53). Amsterdam, the Netherlands: Elsevier.

Kutchai HC (2006). Gastrointestinal secretions. In: Levy MN, Stanton BA, Koeppen BM (Eds.), *Berne & Levy Principles of Physiology*, 4th edition (Chapter 34). Maryland Heights, MO: Elsevier Mosby.

60. E. Secretin decreases gastric emptying.

A. Cholecystokinin, or CCK, is released from glands in the duodenum and jejunum. Gastrin is secreted from G cells in the antrum of the stomach, the duodenum, and the pancreas.

B. Gastrin increases the strength of antral contractions, however, by promoting constriction of the pylorus the overall effect is to reduce gastric emptying.

C. Since the epithelium in the duodenum is more susceptible to damage by acids than the stomach, duodenal pH is tightly regulated by chemoreceptors. If duodenal pH falls, that is to say becomes more acidic, the rate of gastric emptying is reduced by the effect of secretin.

D. Parasympathetic innervation of the pylorus can be either excitatory, as mediated by acetylcholine, or inhibitory, as mediated by vasoactive intestinal peptide, VIP.

E. Correct answer: If duodenal pH falls, secretin is released from glands in the duodenum. This reduces gastric emptying by stimulating constriction of the pyloric sphincter and by inhibiting antral slow wave contractions.

Kutchai HC (2006). Motility of the gastrointestinal tract. In: Levy MN, Stanton BA, Koeppen BM (Eds.), *Berne & Levy Principles of Physiology*, 4th edition (Chapter 33). Maryland Heights, MO: Elsevier Mosby.

Rayner CK, Hebbard GS, Horowitz M (2012). Physiology of the Antral Pump and Gastric Emptying. In: Johnson LR (Ed.), *Physiology of the Gastrointestinal Tract*, 5th edition (Chapter 35). Amsterdam, the Netherlands: Elsevier.

61. C. Muscularis externa.

A. This patient is most likely to be suffering from ileus secondary to his operation. The adventitia, or serosa, is the outermost layer of the gut wall, consisting of connective tissue and squamous mesothelial cells.

B. The epithelium is the innermost layer of the gut wall, varies greatly throughout the GI tract and contains specialized cells to maximize absorption of nutrients and water.

C. Correct answer: The muscularis externa lies external to the submucosa, consisting of an inner layer of circular smooth muscle and an outer layer of longitudinal smooth muscle. It is the layer of the gut wall that generates peristaltic movements of gut contents under control of the myenteric plexus.

D. The muscularis mucosae is a layer of the mucosa, consisting of smooth muscle and does not contribute significantly to peristalsis.

E. The submucosa lies between the muscularis mucosae and the muscularis externa, consists of collagen and elastin fibres and does not contribute to peristalsis.

Kutchai HC (2006). Motility of the gastrointestinal tract. In: Levy MN, Stanton BA, Koeppen BM (Eds.), *Berne & Levy Principles of Physiology*, 4th edition (Chapter 33). Maryland Heights, MO: Elsevier Mosby.

62. E. Submucosa.

This patient is suffering from a volvulus of his large bowel and may have ischaemic bowel, as indicated by the PR blood and fever.

A. The lamina propria is a layer of the mucosa, consisting of loose connective tissue and containing capillaries, lymph nodes, and glands.

B. The mucosa is the innermost layer of the gut wall, consisting of the epithelium, the lamina propria, and the muscularis mucosae.

C. The muscularis externa lies external to the submucosa, consisting of an inner layer of circular smooth muscle and an outer layer of longitudinal smooth muscle.

D. The serosa, or adventitia, is the outermost layer of the gut wall, consisting of connective tissue, and squamous mesothelial cells.

E. Correct answer: The submucosa lies between the muscularis mucosae and the muscularis externa, consists of collagen and elastin fibres and transmits large nerves and blood vessels.

Kutchai HC (2006). Motility of the gastrointestinal tract. In: Levy MN, Stanton BA, Koeppen BM (Eds.), *Berne & Levy Principles of Physiology*, 4th edition (Chapter 33). Maryland Heights, MO: Elsevier Mosby.

63. B. Muscularis mucosae.

This patient is likely to have short gut syndrome, as indicated by the weight loss, history of bowel resection, and multiple surgeries.

A. The lamina propria is a layer of the mucosa, consisting of loose connective tissue and containing capillaries, lymph nodes, and glands.

B. Correct answer: The muscularis mucosae is a layer of the mucosa consisting of smooth muscle and is responsible for increasing gut surface area by throwing the mucosa into folds and ridges.

C. The myenteric plexus is located between the inner and outer layers of the muscularis externa, is part of the enteric nervous system and is responsible for co-ordinating the motor activities of the GI tract.

D. The serosa, or adventitia, is the outermost layer of the gut wall, consisting of connective tissue and squamous mesothelial cells.

E. The submucosal plexus lies within the submucosa, is part of the enteric nervous system and is responsible for co-ordinating the secretory activities of the GI tract.

Kutchai HC (2006). Motility of the gastrointestinal tract. In: Levy MN, Stanton BA, Koeppen BM (Eds.), *Berne & Levy Principles of Physiology*, 4th edition (Chapter 33). Maryland Heights, MO: Elsevier Mosby.

64. E. The longitudinal smooth muscle layer around the large intestine is divided into bands.

A. Mass movements occur one to three times a day and are influenced by factors including gastric filling, which leads to the gastro-colic reflex.

B. The walls of the caecum and proximal colon are divided into segments, or haustrae, where the circular smooth muscle is more prominent than the longitudinal muscle. Here, segmental contractions contribute more to mixing of chyme for maximal reabsorption of water and salts than to propulsion.

C. The defaecation reflex is controlled by the sacral plexus.

D. The internal anal sphincter is under autonomic control, while the external anal sphincter is under both reflex and voluntary control, via the pudendal nerves.

E. Correct answer: The longitudinal smooth muscle layer of the colon is largely divided into three bands, called the taeniae coli. These create the bulging, ovoid appearance of the haustrae and contribute to the periodic mass movements of the colon.

Kutchai HC (2006). Motility of the gastrointestinal tract. In: Levy MN, Stanton BA, Koeppen BM (Eds.), *Berne & Levy Principles of Physiology*, 4th edition (Chapter 33). Maryland Heights, MO: Elsevier Mosby.

65. C. Emulsification of fats.

A. Pancreatic exocrine juice contains both DNase and RNase.

B. Pancreatic acinar cells secrete glycerol ester hydrolase, or pancreatic lipase, which breaks down triglycerides. It also contains cholesterol ester hydrolase, which breaks down lipid carboxyl esters.

C. Correct answer: Bile salts act to emulsify fats and potentiate digestion by lipase enzymes.

D. Pancreatic exocrine juice is rich in bicarbonate, which helps to neutralize acidic gastric contents, thus potentiating enzymatic digestion and protecting the duodenal mucosa.

E. Unlike lipase and amylase, which are secreted as active enzymes, proteases are secreted within zymogens to prevent premature proteolysis that would damage the pancreatic tissue.

Furthermore, pancreatic exocrine juice contains trypsin inhibitor, which prevents activation of trypsinogens, chymotrypsinogens, procarboxypeptidases, and proelastases within the pancreatic ducts.

Kutchai HC (2006). Gastrointestinal secretions. In: Levy MN, Stanton BA, Koeppen BM (Eds.), *Berne & Levy Principles of Physiology*, 4th edition (Chapter 34). Maryland Heights, MO: Elsevier Mosby.

Liddle RA (2012). Regulation of pancreatic secretion. In: Johnson LR (Ed.), *Physiology of the Gastrointestinal Tract*, 5th edition (Chapter 52). Amsterdam, the Netherlands: Elsevier.

66. D. Saliva is primarily hypertonic.

A. The patient in the scenario has xerostomia, or dry mouth, likely an iatrogenic complication of his antidepressant—tricyclics and selective serotonin reuptake inhibitors (SSRIs) are common causes. The primary innervation to the salivary glands is parasympathetic, via acetylcholine and vasoactive intestinal peptide, or VIP.

B. Although primarily parasympathetic, the salivary glands do have sympathetic innervation. Sympathetic stimulation is weaker and shorter, however, and cutting these fibres will not clinically affect saliva production.

C. Saliva contains amylase, which has the same specificity of action on starch as pancreatic amylase. Salivary amylase is normally denatured by gastric acid.

D. Correct answer: Saliva secreted by the acinar cells of the salivary glands is primarily isotonic to plasma. However, sodium and chloride ions are extracted by the ductal system, where bicarbonate is added. The end-product is a hypotonic, alkaline saliva.

E. There is a complex relationship between taste and saliva, where taste and smell stimulate saliva production, while saliva is an important carrier for taste molecules and keeps taste receptors moist.

Herness S (2012). The neurobiology of gustation. In: Johnson LR (Ed.), *Physiology of the Gastrointestinal Tract*, 5th edition (Chapter 26). Amsterdam, the Netherlands: Elsevier.

Kutchai HC (2006). Gastrointestinal secretions. In: Levy MN, Stanton BA, Koeppen BM (Eds.), *Berne & Levy Principles of Physiology*, 4th edition (Chapter 34). Maryland Heights, MO: Elsevier Mosby.

67. C. Enterocytes absorb Fe^{2+} ions via the DCT1 co-transporter.

A. This is incorrect, because only approximately 5% of ingested iron is absorbed. Iron is poorly absorbed in the GI tract due to the formation of insoluble salts. By contrast, iron ingested in the form of haem groups is readily absorbed.

B. Ascorbic acid, or vitamin C, promotes iron absorption in two ways. It binds with iron to form a soluble complex and promotes the reduction of Fe^{3+} to Fe^{2+}.

C. Correct answer: The DCT1 brush border protein transports Fe^{2+} and H^+ from the gut lumen into the enterocyte by using the electrochemical gradient of H^+ to provide energy. Fe^{3+} cannot be transported, but can be reduced by iron reductase, a brush border enzyme.

D. Patients with chronic iron deficiency secondary to haemorrhage have an increased capacity to absorb iron. This change takes place within three to four days of the haemorrhage, which is the time from cell formation in the crypts of Lieberkuhn to migration to the tips of the microvilli.

E. Transferrin is found in the bloodstream.

Kutchai HC (2006). Motility of the gastrointestinal tract. In: Levy MN, Stanton BA, Koeppen BM (Eds.), *Berne & Levy Principles of Physiology*, 4th edition (Chapter 33). Maryland Heights, MO: Elsevier Mosby.

68. A. Secondary peristalsis occurs if a food bolus does not completely pass down the oesophagus.

A. Correct answer: Primary peristalsis occurs when a food bolus first enters the oesophagus and begins at the level of the upper oesophageal sphincter. Secondary peristalsis occurs from the level of the obstruction, and is mediated by stretch receptors at this level.

B. This is incorrect, as oesophageal peristalsis occurs at approximately 3–5 cm/second. As such, the oesophageal phase can last for up to ten seconds, while it is the pharyngeal phase that takes place in under one second.

C. This is incorrect, as the upper third of the oesophagus contains skeletal muscle only, the lower third contains smooth muscle only, while the middle third contains both.

D. The pharyngeal phase is controlled by the swallowing centre in the lower pons and medulla of the brainstem by a reflex arc, the afferent limb of which is stimulated by touch receptors in the pharynx. The efferent limb is formed by the cranial nerves that control pharyngeal muscle contraction to pass the food bolus into the open upper oesophageal sphincter. By contrast, the oral phase is under voluntary control.

E. This is incorrect, as the upper oesophageal sphincter is under reflex control to open during the pharyngeal phase of swallowing, at which point the vocal cords close and the larynx is lifted superiorly and anteriorly to prevent aspiration of food or gastric contents.

Kutchai HC (2006). Motility of the gastrointestinal tract. In: Levy MN, Stanton BA, Koeppen BM (Eds.), *Berne & Levy Principles of Physiology*, 4th edition (Chapter 33). Maryland Heights, MO: Elsevier Mosby.

Mittal RK (2012). Motor function of the pharynx, the esophagus, and its sphincters. In: Johnson LR (Ed.), *Physiology of the Gastrointestinal Tract*, 5th edition (Chapter 33). Amsterdam, the Netherlands: Elsevier.

69. E. Surgery has resulted in pernicious anaemia due to removal of parietal cells.

A. While it is true that B12 absorption is dependent on intrinsic factor, the latter is produced by the parietal cells of the stomach, not the chief cells which are responsible for secreting pepsinogen.

B. B12 is a fat-soluble vitamin; however the main source of lipase in digestion is from the pancreas which should not be affected by gastric bypass surgery. In addition, B12 is chaperoned by intrinsic factor through the small intestine, and then endocytosed by receptors found on ileal cells.

C. Bariatric surgery reduces the size of space that a food bolus can be digested in, and as such should, over time, reduce the amount of food being consumed per sitting. The proportion of food groups ingested however should be maintained. B12 is found in animal products such as eggs, meat, and milk.

D. This patient is not expected to have a deficiency in R-binder protein (also known as transcobalamin-1), as it is mostly found in saliva. It is not until R-binder and B12 both reach the acidic and pepsin containing environment of the stomach where R-binder's affinity for B12 peaks, and B12 can be chaperoned into the duodenum. Medication that reduces the pH of the stomach (such as H_2 antagonists or proton pump inhibitors (PPI)) can cause B12 deficiency as a side effect.

E. Correct answer: Gastric surgery which involves removal of part/all of the stomach can result in a depletion of parietal cells from where the glycoprotein intrinsic factor is released. Intrinsic factor has a higher affinity for B12 in the environment of the duodenum than R-binder protein, and displaces the protein as a chaperone. R-binder protein is also degraded by pancreatic proteases. The B12-intrinsic factor complex travels to the terminal ileum where it is endocytosed from the apical membrane and enters the hepatic portal circulation.

Costanzo LS (Ed.) (2014). Digestion of vitamins, digestion and absorption. In: *Physiology*, 5th edition. Philadelphia, PA: Saunders Elsevier.

70. A. Fructose.

A. Correct answer: Alongside glucose and galactose, fructose is a monosaccharide produced by intestinal digestion of carbohydrates. Fructose and glucose together form sucrose, and is absorbed by the intestinal brush border by the GLUT 5 transporter. All three monosaccharides (fructose, galactose, and glucose) are transported across the basolateral membrane and into the blood by GLUT 2.

B. Lactose is an example of a naturally occurring disaccharide formed from galactose and glucose. It is cleaved by the pancreatic enzyme lactase. Those individuals who lack or have defective lactase suffer from lactose intolerance, characterized by bloating and diarrhoea after the ingestion of lactose-containing products such as milk.

C. Maltose is a disaccharide formed from glucose. It is a product of salivary and pancreatic carbohydrate digestion, in which α-amylase breaks down complex carbohydrates to three disaccharides, including maltose. Maltase is an intestinal brush border enzyme, which cleaves maltose into its glucose counterparts to be absorbed from the lumen by Na+-glucose SGLT 1 symporter.

D. Sucrose is a naturally occurring disaccharide, cleaved into fructose and glucose by enzyme sucrase. Sucrase also digests one of the initial disaccharides produced from starch, maltotriose into its glucose components.

E. Trehalose is another naturally occurring disaccharide which is comprised of two glucose molecules, broken down my enzyme trehalase. All three naturally occurring disaccharides (trehalose, sucrose and lactose) do not require amylase dependent digestion, and pass unaltered into the small intestine.

Costanzo LS (Ed.) (2014). Digestion of vitamins, digestion and absorption. In: *Physiology*, 5th edition. Philadelphia, PA: Saunders Elsevier.

Hall JE (2010). Digestion and absorption in the gastrointestinal tract, Unit XII. In: *Guyton and Hall: Textbook of Medical Physiology*, 12th edition. Philadelphia, PA: Saunders Elsevier Ltd.

71. C. Non-absorbable solutes in the intestine cause retention of water in the lumen.

A. Diarrhoea, in general, results in loss of HCO3- and K+; bicarbonate content is high due to gastric, pancreatic and salivary secretions, and potassium loss is dependent on the rate of flow of luminal contents. In most cases, chlorine is not excreted as quickly as HCO3- and this results in a hyperchloraemic metabolic acidosis with a normal anion gap. Loss of chloride is a particular feature of Vibrio Cholera infection, which results in secretory diarrhoea. The cholera toxin permanently activates adenyl cyclase which increases intracellular cAMP levels and keeps apical chloride channels open. Chloride loss is followed by sodium and water loss at a rate faster than what the bowel wall can reabsorb.

B. This correctly describes the method in which water is lost from the interstitium to the lumen in secretory diarrhoea.

C. Correct answer: Lactose intolerance is an example of this, whereby lactose molecules cannot be hydrolysed by lactase due to deficiency of the enzyme. As carbohydrates can only be absorbed from the intestine as monosaccharides fructose, galactose, and glucose, lactose passes through the lumen unchanged but altering the osmotic gradient and therefore drawing water out of intestinal tissue.

D. This describes the primary mechanism for secretory diarrhoea, resulting in an overgrowth of pathogenic bacteria which usually reside in the gut such as E. *Coli*.

E. A shorter gut reduces the surface area available for absorption of water leading to excess excretion of water. Inflammation and infection of the gut mucosa can also cause this due to impaired absorption.

Costanzo LS (Ed.) (2014). Intestinal fluid and electrolyte transport. In: *Physiology*, 5th edition. Philadelphia, PA: Saunders Elsevier.

72. A.   Excessive absorption of bile salts and water results in cholesterol precipitating into crystals.

A. Correct answer.

B. Bile salts are formed in hepatocytes from cholesterol extracted from circulating plasma and from the liver's metabolism of fats. Approximately 1–2 g of cholesterol is removed from blood daily. Circulating cholesterol does not contribute to gallstone formation, but can impact on atherosclerotic activity in blood vessels. A high fat diet results in a higher circulating cholesterol concentration, but also a greater amount of cholesterol metabolism by hepatocytes therefore increasing the chance of gallstone formation.

C. Cholesterol is strongly hydrophobic and requires physical mixing with bile salts and lecithin to form ultramiscroscopic micelles which can exist in a water-based medium. When bile is concentrated in the gall bladder, water is removed leaving a solution of bile salts, lecithin, and cholesterol. Excessive water absorption can result in precipitation of cholesterol.

D. Inflammation of the epithelium can result in a low-grade chronic infection and changes the absorption characteristics of the mucosa. Water and bile salts can be excessively absorbed, leaving behind solid crystals of cholesterol which then develop and build into stones.

E. Most gallstones are radiolucent on plain abdominal radiographs, as they are comprised of cholesterol. Calcium containing products are characteristically radio-opaque, as evidenced by renal stones and bones.

Hall JE (2010). Secretory functions of the alimentary tract, Unit XII. In: *Guyton and Hall: Textbook of Medical Physiology*, 12th edition. Philadelphia, PA: Saunders Elsevier Ltd.

73. E.   Secretin.

A. Acetylcholine is the main parasympathetic neurotransmitter in the peripheral nervous system, and is released by the branches of the Vagus nerve during the cephalic and gastric phases of secretion. It binds to muscarinic M2 receptors to stimulate release of pepsinogen from chief cells, hydrochloric acid from parietal cells and mucous from goblet cells.

B. Gastrin is the principal hormone released by the endocrine G cells to stimulate hydrochloric secretion from parietal cells.

C. Ghrelin stimulates appetite and therefore forms a component of the cephalic phase.

D. Histamine release from enterochromaffin cells is triggered by acetylcholine. Histamine binds to H_2 receptors to stimulate acid secretion from parietal cells.

E. Correct answer: The presence of the broken-down products of gastric digestion in the duodenum can cause irritation and subsequent release of several intestinal hormones. Secretin has an important role in pancreatic secretions, but also inhibits stomach secretion by:
- Stimulating release of somatostatin from the D cells in the stomach
- Inhibiting release of gastrin in the pyloric antrum
- Directly inhibiting the parietal cells from further acid production.

Boron, WF, Boulpaep, EL (Eds.) (2012). Acid secretion. In: *Medical Physiology*, 2nd edition. Philadelphia, PA: Elsevier Saunders.

Hall JE (2010). Gastric secretion, Unit XII. In: *Guyton and Hall: Textbook of Medical Physiology*, 12th edition. Philadelphia, PA: Elsevier Saunders.

74. E.   Triglycerides are broken down into free fatty acids and monoglycerides by lipase.

A. Emulsification is the first step to the digestion of dietary fats, and starts in the stomach with agitation of stomach contents to allow the fat to mix into chyme. Most emulsification is carried out in the duodenum under the influence of bile.

B. The diameters of the fat globules are decreased due to agitation in the small intestine, and this radically increases the surface area available for digestion. The emulsification process can increase this area by 1,000-fold.

C. While bile salts are an important component of bile, the phospholipid lecithin is also present in bile in large quantities. Bile salts and lecithin are polar molecules and therefore result in hydrophobic and hydrophobic parts, interacting with both fat and the water-containing intestinal contents. This decreases the surface tension of the fat and increases its solubility.

D. Pancreatic lipases are water-soluble hydrophilic compounds that can interact with only the surface of fat globules. Hence the importance of emulsification and subsequent increase in surface area of fats.

E. Correct answer: Pancreatic lipase is secreted in its active form to hydrolyse one triglyceride molecule into two free fatty acids and one monoglyceride, although salivary and gastric lipases also have a small role. One issue is that lipase is inactivated by bile salts. To overcome this, the pancreas releases pro-enzyme procolipase which is activated in the duodenal lumen by trypsin to colipase, and displaces bile salts at the lipid-water interface to allow lipase to continue its digestive processes.

Costanzo LS (Ed.) (2014). Digestion of lipids, digestion and absorption. In: *Physiology*, 5th edition. Philadelphia, PA: Saunders Elsevier.

Hall JE (2010). Digestion and absorption in the gastrointestinal tract, Unit XII. In: *Guyton and Hall: Textbook of Medical Physiology*, 12th edition. Philadelphia, PA: Saunders Elsevier Ltd.

75. D.   Splitting proteins into smaller polypeptides.

A. Carboxylpolypeptidase is one of the major proteolytic enzymes released by the pancreas and is responsible for dismantling proteins one amino acid at a time from the carboxyl end.

B. This described the action of pepsin. Chief cells in the stomach release pepsinogen which is converted to active enzyme pepsin by an acidic environment in the stomach. Pepsin digests collagen found the connective tissue in meat, therefore initiating protein digestion.

C. Elastin fibres form part of the connective tissue of meat, and is broken down in the duodenum and jejunum by enzyme elastase. The zymogen proelastase is released from the pancreas, which is then converted to elastase.

D. Correct answer: This correctly describes the hydrolysing action of trypsin, which also starts catabolizing proteins from the carboxyl terminus. Trypsin is derived from trypsinogen by the enzyme enterokinase. Trypsin, in turn, catalyses further conversion of trypsinogen (to more trypsin), procarboxylpeptidase (to carboxylpeptidase) and increases the concentration of chymotrypsin which has a similar action to trypsin in the digestion of proteins.

Hall JE (2010). Digestion and absorption in the gastrointestinal tract, Unit XII. In: *Guyton and Hall: Textbook of Medical Physiology*, 12th edition. Philadelphia, PA: Saunders Elsevier Ltd.

76. D. Noradrenaline.

A. Acetylcholine is a ubiquitous neurotransmitter in the CNS. Muscarinic receptors are found in the Vomiting Centre in the medulla which is stimulated by vagal sensory nerves, the chemoreceptor trigger zone, and the vestibular nucleus in the pons, to initiate the action of vomiting.

B. Dopamine is released by the Chemoreceptor Trigger Zone in the medulla. Of note, this zone is found outside the blood brain barrier and therefore is more permeable to circulating substances such as drugs and toxins, including alcohol.

C. Histamine and muscarinic receptors are found in the vestibular nucleus which lies in the pons. It is the mediator of motion sickness after hyperstimulation of the vestibulocochlear nerve from fluid movement in the labyrinth. Antihistamines are therefore particularly effective in motion sickness.

D. Correct answer: Noradrenaline has no role in direct role in vomiting.

E. Serotonin is produced by the Chemoreceptor Trigger Zone, in a similar way to dopamine.

Hall JE (2010). Physiology of gastrointestinal disorders, Unit XII. In: *Guyton and Hall: Textbook of Medical Physiology*, 12th edition. Philadelphia, PA: Saunders Elsevier Ltd.

77. C. Cyanide intoxication.

A. This patient is presenting with a high anion gap metabolic acidosis. Anion gap is calculated as follows, with a normal range of 8–16 mEq/L:

$$([Na^+] + [K^+]) - ([Cl^-] + [HCO_3^-])$$

Potassium is often omitted as negligible, and corrections for hypoalbuminaemia should be considered in chronically unwell patients. Addison's disease is generally a cause of a normal anion gap metabolic acidosis.

B. Chloride administration, for instance, in prolonged fluid resuscitation with 0.9% sodium chloride, is a cause of normal anion gap metabolic acidosis, as the high Cl⁻ compensates for loss of HCO_3^-.

C. Correct answer: Cyanide intoxication is a cause of high anion gap metabolic acidosis, the causes of which are listed by the mnemonic CAT MUDPILES. These include, but are not limited to, carbon monoxide, alcoholic ketoacidosis, toluene ingestion, methanol, and uraemia.

D. Diarrhoea is a cause of normal anion gap metabolic acidosis.

E. Renal tubular acidosis is a cause of normal anion gap acidosis, as HCO_3^- is lost.

Koeppen BM, Stanton BA (2006). Role of the kidneys in acid-base balance. In: Levy MN, Stanton BA, Koeppen BM (Eds.), *Berne & Levy Principles of Physiology*, 4th edition (Chapter 40). Maryland Heights, MO: Elsevier Mosby.

78. D. Respiratory acidosis.

A. This is incorrect, as a fully compensated sample would have a normal pH value.

B. This is incorrect, as the bicarbonate and base excess values are both normal.

C. This is incorrect, as a partially compensated sample would be likely to demonstrate a raised bicarbonate or base excess value with an acidotic pH value.

D. Correct answer: The pH value is acidotic, the arterial partial pressure of carbon dioxide is elevated and there is no evident metabolic disturbance.

E. This may be more or less likely, depending on your confidence in the medical student.

Koeppen BM, Stanton BA (2006). Role of the kidneys in acid-base balance. In: Levy MN, Stanton BA, Koeppen BM (Eds.), *Berne & Levy Principles of Physiology*, 4th edition (Chapter 40). Maryland Heights, MO: Elsevier Mosby.

79. D. Partially compensated metabolic alkalosis.

A. This is incorrect, as a fully compensated sample would have a normal pH value.
B. This is partly correct; however, the arterial CO_2 is slightly elevated, suggesting a degree of compensation.
C. This is incorrect, as the values shown are out of range.
D. Correct answer: The pH value is alkalotic with a high base excess and normal bicarbonate, indicating the presence of an unknown base. However, the arterial partial pressure of carbon dioxide is slightly elevated, indicating a degree of CO_2 retention in order to compensate.
E. This is incorrect, as the arterial partial pressure of carbon dioxide is not low.

Koeppen BM, Stanton BA (2006). Role of the kidneys in acid-base balance. In: Levy MN, Stanton BA, Koeppen BM (Eds.), *Berne & Levy Principles of Physiology*, 4th edition (Chapter 40). Maryland Heights, MO: Elsevier Mosby.

80. A. Aldosterone.

A. Correct answer: Aldosterone secretion from the zona glomerulosa of the adrenal glands is stimulated by angiotensin II. Inhibition of ACE reduces the level of angiotensin II and thereby the level of aldosterone.
B. Angiotensin I is not converted to angiotensin II due to ACE inhibition and will be either elevated or unaffected.
C. ACE degrades bradykinin, a potent vasodilator. Inhibition of ACE therefore increases bradykinin levels and can cause the side effect of dry cough in 15% of patients.
D. Angiotensin II reduces renin levels by negative feedback. In the absence of angiotensin II, renin levels remain elevated.
E. ACE inhibitors do not affect serum albumin levels.

Koeppen BM, Stanton BA (2006). Control of body fluid osmolality and extracellular fluid volume. In: Levy MN, Stanton BA, Koeppen BM (Eds.), *Berne & Levy Principles of Physiology*, 4th edition (Chapter 38). Maryland Heights, MO: Elsevier Mosby.

81. B. Apical aquaporin 2.

A. This protein is found in the thick ascending limb of the loop of Henle and is inhibited by loop diuretics, such as furosemide.
B. Correct answer: In the absence of ADH, aquaporin 2 is stored in cytoplasmic vesicles. When ADH binds to V2 receptors in the cells lining the collecting duct of the nephron, intracellular cAMP increases and activates protein kinase A. The vesicles then bind and insert aquaporin 2 by exocytosis into the apical membrane of the cell. When ADH is removed, aquaporin 2 is retrieved for storage and the apical membrane becomes impermeable to water.
C. Aquaporin 3 and 4 are always present in the basolateral membranes of the cells in the collecting duct.
D. This protein acts to increase Na^+ reabsorption across the basolateral membrane in the thick ascending limb of the loop of Henle.
E. This protein is inhibited by thiazide diuretics in the thick ascending limb.

Koeppen BM, Stanton BA (2006). Control of body fluid osmolality and extracellular fluid volume. In: Levy MN, Stanton BA, Koeppen BM (Eds.), *Berne & Levy Principles of Physiology*, 4th edition (Chapter 38). Maryland Heights, MO: Elsevier Mosby.

82. D.   Thirst is more responsive to changes in plasma osmolality than blood volume.

A. ADH binds to V_2 receptors in the cells lining the collecting duct. This stimulates fusion of intracellular vesicles containing aquaporin 2 with the apical membrane of the cell. Aquaporin 2 is inserted into the membrane by exocytosis and the apical membrane becomes permeable to water.

B. ADH is produced by the supraoptic and paraventricular nuclei of the hypothalamus, but is secreted by nerve terminals in the posterior pituitary gland, or neurohypophysis.

C. Increasing plasma osmolality means more concentrated blood, which is detected by osmoreceptors in the hypothalamus and stimulates ADH secretion.

D. Correct answer: Both blood volume and plasma osmolality are important regulators of thirst. However, small increases in plasma osmolality—as little as 2–3%—will generate a thirst response, while one can lose as much as 10% of their blood volume before any sensation of thirst is initiated.

E. This gentleman has syndrome of inappropriate antidiuretic hormone (SIADH), which is a common paraneoplastic phenomenon and also associated with chemotherapeutic agents. In central diabetes insipidus, the gentleman would have polydipsia with dilute urine, due to insufficient secretion of ADH. This is treated with exogenous vasopressin.

Koeppen BM, Stanton BA (2006). Control of body fluid osmolality and extracellular fluid volume. In: Levy MN, Stanton BA, Koeppen BM (Eds.), *Berne & Levy Principles of Physiology*, 4th edition (Chapter 38). Maryland Heights, MO: Elsevier Mosby.

83. D.   Stimulation of Na^+ entry across the apical membranes of the cells of the distal convoluted tubule.

Feedback:

A. This is a function of ACE.

B. This is one of the functions of the atrial natriuretic peptide (ANP).

C. This is one of the functions of ADH.

D. Correct answer: This occurs via activation and up-regulation of Na^+-selective channels. Aldosterone also increases Na^+ transport across the basolateral membrane and into the bloodstream via the Na^+,K^+-ATPase pump. These actions increase water reabsorption.

E. These are functions of angiotensin II.

Koeppen BM, Stanton BA (2006). Control of body fluid osmolality and extracellular fluid volume. In: Levy MN, Stanton BA, Koeppen BM (Eds.), *Berne & Levy Principles of Physiology*, 4th edition (Chapter 38). Maryland Heights, MO: Elsevier Mosby.

84. B.   Autoregulation is absent at this blood pressure.

A. Angiotensin II is a vasoconstrictor, acting to reduce renal blood flow and thereby glomerular filtration rate.

B. Correct answer: As renal autoregulation can only occur between arterial blood pressures of 90–180 mmHg. In this gentleman, the capacity of the kidneys to maintain glomerular filtration will be exceeded leading to an insult of the renal tissue.

C. Haemorrhage decreases arterial blood pressure, detected by baroreceptors in the carotid sinus, aortic arch, and juxtaglomerular apparatus. This results in sympathetic stimulation to the renal arterioles and increased activity of the renin-angiotensin-aldosterone pathway, all of which act to reduce renal blood flow and glomerular filtration.

D. Nitric oxide is one of the major vasodilators in the body.

E. As described, sympathetic stimulation of the renal arterioles causes vasoconstriction, reduces renal blood flow and thereby glomerular filtration.

Koeppen BM, Stanton BA (2006). Elements of renal function. In: Levy MN, Stanton BA, Koeppen BM (Eds.), Berne & Levy Principles of Physiology, 4th edition (Chapter 36). Maryland Heights, MO: Elsevier Mosby.

85. A.   Collecting duct.

A. Correct answer: The collecting duct has limited reabsorptive capacity but is a site of adjustments to urine composition, mediated by the activity of several hormones, including ADH and aldosterone. Aldosterone acts on the nephron from the thick segment to the collecting duct, stimulating NaCl reabsorption and secretion of K^+ and H^+ to modify the urine composition.

B. The descending loop of Henle reabsorbs approximately 15% of the water in the glomerular filtrate via aquaporin 1 channels. It forms part of the countercurrent multiplier mechanism that maximizes NaCl and water reabsorption.

C. The juxtaglomerular apparatus is the site of renin release in response to reduced circulating volume. This leads to aldosterone release from the zona glomerulosa of the adrenal glands and salt conservation.

D. The proximal convoluted tubule is the site of approximately 2/3 of the reabsorption of the glomerular filtrate. It is the main site of reabsorption of glucose, HCO_3^-, amino acids, and organic anions.

E. The ascending loop of Henle is the site of approximately 25% of the NaCl reabsorption from the glomerular filtrate, occurring in both thin and thick segments. The thick segment is impermeable to water, preventing urine dilution as the concentration of the interstitial decreases.

Koeppen BM, Stanton BA (2006). Solute and water trasport along the nephron: Tubular function. In: Levy MN, Stanton BA, Koeppen BM (Eds.), Berne & Levy Principles of Physiology, 4th edition (Chapter 37). Maryland Heights, MO: Elsevier Mosby.

86. D. HCO_3^-.

Many people mistake the Henderson–Hasselbalch equation for the equilibrium reaction between CO_2 and H_2O, but it is actually a means of calculating pH, PCO_2, or the concentration of bicarbonate when given the other two variables. See the following equation:

$$pH = 6.1 + \log ([HCO_3^-]/0.03PCO_2)$$

A. Chloride is a factor in calculating anion gap, but does not feature in the Henderson–Hasselbalch equation.

B. Partial pressure of O_2, or PO_2, is not a factor.

C. pH is calculated as the negative log of H^+ concentration, but H^+ itself is not in the equation.

D. Correct answer: As shown, bicarbonate is a factor in this equation.

E. Sodium ions are used to calculate anion gap in practice, but do not feature in this equation.

Koeppen BM, Stanton BA (2006). Role of the kidneys in acid-base balance. In: Levy MN, Stanton BA, Koeppen BM (Eds.), *Berne & Levy Principles of Physiology*, 4th edition (Chapter 40). Maryland Heights, MO: Elsevier Mosby.

87. C. Na⁺ reabsorption increases.

   A. The opposite occurs, as reduced circulating volume stimulates central and renal baroreceptors to increase sympathetic tone to maintain blood pressure and renal perfusion.

   B. With renal blood flow reduced by arteriolar vasoconstriction, glomerular filtration rate is reduced.

   C. Correct answer: Activation of the renin-angiotensin-aldosterone system stimulates reabsorption of Na⁺ in the proximal and distal tubules and the collecting duct. This increases the osmolality of the ECF, drives the thirst response, and increases water reabsorption in the nephron.

   D. The opposite occurs, as ANP and brain natriuretic peptide (BNP) are released in hypervolaemia.

   E. The opposite occurs, as the juxtaglomerular apparatus release renin in response to hypovolaemia.

Koeppen BM, Stanton BA (2006). Control of body fluid osmolality and extracellular fluid volume. In: Levy MN, Stanton BA, Koeppen BM (Eds.), *Berne & Levy Principles of Physiology*, 4th edition (Chapter 38). Maryland Heights, MO: Elsevier Mosby.

88. E. Stimulation of parasympathetic fibres causes detrusor contraction.

   A. The detrusor muscle is composed of a syncytium of smooth muscle.

   B. The external sphincter relaxes voluntarily when cortical inhibition of the pudendal nerve occurs.

   C. Sympathetic innervation via the hypogastric nerves does not affect the micturition reflex, but loss of parasympathetic innervation causes bladder dysfunction.

   D. The pudendal nerve provides efferent innervation to the external urinary sphincter.

   E. Correct answer: As bladder filling occurs, stretch receptors send sensory information via the afferent arm of a spinal reflex loop. Efferent innervation via parasympathetic fibres causes contraction of the detrusor muscle, allows urine into the posterior urethra.

Koeppen BM, Stanton BA (2006). Elements of renal function. In: Levy MN, Stanton BA, Koeppen BM (Eds.), *Berne & Levy Principles of Physiology*, 4th edition (Chapter 36). Maryland Heights, MO: Elsevier Mosby.

89. C. Juxtaglomerular apparatus.

   A. This is incorrect, as the Bowman's capsule is an envelope of membrane surrounding the glomerular capillaries where the filtration of water and salts begins.

   B. This is incorrect, as the descending loop of Henle is a thin tubule traversing the cortex into the medulla across which the reabsorption of water occurs.

   C. Correct answer: The juxtaglomerular apparatus is formed of the macula densa of the thick ascending limb, the extraglomerular mesangial cells, and the granular cells of the afferent arteriole. The latter cells are modified smooth muscle cells that release renin in response to falling pressure in the afferent arteriole.

   D. This is incorrect, as podocytes are the epithelial cells that form the visceral layer of the Bowman's capsule.

E. This is incorrect, as the vasa recta are the capillaries that descend into the medulla to supply the loop of Henle, return reabsorbed water, and modulate urine concentration.

Koeppen BM, Stanton BA (2006). Elements of renal function. In: Levy MN, Stanton BA, Koeppen BM (Eds.), *Berne & Levy Principles of Physiology*, 4th edition (Chapter 36). Maryland Heights, MO: Elsevier Mosby.

90. E. Proteinuria > 3.5 g/day/1.73 m².

A. Haematuria is a feature of nephritic syndrome, indicating that glomerular damage is so significant that red cells are not being filtered.

B. Recent upper respiratory tract infection is a feature in post-streptococcal glomerulonephritis and IgA nephropathy.

C. Hypertension can be a feature of nephrotic syndrome, but is more indicative of nephritic syndrome. Many signs and symptoms in these conditions do overlap considerably, and there is some discussion in the literature as to whether the conditions are part of a single spectrum.

D. Oliguria is a feature of nephritic syndrome, indicating impaired renal function.

E. Correct answer: Proteinuria to this degree is one of the criteria of nephrotic syndrome. In nephritic syndrome, proteinuria is often mild due to reduced urine output and glomerular filtration rate. This patient presents with oedema and lipids in her urine. Her serum albumin is likely to be low, leading hepatic production of albumin to increase. This causes hyperlipidaemia as a by-product. The likely aetiology in this case is systemic lupus erythematosus (SLE), demonstrated by the butterfly facial rash. Other causes of nephrotic syndrome include minimal change disease, diabetes mellitus, and malignancy.

Koeppen BM, Stanton BA (2006). Role of the kidneys in acid-base balance. In: Levy MN, Stanton BA, Koeppen BM (Eds.), *Berne & Levy Principles of Physiology*, 4th edition (Chapter 40). Maryland Heights, MO: Elsevier Mosby.

91. A. Potassium is secreted by principal cells in the distal tubule and collecting duct.

A. Correct answer: This is the chief mode of potassium secretion into the urine and occurs by channel diffusion down the electrochemical gradient in the distal parts of the nephron.

B. Potassium is reabsorbed in the distal tubule and collecting duct by an antiporter that exchanges K^+ for H^+.

C. Renal failure causes hyperkalaemia due to reduced tubular fluid flow and impaired acid-base balance. In the latter, potassium reabsorption is decreased due to impaired H^+ excretion and acidaemia.

D. Approximately 90% of daily potassium intake is excreted in the urine, while the remainder is excreted in the stool and the sweat.

E. The initial treatments for hyperkalaemia, including calcium gluconate, insulin-dextrose, and nebulized salbutamol do not increase net potassium excretion. Calcium gluconate stabilizes the myocardium, preventing tachyarrhythmias, while insulin-dextrose and salbutamol nebulizers drive potassium from the extracellular into the intracellular compartments.

Koeppen BM, Stanton BA (2006). Potassium, calcium and phosphate homeostasis. In: Levy MN, Stanton BA, Koeppen BM (Eds.), *Berne & Levy Principles of Physiology*, 4th edition (Chapter 39). Maryland Heights, MO: Elsevier Mosby.

92. D. Prostaglandins.

A. Angiotensin II is a vasoconstrictor, causing constriction of the renal arteries and afferent arterioles, resulting in reduced GFR.

B. Endothelin is a vasoconstrictor released by the endothelial cells of the renal arteries and the juxtaglomerular apparatus.

C. Noradrenaline is a vasoconstrictor.

D. Correct answer: Prostaglandins are vasodilators and act to maintain renal blood flow in dehydration and haemorrhage. The history states the patient takes regular non-steroidal anti-inflammatory drugs (NSAIDs), which inhibit the synthesis of prostaglandins.

E. Sympathetic nerves innervating the afferent and efferent renal arterioles release noradrenaline and stimulate vasoconstriction if circulating volume falls.

Koeppen BM, Stanton BA (2006). Elements of renal function. In: Levy MN, Stanton BA, Koeppen BM (Eds.), *Berne & Levy Principles of Physiology*, 4th edition (Chapter 36). Maryland Heights, MO: Elsevier Mosby.

93. E. Proximal convoluted tubule.

A. The ascending loop of Henle is the site of approximately 25% of the NaCl reabsorption from the glomerular filtrate, mediated largely by the $1Na^+,1K^+,2Cl^-$ symporter and inhibited by the action of loop diuretics.

B. The collecting duct is a site of adjustments to urine composition, mediated by the activity of several hormones, including ADH and aldosterone.

C. The descending loop of Henle reabsorbs approximately 15% of the water in the glomerular filtrate via aquaporin 1 channels. It forms part of the countercurrent multiplier mechanism that maximizes NaCl and water reabsorption.

D. The distal convoluted tubule has limited reabsorptive capacity but secretes K^+ and H^+ to modify the urine composition.

E. Correct answer: The proximal convoluted tubule is the site of approximately two-thirds of the reabsorption of the glomerular filtrate. It is the main site of reabsorption of glucose, HCO_3^-, amino acids, and organic anions.

Koeppen BM, Stanton BA (2006). Solute and water transport along the nephron: Tubular function. In: Levy MN, Stanton BA, Koeppen BM (Eds.), *Berne & Levy Principles of Physiology*, 4th edition (Chapter 37). Maryland Heights, MO: Elsevier Mosby.

94. B. Dilution occurs in the thick ascending limb.

A. This patient is likely to have psychogenic polydipsia, which may have caused a seizure by electrolyte disturbance. As such, their plasma osmolality will be very low and the osmoreceptors of the hypothalamus will suppress release of ADH from the posterior pituitary.

B. Correct answer: The thick ascending limb of the loop of Henle is sometimes called the diluting segment. It is impermeable to water and urea, but the apical membrane of the cells contain the $Na^+,K^+,2Cl^-$ symporter actively transports NaCl from the lumen.

C. Water reabsorption in the loop of Henle occurs in the descending loop, which is highly permeable to water. This is driven by the increasing osmolality of the interstitium within the medulla, which is maintained by the countercurrent mechanism and the vasa recta.

D. Within the plasma, urea is considered an ineffective osmole. However, within the interstitium of the medulla urea and NaCl are present in high concentrations to aid water reabsorption. As such, urea is considered an effective osmole in the medulla.

E. Plasma osmolality is approximately 290 mOsm/kg H_2O in health. In this patient the urine will be very dilute, as low as 50 mOsm/kg H_2O. In dehydration, the effects of various hormones such as ADH can concentrate the urine up to 1,200 mOsm/kg H_2O.

Koeppen BM, Stanton BA (2006). Control of body fluid osmolality and extracellular fluid volume. In: Levy MN, Stanton BA, Koeppen BM (Eds.), *Berne & Levy Principles of Physiology*, 4th edition (Chapter 38). Maryland Heights, MO: Elsevier Mosby.

95. C. Increased Ca^{2+}; decreased PO_4^-.

A. This patient is presenting with the classic symptomology of hypercalcaemia: bones, stones, groans, and psychiatric overtones. Hyperparathyroidism often presents in this way.
B. This is incorrect, as PTH decreases PO_4^- reabsorption in the proximal convoluted tubule.
C. Correct answer: These bloods results are consistent with hyperparathyroidism. The main cause of primary hyperparathyroidism is benign PTH-secreting adenoma in one of the parathyroid glands. Hyperplasia of two or more of the parathyroid glands is the next most common cause.
D. This is incorrect.
E. This is incorrect, as PTH increases Ca^{2+} reabsorption in the distal convoluted tubule.

Koeppen BM, Stanton BA (2006). Potassium, calcium and phosphate homeostasis. In: Levy MN, Stanton BA, Koeppen BM (Eds.), *Berne & Levy Principles of Physiology*, 4th edition (Chapter 39). Maryland Heights, MO: Elsevier Mosby.

96. D. Calcium reabsorption is increased in the distal tubule AND phosphate reabsorption is decreased in the proximal tubule.

A. Parathyroid hormone (PTH) does activate α-hydroxylase to activate vitamin D from calcidiol to calcitriol. This acts to reduce excretion of both calcium and phosphate in the kidney. It also increases absorption of calcium within the intestines.
B. This is incorrect.
C. This is incorrect.
D. Correct answer: The patient is hypercalcaemic due to decreased calcium excretion. Approximately 70% of calcium ions are reabsorbed in the proximal convoluted tubule, with a further 20% reabsorbed in the thick ascending limb and approximately 9% in the distal convoluted tubule. Less than 1% is excreted in health. In hyperparathyroidism, PTH increases reabsorption despite hypercalcaemia. The greatest change is in the distal convoluted tubule, where reabsorption can increase significantly. Similarly, phosphate excretion increases in hyperparathyroidism, the main change occurring in the proximal convoluted tubule.
E. This is incorrect.

Koeppen BM, Stanton BA (2006). Potassium, calcium and phosphate homeostasis. In: Levy MN, Stanton BA, Koeppen BM (Eds.), *Berne & Levy Principles of Physiology*, 4th edition (Chapter 39). Maryland Heights, MO: Elsevier Mosby.

97. E. Removal of negative feedback to ACTH secretion.

A. This describes normal tanning and occurs in health.
B. This is the mechanism for acanthosis nigricans, which is the hyperpigmentation seen mostly in skin folds and associated with various endocrine and oncological conditions. This is unlikely to be correct as most patients with acanthosis nigricans are insulin resistant, which does not explain the hypoglycaemia in this patient.

C. This is the pathophysiology of hereditary haemochromatosis, which can cause hyperpigmentation due to iron overload. Bronzing of the skin is seen, but typical presentations are related to cirrhosis of the liver, diabetes secondary to pancreatic haemosiderosis and cardiomyopathy.

D. This is the autosomal dominant mutation associated with Peutz-Jeghers syndrome. These patients have perioral pigmented macules and gastrointestinal polyps. They often present with intussusception or volvulus.

E. Correct answer: This patient is most likely to be suffering from an Addisonian crisis. In Addison's disease, the adrenal cortex is damaged or impaired, decreasing secretion of aldosterone and cortisol. Since cortisol is the only adrenal hormone that suppresses ACTH secretion, this patient will have high levels of ACTH. ACTH is a product of proopiomelanocortin (POMC) which also synthesizes melanocyte-stimulating hormone as a co-product. The hyperpigmentation typically occurs in skin creases and around the lips and is not seen in secondary or tertiary forms of Addison's disease, as ACTH is not increased.

Genuth SM (2006). Adrenal cortex. In: Levy MN, Stanton BA, Koeppen BM (Eds.), *Berne & Levy Principles of Physiology*, 4th edition (Chapter 47). Maryland Heights, MO: Elsevier Mosby.

98. A. Capsule produces no hormones.

A. Correct answer: The capsule consists only of connective tissue.

B. The medulla is the site of production of catecholamines, including adrenaline and noradrenaline. It constitutes 10–20% of the total mass of the adrenal gland.

C. The cortex of the adrenal gland is divided into the zona glomerulosa, zona fasciculata and zona reticularis (superficial to deep). All the hormones produced in the cortex are derived from cholesterol. While there is a small degree of overlap, the zona fasciculata is the chief site of cortisol production.

D. The zona glomerulosa is the only site of aldosterone production.

E. The zona reticularis produces weak androgens, including dehydroepiandrosterone (DHEA) and androstenedione. In women, the adrenals supply approximately half the body's androgen requirement. In men, this is largely redundant due to the function of the testes.

Genuth SM (2006). Adrenal cortex. In: Levy MN, Stanton BA, Koeppen BM (Eds.), *Berne & Levy Principles of Physiology*, 4th edition (Chapter 47). Maryland Heights, MO: Elsevier Mosby.

99. C. Hydroxyproline and hydroxylysine concentrations in the urine reflect bone turnover rate.

A. Osteocytes embedded with bone detect fatigue and areas of weakness. They signal to resting or lining cells, which recruit osteoclasts to the area. Osteoclasts contain copious mitochondria and lysosomes for bone resorption. The cavity generated by the osteoclasts becomes the site for new bone formation by the osteoblasts. With age, bone resorption exceeds formation and bone density falls, increasing the risk of fractures.

B. Collagen fibres form the organic matrix, also called osteoid. Calcium and phosphate ions are deposited and modified by osteocalcin and osteonectin, both osteoblast products, which add hydroxy and bicarbonate groups to produce hydroxyapatite. This is the mineral phase of bone.

C. Correct answer: Hydroxyproline and hydroxylysine are amino acids specific to collagen. Their concentration in the urine is reflective of the activity of osteoclasts in bone resorption. Other products of bone resorption include pyridinolines, pyridiniums, and N-telopeptides.

D. Active osteoblasts have a lifespan of 3 months. However, if the osteoblast becomes completely enveloped in mineralized bone, it becomes an osteocyte with a lifespan of 20 years. Osteocytes represent 90% of all bone cells.

E. Osteoblasts arise from pluripotential mesenchymal cells, while osteoclasts are derived from haematopoietic stem cells. This is the same precursor cell that gives rise to circulating monocytes.

Genuth SM (2006). Endocrine regulation of the metabolism of calcium and phosphate. In: Levy MN, Stanton BA, Koeppen BM (Eds.), *Berne & Levy Principles of Physiology*, 4th edition (Chapter 44). Maryland Heights, MO: Elsevier Mosby.

100. C. Hypokalaemia.

A. Conn syndrome describes primary hyperaldosteronism, which is now being recognized as a cause of treatment-resistant hypertension in 10–15% of cases. Most cases are the result of a unilateral aldosterone-secreting adrenal adenoma, but bilateral adrenal hyperplasia may cause a similar picture. Due to increased water and salt conservation in the distal tubule and collecting duct of the nephron, volume expansion takes place rather than dehydration, which is a feature of Addison's disease.

B. Hyperchloraemic acidosis is another feature of Addison's disease.

C. Correct answer: Aldosterone acts to increase reabsorption of water, Na^+ and Cl^- in the distal nephron where it also stimulates secretion of K^+. This results in hypokalaemia that is responsive to treatment with aldosterone antagonists, such as spironolactone.

D. Natriuresis is a feature of Addison's disease, which is the result of aldosterone deficiency.

E. Despite the volume expansion that occurs in Conn syndrome, the high osmolality of plasma due to salt conservation prevents peripheral oedema.

Genuth SM (2006). Adrenal cortex. In: Levy MN, Stanton BA, Koeppen BM (Eds.), *Berne & Levy Principles of Physiology*, 4th edition (Chapter 47). Maryland Heights, MO: Elsevier Mosby.

101. C. Cortisol increases proteolysis.

A. This woman has presented with signs and symptoms of Cushing's syndrome, which is the result of excessive cortisol. Cortisol is described as a permissive hormone, in that the presence of cortisol potentiates several effects that cortisol does not directly stimulate. One such example is the maintenance of blood pressure, where cortisol enhances the activity of adrenergic receptors and angiotensin II without directly stimulating vasoconstriction.

B. A symptom of Cushing's syndrome is osteoporosis and resulting fragility fractures. This is because cortisol decreases bone density in two ways. Primarily, cortisol reduces osteogenesis, however, it also slightly increases bone resorption.

C. Correct answer: This is one of the major effects of the stress response and prevent hypoglycaemia when glycogen stores have been exhausted. By breaking down protein in muscle, skin, and vessel walls cortisol causes several of the signs and symptoms seen in Cushing's syndrome. For example, the thin and wasted limbs that contribute to the classical 'lemon on sticks' appearance.

D. Cortisol and insulin oppose each other in several ways, but the promotion of glycogen formation in the liver is not one of them. Cortisol potentiates the activity of glycogen synthase in hepatocytes.

E. Cortisol has a complex range of actions on inflammatory and immune pathways, but one of the main ways in which cortisol impairs the immune response is by blocking the secretion of cytokines, such as the interleukins, that generate fever and stimulate lymphocyte proliferation.

Genuth SM (2006). Adrenal cortex. In: Levy MN, Stanton BA, Koeppen BM (Eds.), *Berne & Levy Principles of Physiology*, 4th edition (Chapter 47). Maryland Heights, MO: Elsevier Mosby.

102. B. Galactorrhoea.

A. This man has presented with signs of glucocorticoid excess, the clinical picture of which described as Cushing syndrome. This diagnosis incorporates all causes of hypercortisolism. Cushing's disease presents as Cushing syndrome, but is caused by an ACTH-secreting pituitary adenoma. As such, a reduced level of ACTH suggests a primary cause of hypercortisolism rather than a secondary, or pituitary, cause.

B. Correct answer: Galactorrhoea is a symptom of hyperprolactinaemia, which may be caused by compression of the pituitary stalk in Cushing's disease. Other such symptoms include polyuria and nocturia, resulting from reduced ADH secretion central diabetes insipidus. Symptoms such as headache or visual disturbance reflect the presence of an intracranial space-occupying lesion.

C. Cushing syndrome has a 5:1 female-to-male prevalence. Ectopic ACTH-secreting tumours include small-cell lung carcinoma and are more common among men. Ectopic tumours comprise 20% of ACTH-dependent Cushing syndrome cases. The remainder are caused by Cushing's disease.

D. Low-dose dexamethasone suppression test involves administration of 1 mg dexamethasone overnight and measuring 8AM cortisol levels, where a level below 2 mcg/dL excludes Cushing syndrome with a 98.5% negative predictive value. A positive test result may suggest Cushing syndrome but cannot differentiate Cushing's disease. The high-dose dexamethasone suppression test with 8 mg dexamethasone overnight is deemed positive where 8AM cortisol is more than 50% below the baseline, which suggests Cushing's disease is the cause.

E. The most common cause of Cushing syndrome is iatrogenic, or exogenous glucocorticoid administration.

Genuth SM (2006). Adrenal cortex. In: Levy MN, Stanton BA, Koeppen BM (Eds.), *Berne & Levy Principles of Physiology*, 4th edition (Chapter 47). Maryland Heights, MO: Elsevier Mosby.

103. E. Serum triglyceride level.

A. Kussmaul breathing describes the rapid, deep breaths taken by patients with profound acidosis. This patient is clearly in diabetic ketoacidosis, DKA, due to lack of insulin administration and presumed alcohol excess. As such, CO_2 will be eliminated and hypocapnia may result.

B. Glucokinase is the enzyme responsible for phosphorylation of glucose into glucose-6-phosphate. The action of glucokinase is stimulated by insulin as the first step of glycogen synthesis and will be reduced in this patient.

C. Lipoprotein lipase is the enzyme responsible for liberating fatty acids from circulating triglycerides prior to esterification in the adipose tissue. Insulin stimulates the activity of this enzyme.

D. C-peptide is the inactive by-product of insulin secretion. The serum level will be reduced in this patient, even in health, since he will have no significant endogenous insulin or C-peptide production.

E. Correct answer: Serum triglyceride will be elevated in this patient due to the increased lipolysis of adipose tissue promoted by glucagon and the reduced activity of lipoprotein lipase, as discussed.

Genuth SM (2006). Hormones of the pancreatic islets. In: Levy MN, Stanton BA, Koeppen BM (Eds.), *Berne & Levy Principles of Physiology*, 4th edition (Chapter 43). Maryland Heights, MO: Elsevier Mosby.

104. C. Serum C-peptide level.

A. Basal metabolic rate will certainly increase in this patient, as he has been exercising. O_2 consumption has increased at a cellular level, cardiac output and respiratory rate have increased to meet the increased demand and stores of glucose will be broken down for use.

B. Cortisol is the stress hormone, secreted when the body is under stress due to illness or trauma in order to prevent hypoglycaemia and inhibit inflammation. It will be elevated in this patient.

C. Correct answer: C-peptide is a by-product of insulin secretion, which will be reduced in this patient due to the increased demand for glucose in the skeletal muscle. Since insulin inhibits glycogenolysis, gluconeogenesis and lipolysis, insulin secretion falls during periods of prolonged exercise.

D. Conversely, glucagon acts reciprocally to insulin, therefore glucagon secretion will be increased.

E. The sympathetic nervous system response is colloquially termed the 'fight or flight' response. In this case, the patient has done both.

Genuth SM (2006). Hormones of the pancreatic islets. In: Levy MN, Stanton BA, Koeppen BM (Eds.), *Berne & Levy Principles of Physiology*, 4th edition (Chapter 43). Maryland Heights, MO: Elsevier Mosby.

105. E. Somatostatin analogues.

A. Dopamine tonically inhibits the release of prolactin, a hormone structurally-similar to growth hormone and released from mammotroph cells in the anterior pituitary. Prolactin promotes differentiation and breast tissue and lactogenesis. Through inhibition of gonadotropin-releasing hormone, prolactin also modulates the reproductive axis.

B. While this gentleman's blood glucose is indicative of a new diagnosis of diabetes mellitus, insulin therapy is unlikely to be effective due to the underlying aetiology.

C. This gentleman is likely to have high circulating levels of insulin growth factors (IGF). Further supplementation will exacerbate his symptoms.

D. A ketogenic diet is employed in certain metabolic disorders to maintain energy supplies for brain tissue and prevent seizures. There is also some evidence to recommend its use in autistic spectrum disorders. However, it will not help this gentleman.

E. Correct answer: The history of enlargement of the hands and muscles such as the tongue is indicative of acromegaly, literally meaning 'great extremities' in ancient Greek. This condition can be associated with coarsening facial features, decreased subcutaneous fat, increased cardiac output, accelerated atherosclerotic disease, and insulin resistance. The condition is caused by hypersecretion of growth hormone, most likely from a pituitary tumour of the somatotroph cells. Growth hormone secretion is stimulated by growth hormone releasing hormone and inhibited by somatostatin. If surgical resection is unsuccessful or unfeasible, somatostain analogues can be effective treatment.

Genuth SM (2006). Hypothalamus and pituitary gland. In: Levy MN, Stanton BA, Koeppen BM (Eds.), *Berne & Levy Principles of Physiology*, 4th edition (Chapter 45). Maryland Heights, MO: Elsevier Mosby.

106. B. Cortisol is the only product of the adrenal cortex that participates in negative feedback to CRH and ACTH.

A. Patients on long-term steroids can experience an iatrogenic form of adrenal insufficiency when they finish their course. This is because the adrenal cortex is ACTH-dependent and atrophies in the absence of this stimulation. As such, the patient is deficient in minerallocorticoids, glucocorticoids, and androgenic steroids.

B. Correct answer: Aldosterone and androgens do not suppress CRH or ACTH release.

C. CRH is produced in the paraventricular nucleus, also known as the median eminence of the hypothalamus, and is transported to the anterior pituitary via the portal venous system. ACTH is produced by corticotrophs in the anterior pituitary gland from the precursor, POMC.

D. Exogenous steroids, such as dexamethasone and prednisolone, also act to suppress CRH and ACTH release in a similar manner to cortisol. Therefore, exogenous steroids must be stopped for a period prior to cortisol testing.

E. Serotonin is one of the neurotransmitters that stimulates CRH release, along with acetylcholine, GABA, and noradrenaline. Endorphin acts to inhibit CRH release.

Genuth SM (2006). Adrenal cortex. In: Levy MN, Stanton BA, Koeppen BM (Eds.), *Berne & Levy Principles of Physiology*, 4th edition (Chapter 47). Maryland Heights, MO: Elsevier Mosby.

107. D.   PTH synthesis will be suppressed in this patient.

A. Calcitonin is synthesized by neuroendocrine C cells in the thyroid glands and is secreted in response to hypercalcaemia. It acts as a PTH antagonist to inhibit bone resorption and lower plasma calcium concentration.

B. On the contrary, intracellular $[Ca^{2+}]$ varies greatly to perform the multiple functions that involve calcium, such as muscle contraction, neuronal signalling, and coagulation. Extracellular $[Ca^{2+}]$ is approximately 10,000 times greater than intracellular $[Ca^{2+}]$, but is tightly controlled to allow these functions to take place.

C. This is incorrect, as the ratio of bone mineral:matrix content is normal in osteoporosis with overall reduced bone density. In osteomalacia, bone mineral content is resorbed, normally as the result of vitamin D deficiency, while bone matrix is maintained.

D. Correct answer: Calcium forms a negative feedback loop with PTH synthesis. The four parathyroid glands contain calcium receptors in their plasma membranes. This receptor is a G protein coupled to promote or prevent exocytosis of PTH-containing vesicles and synthesis of PTH.

E. Vitamin D_3 binds to cytosolic receptors in the enterocytes. The hormone-receptor complex enters the nucleus to increase production of calcium-binding protein such as calbindin. This potentiates increased intestinal absorption of calcium.

Genuth SM (2006). Endocrine regulation of the metabolism of calcium and phosphate. In: Levy MN, Stanton BA, Koeppen BM (Eds.), *Berne & Levy Principles of Physiology*, 4th edition (Chapter 44). Maryland Heights, MO: Elsevier Mosby.

108. E.   Thyroid peroxidase activity.

A. Basal metabolic rate is increased in hyperthyroidism, leading affected individuals to increase daily calorie intake despite losing weight.

B. Cardiac output is the product of heart rate and stroke volume. Triiodothyronine, or T_3, increases the cardiovascular response to adrenaline by up-regulating α-adrenergic receptors, which potentiates an increase in heart rate. By increasing myocardial uptake of Ca^{2+} and reducing the afterload via arteriolar vasodilatation, T_3 also increases stroke volume.

C. Minute ventilation is the volume of air inspired or expired within one minute. Due to increased basal metabolic rate, O_2 consumption is increased and respiratory rate follows.

D. Reverse triiodothyronine, or rT$_3$, is a product of peripheral monodeiodination of thyroxine (T$_4$) that has no recognized hormonal activity. It should be present at higher levels due to the higher levels of T$_4$ being converted.

E. Correct answer: Thyroid peroxidase is the enzyme that catalyses the synthesis of T$_3$ and T$_4$ from tyrosine and iodine. The activity of the enzyme is related to thyroid stimulating hormone (TSH) levels, which will be reduced in this patient. Similarly, thyroglobulin synthesis, iodine trapping, and the height of the thyroid epithelial cells will be reduced.

Genuth SM (2006). Thyroid gland. In: Levy MN, Stanton BA, Koeppen BM (Eds.), *Berne & Levy Principles of Physiology*, 4th edition (Chapter 46). Maryland Heights, MO: Elsevier Mosby.

109. C. Reduced number of cardiac α adrenergic receptors.

A. Cardiac output is the product of heart rate and stroke volume. With reduced circulating levels of triiodothyronine and tetraiodothyronine, or T$_3$ and T$_4$ heart rate would be expected to fall. These hormones are also responsible for reducing peripheral vascular resistance as a means of increasing tissue perfusion, but the effect on cardiac output is not as significant.

B. Thyroid hormones potentiate several of the actions of the sympathetic nervous system, one of which is catecholamine-stimulated gluconeogenesis.

C. Correct answer: T$_3$ increases the cardiovascular response to catecholamines by binding to nuclear receptors to up-regulate production of α-adrenergic receptors, which potentiates an increase in heart rate. By increasing myocardial uptake of Ca^{2+} and reducing the afterload via arteriolar vasodilatation, T$_3$ also increases stroke volume.

D. Thyrotropin, or TSH, has a trophic effect on the thyroid gland, seen clinically as a goitre. This occurs due to increased height of the thyroid epithelial cells, synthesis of colloid, and follicular enlargement. While TSH is not always elevated in hypothyroidism, the presence of goitre suggests this is true.

E. The quantity of colloid is related to TSH levels, which will be elevated in this patient. Thyroglobulin synthesis, iodine trapping, and the rate of colloid resorption will also be increase.

Genuth SM (2006). Thyroid gland. In: Levy MN, Stanton BA, Koeppen BM (Eds.), *Berne & Levy Principles of Physiology*, 4th edition (Chapter 46). Maryland Heights, MO: Elsevier Mosby.

110. E. Muscle glucose uptake.

A. Insulin is the major anabolic hormone in the body. It is composed of two peptide chains linked by a disulphide bond.

B. Insulin stimulates glycogen synthase and thereby inhibits hepatic glycogenolysis. Essentially, insulin stimulates the removal of glucose from the ECF for storage, which is why it causes hypoglycaemia in cases such as this.

C. Insulin is strongly antiketogenic, due to its stimulatory action on lipoprotein lipase activity. This enzyme is involved in storing free fatty acids as adipose tissue, which prevents their conversion in fasting states into ketones such as α-hydroxybutyrate and acetoacetate.

D. In addition to stimulating lipoprotein lipase, insulin inhibits the action of adipose tissue lipase, which inhibits the liberation of free fatty acids from adipose tissue.

E. Correct answer: Insulin upregulates the presence of GLUT4 receptors in the plasma membranes of striated muscle cells. This potentiates the shift of plasma glucose into glycogen and pyruvate pathways.

Genuth SM (2006). Hormones of the pancreatic islets. In: Levy MN, Stanton BA, Koeppen BM (Eds.), *Berne & Levy Principles of Physiology*, 4th edition (Chapter 43). Maryland Heights, MO: Elsevier Mosby.

111. C. Serum insulin levels are an inaccurate proxy of α cell function in diabetic patients.

A. This is the pathophysiology of type 1 diabetes mellitus, an autoimmune condition in which the α cells of the islets of Langerhans are destroyed by apoptosis. This results in absent or negligible insulin production, while this gentleman will have inadequate insulin production for his total body requirement due to peripheral tissue insulin resistance or increased body mass.

B. Within the pancreatic islets, glucagon-secreting α and insulin-secreting β cells exist in close proximity and communicate with each other via tight junctions and gap junctions. This allows the secretion of one hormone to influence the secretion of the other, which is beneficial since they have reciprocal actions.

C. Correct answer: Insulin is secreted into the pancreatic veins in granules with C-peptide, an inactive by-product of insulin synthesis. These granules enter the portal vein and mix with the substrates of digestion from the mesenteric circulation. The liver is the first organ to process the insulin and hepatocytes account for approximately 50% of total insulin use, though this is dependent on the carbohydrate load of the meal. As such, serum insulin levels are a poor proxy of α cell function in patients and C-peptide, which is not taken up by hepatocytes, is the recommended test.

D. Since C-peptide is the product of endogenous insulin synthesis, serum levels will not be elevated in patients taking exogenous insulin. Although this gentleman would initially have increased endogenous insulin production as the result of insulin resistance and the metabolic syndrome, administration of exogenous insulin would reduce this by negative feedback.

E. Zinc joins insulin molecules into hexamers within the secretory granules. These dissociate peripherally into the active monomer form.

Genuth SM (2006). Hormones of the pancreatic islets. In: Levy MN, Stanton BA, Koeppen BM (Eds.), *Berne & Levy Principles of Physiology*, 4th edition (Chapter 43). Maryland Heights, MO: Elsevier Mosby.

112. A. Adipose tissue.

A. Correct answer: Leptin is a secreted product of adipose tissue, acting on receptors in the hypothalamus to reduce appetite, or in other words, to induce satiety. Leptin also increases the basal metabolic rate, partly by increasing sympathetic tone to the body. Plasma leptin levels are proportionate to BMI, but there has been no proven genetic link between mutations in the leptin pathway and obesity.

B. Duodenal epithelium secretes cholecystokinin and secretin in response to low pH or fatty gastric contents. Brunner's glands in the duodenum secrete mucus and bicarbonate.

C. The endocrine pancreas secretes insulin and glucagon.

D. The exocrine pancreas secretes digestive enzymes and bicarbonate.

E. Leptin stimulates receptors in the hypothalamus that modulate our food seeking or food avoidance behaviours.

Genuth SM (2006). Whole-body metabolism. In: Levy MN, Stanton BA, Koeppen BM (Eds.), *Berne & Levy Principles of Physiology*, 4th edition (Chapter 42). Maryland Heights, MO: Elsevier Mosby.

113. B. Cholinergic preganglionic fibres stimulate catecholamine release.

A. Adrenaline and noradrenaline are synthesized from tyrosine. Steroid hormones are synthesized from cholesterol.

B. Correct answer: This patient in this case has a phaeochromocytoma, a tumour of the adrenal medulla. The adrenal medulla is essentially a large, specialized ganglion of the sympathetic nervous system. Innervation to the adrenal medulla is via preganglionic sympathetic nerves in which transmission is via acetylcholine. Since catecholamines are not stored, synthesis occurs following sympathetic stimulation in response to stress.

C. Stressors that activate this sympathetic response include hypovolaemia, hypotension, exercise, psychological stress, and hypoglycaemia.

D. Phaeochromocytoma is a tumour of the chromaffin cells of the adrenal medulla.

E. Many of the triggers that stimulate sympathetic stimulation of the adrenal medulla also stimulate release of CRH. This stimulates secretion of adrenocorticotrophic hormone (ACTH) which in turn stimulates cortisol secretion. These pathways are functionally and physiologically overlapping, as activation of one stimulates the other.

Genuth SM (2006). Adrenal medulla. In: Levy MN, Stanton BA, Koeppen BM (Eds.), *Berne & Levy Principles of Physiology*, 4th edition (Chapter 48). Maryland Heights, MO: Elsevier Mosby.

114. A. Adrenal crisis secondary to pituitary ischaemic necrosis.

A. Correct answer: Sheehan syndrome, also known as post-partum hypopituitarism, is a rare complication of significant blood loss or hypotension during labour. Symptoms commonly include agalactorrhoea, amenorrhoea, fatigue, and features of hypothyroidism such as cold intolerance and bradycardia. Rarely, adrenal crisis can be provoked, often by significant illness or surgery. In these patients, severe hypotension can lead to coma and death. During pregnancy, hyperplasia of prolactin-producing cells called lactotrophs occurs. Furthermore, the low-pressure portal venous supply to the anterior pituitary gland from the hypothalamus leave the anterior pituitary vulnerable to ischaemia. The posterior pituitary receives direct arterial supply.

B. Bilateral adrenal haemorrhage may occur during severe sepsis, particularly in meningococcal infection, and is known as Waterhouse-Friderichsen syndrome. In this case the patient is afebrile and previously well.

C. Hypothalamic ischaemia in hypotension is uncommon due to direct arterial supply.

D. Tachycardia-induced cardiomyopathy can occur at any age; however, the ECG shows no evidence of ventricular strain or hypertrophy.

E. Thyroid storm is likely to present with hyperpyrexia, tachycardia, and hypertension rather than hypotension.

Genuth SM (2006). Hypothalamus and pituitary gland. In: Levy MN, Stanton BA, Koeppen BM (Eds.), *Berne & Levy Principles of Physiology*, 4th edition (Chapter 45). Maryland Heights, MO: Elsevier Mosby.

115. B. Steroid hormones are produced from cholesterol.

A. Steroid hormones act on nuclear receptors to alter gene expression. Peptides (e.g. ADH), proteins (e.g. insulin) and catecholamines (e.g. noradrenaline) act on plasma membrane receptors and stimulate intracellular signalling pathways.

B. Correct answer: Steroid hormones including cortisol, aldosterone, androgens, and oestrogens are produced by a multienzyme pathway from cholesterol.

C. Steroid hormones are released by diffusion when they are produced. Peptides and catecholamines are released by exocytosis.

D. Steroid hormones are not stored in the gland of production, but produced from an intracellular store of cholesterol when the gland is stimulated. Peptides and catecholamines are stored in secretory granules.

E. Tyrosine is a key building block for thyroid hormones and catecholamines.

Genuth SM (2006). General principles of endocrine physiology. In: Levy MN, Stanton BA, Koeppen BM (Eds.), *Berne & Levy Principles of Physiology*, 4th edition (Chapter 41). Maryland Heights, MO: Elsevier Mosby.

116. A. G-cell activity is reduced compared to normal state.

A. Correct answer: This question requires you to know that Zollinger–Ellison syndrome describes a patient with a gastrin-secreting tumour and high circulating levels of gastrin. The normal parasympathetic response to peptides in the stomach and duodenum stimulates the G cells of the gastric antrum to release gastrin, which triggers the parietal cells to secrete stomach acid (HCl) via CCK_B or gastrin receptors. In Zollinger–Ellison, ectopic gastrin secretion inhibits G-cell activity by negative feedback.

B. The opposite is true, as gastrin levels are persistently elevated despite the usual physiological stimuli to promote secretion.

C. Gastrin is a trophic hormone that upregulates the production of parietal cells in the gastric mucosa.

D. Histamine also triggers HCl secretion via H_2 receptors, which explains the efficacy of H_2-receptor antagonists such as ranitidine in many cases of peptic ulcer disease. In Zollinger–Ellison syndrome, however, H_2-receptor antagonists are ineffective due to high circulating levels of gastrin. PPI are the medical treatment of choice.

E. Gastrin triggers D cells in the gastric antrum to secrete somatostatin, which inhibits HCl release via an inhibitory G-protein pathway. In Zollinger–Ellison syndrome, somatostatin levels are likely to be elevated but remain insufficient to negate the increase in gastrin levels.

Kutchai HC (2006). Gastrointestinal secretions. In: Levy MN, Stanton BA, Koeppen BM (Eds.), *Berne & Levy Principles of Physiology*, 4th edition (Chapter 34). Maryland Heights, MO: Elsevier Mosby.

1. **A 19-year-old backpacker has had fever, muscle pain, headaches, and a blanching rash having returned to the United Kingdom seven days ago. You suspect he may have dengue fever. Which single statement regarding dengue fever is most accurate?**
   A. Can be spread by tick bites
   B. Endemic to Northern Africa
   C. Mortality rate is 1–5% when adequately treated
   D. Spread by the Aedes mosquito
   E. The dengue virus is a DNA virus

2. **A four-day-old baby is pre-alerted to the emergency department (ED) with a history of poor feeding, low tone, and tachycardia. The mother had group B streptococcus (GBS) colonization in her last pregnancy. Which is the single most appropriate antibiotic therapy?**
   A. Amoxicillin
   B. Benzylpenicillin and gentamicin
   C. Cefotaxime
   D. Ceftriaxone and amoxicillin
   E. Clindamycin

3. **A 94-year-old man from a nursing home has had worsening productive cough, fever, and increased confusion. He had previous stroke, dementia, and ischaemic heart disease. His heart rate (HR) is 116 bpm, respiratory rate (RR) 30 breaths/min and T 38.8°C. The chest X-ray (CXR) was normal two weeks ago. His CXR today shows multiple cavitating lesions in his right upper lobe. Which single organism is most likely to have caused the symptoms?**
   A. *Bacillus anthracis*
   B *Haemophilus influenzae*
   C. *Kleibsiella pneumoniae*
   D. *Staphylococcus aureus*
   E. *Streptococcus pneumoniae*

4. **A 27-year-old female has had lower abdominal pain, vaginal discharge, and dyspareunia. Cervical swabs reveal an ovoid Gram-negative bacterium. Which is the single most likely causative organism?**
   A. *Chlamydia trachomatis*
   B. *Escherichia coli*
   C. *Neisseria gonorrhoeae*
   D. *Treponema pallidum*
   E. *Trichomonas vaginalis*

5. **A 47-year-old female has had dysuria and urinary frequency for 48 hours. Her urine dipstick is positive for leucocytes and nitrites. She has a negative pregnancy test. She is otherwise well with no known drug allergies. Which single antibiotic choice is most appropriate?**
   A. Cefalexin 500 mg twice daily orally
   B. Ciprofloxacin 500 mg twice daily orally
   C. Co-amoxiclav 625 mg three times a day orally
   D. Gentamicin 5 mg/kg single dose intravenously
   E. Trimethoprim 200 mg twice a day orally

6. **A 52-year-old man has had unilateral leg swelling and redness. He has normal clinical observations and blood tests. The provisional diagnosis is uncomplicated cellulitis. Which single organism is most likely to have caused the symptoms?**
   A. *Clostridium perfringens*
   B. *Staphylococcus aureus*
   C. *Streptococcus pyogenes*
   D. *Pasteurella multocida*
   E. *Pseudomonas aeruginosa*

7. **A 77-year-old man with a previous anaphylactic reaction to amoxicillin has had symptoms and signs of pneumonia with a CURB-65 score of 4. His blood cultures grew Mycoplasma pneumoniae. Which single antibiotic is most appropriate for this patient?**
   A. Co-amoxiclav
   B. Ciprofloxacin
   C. Clarithromycin
   D. Meropenem
   E. Tazocin

8. **A five-year-old boy has had fever, headache, photophobia, and vomiting. A lumbar puncture is performed and the cerebrospinal fluid (CSF) shows a lymphocytosis, raised protein, and normal glucose. Which is the most likely organism causing the symptoms?**

   A. *Coxsackievirus*

   B. Group B streptococci

   C. *Haemophilus* influenzae type B

   D. HSV-1

   E. *Neisseria meningitidis*

9. **A 33-year-old man with recurrent cold sores has had worsening fever, headache, and confusion for three days. Viral encephalitis secondary to herpes simplex infection is suspected. Which statement regarding Herpes Simplex encephalitis is the most accurate?**

   A. Diagnosed by blood polymerase chain reaction (PCR)

   B. Mortality of less than 5% if treated

   C. Predominantly affects the frontal lobe

   D. Treatment of choice is acyclovir

   E. Typically caused by HSV-2

10. **A 24-year-old male has had fever after arriving to the United Kingdom from abroad. He has been unwell with headaches, lethargy, occasional diarrhoea, and malaise. Which single disease is notifiable in the United Kingdom according to Public Health England?**

    A. *Clostridium difficile*

    B. Dengue fever

    C. Haemolytic uraemic syndrome

    D. Human immunodeficiency virus (HIV)

    E. Middle East respiratory syndrome coronavirus (MERS-CoA)

11. **A 57-year-old known Intravenous drug user has had a fever, malaise, weight loss, and new systolic murmur. Her initial blood culture is positive. Endocarditis is suspected. Which single most likely organism is grown?**

    A. *Candida albicans*

    B. *Cardiobacterium hominis*

    C. *Coxiella burnetii*

    D. *Staphylococcus aureus*

    E. *Streptococcus viridans*

12. **A seven-month-old baby has had a cough and poor feeding for the last couple of days. There is scattered crepitations and wheeze throughout the chest. The RR is 50 breaths per minute with mild intercostal recession. Bronchiolitis is suspected. Which single organism is the most likely to cause the symptoms?**

A. Bordetella pertussis

B. *Haemophilus influenzae*

C. Parainfluenza

D. Respiratory syncytial virus

E. *Streptococcus pneumoniae*

13. **A 40-year-old man sustained a laceration on his right thigh after falling in a park a week ago. He is now unwell and in considerable pain. His HR is 130 bpm and T 38.9°C. The skin around the wound is swollen and discoloured, discharging a serous fluid with sweet odour. Which single most likely causative organism?**

A. *Clostridium botulinum*

B. *Clostridium histolyticum*

C. *Clostridium perfringens*

D. *Clostridium septicum*

E. *Clostridium tetani*

14. **A 21-year-old student has just returned from travelling South East Asia. He has fevers, headaches, and myalgia. His blood film confirms malarial parasites. Which single Plasmodium species is he most likely to be infected with?**

A. *Plasmodium Falciparum*

B. *Plasmodium Knowlesi*

C. *Plasmodium Malariae*

D. *Plasmodium Ovale*

E. *Plasmodium Vivax*

15. **A 33-year-old man recently returned from India has had weight loss, anal itching, rash, and nausea. He is diagnosed with roundworm. Which single species is the most likely cause of his symptoms?**

A. *Ascaris Lumbricoides*

B. *Enterobius Vernicularis*

C. *Necator Americanus*

D. *Taenia Saginata*

E. *Taenia Solium*

16. **A 14-year-old girl currently taking methotrexate for juvenile arthritis has had fever. She is concerned as she recently received a series of vaccinations from her GP. Which single vaccine listed is contraindicated in this patient?**

    A. Diphtheria, pertussis, and tetanus
    B. Human papillomavirus (HPV)
    C. Intranasal influenza vaccine
    D. Meningitis C conjugate
    E. Pneumococcal conjugate (PCV)

17. **A 15-year-old boy has a sore throat and has had difficulty in swallowing for three days. His temperature is 38.6°C. His tonsils are enlarged, red, and have white spots on the surface. The cervical lymph nodes are tender. The WCC 12.0 × 10⁹/L, neutrophils 6.0 x 10⁹/L, and lymphocytes 7.5 × 10⁹/L with a few atypical cells. Which is the single most likely causative organism?**

    A. Cytomegalovirus (CMV)
    B. Epstein–Barr virus (EBV)
    C. GBS
    D. HSV
    E. *Toxoplasmosis gondii*

18. **A 21-year-old female has had green cervical discharge, dysuria, and intermenstrual bleeding. An endocervical swab reveals Gram-negative diplococci. Which single antibiotic is the most appropriate?**

    A. Benzylpenicillin
    B. Ceftriaxone
    C. Co-amoxiclav
    D. Doxycycline
    E. Metronidazole

19. **A 55-year-old patient has had a cough, fever, night sweats, and haemoptysis. His CXR reveals small left sided pleural effusion and cavitation in the left upper zone. He has recently returned from visiting family in India. You decide to investigate for tuberculosis (TB). Which single statement regarding TB is the most accurate?**

    A. Culture using Lowenstein–Jensen agar will provide results within two weeks
    B. Microscopy and staining with Ziehl–Neelsen stain provides definitive diagnosis
    C. Mycoplasma TB is a Gram-negative acid-fast bacilli
    D. This patient requires barrier nursing and full respiratory precautions
    E. Treatment is with rifampicin alone as first line

20. A 28-year-old farmer has impaled himself on a pitchfork while shovelling manure. He has a puncture wound to his right foot. He is fully immunized. You decide that this patient is at risk of tetanus and decide to treat accordingly. Which single answer describes the treatment he requires?

A. Human tetanus immunoglobulin

B. Human tetanus immunoglobulin and tetanus vaccination

C. Human tetanus immunoglobulin immediately and tetanus vaccination after three months

D. Tetanus vaccination

E. Tetanus vaccination followed by full immunization schedule for tetanus

21. A 55-year-old vet has a dog bite to his right hand that was sustained while examining a recently imported dog from a rabies endemic region. He received a full course of rabies vaccine 20 years ago. Which single statement regarding rabies is the most accurate?

A. Once symptoms develop treatment with Human Rabies Immunoglobulin is required

B. Rabies symptoms in humans include hydrophobia, aerophobia, confusion, paranoia, delirium, and fever

C. Rabies is exclusively caused by bat lyssavirus

D. This patient does not require any post-exposure treatment

E. This patient requires treatment with rabies vaccine and human rabies immunoglobulin

22. A three-year-old child has had a high fever, coryza, red eyes, and a rash, which started on the face and has now spread. There are small white spots inside the mouth. He has not received any of his routine childhood vaccinations. Which is the single most likely diagnosis?

A. Chickenpox

B. Erythema infection

C. Measles

D. Mumps

E. Rubella

23. A 20-year-old woman has attended the ED asking for an HIV test. She had unprotected intercourse with an unknown man the night before. Which is the single most important mode of possible transmission of HIV infection from the man?

A. Alveolar fluid

B. Salivary secretions

C. Semen

D. Sweat

E. Vaginal fluid

24. **A 38-year-old female who is known to be HIV positive has had a fever and persistent cough. Her last CD4 count was 180 and she has been non-compliant with her medications. Which single statement regarding HIV is the most accurate?**

A. HIV is most commonly acquired by vertical transmission
B. HIV is a single-stranded ribonucleic acid (RNA) retrovirus
C. This patient can be diagnosed with acquired immunodeficiency syndrome (AIDS) on the basis of her CD4 count alone
D. This patient should not be on any prophylaxis against opportunistic infection
E. Treatment is aimed at preventing viral replication usually with a single antiretroviral agent

25. **A 70-year-old lady has had a high fever, sore throat, myalgia, rhinitis, and headaches for two days. A diagnose of flu is suspected but the patient disagrees as she had a flu immunization three years ago. Which single statement regarding influenza is the most accurate?**

A. Antigenic drift occurs only in influenza type A
B. Antigenic shift is influenza viruses lead to yearly changes in surface antigens and the need for yearly flu vaccines
C. Ribavarin is commonly used to treat all elderly patients with flu symptoms
D. The incubation period is four to five days
E. Transmission is via respiratory droplets

26. **The on-call surgical trainee has sustained a needle-stick injury from a high-risk patient while in theatre. Her vaccinations are up to date. Which of the single statements is the most accurate?**

A. The risk of hepatitis B infection is approximately 0.03%
B. The risk of hepatitis C infection is approximately 30%
C. The risk of HIV infection is approximately 0.3%
D. The risk of infection is less with a hollow bore needle than a solid needle
E. This patient should not be offered post-exposure prophylaxis

27. **A 48-year-old male who works at a bird sanctuary has had a cough, fever, pleuritic chest pain, and shortness of breath. He received a kidney transplant three years ago and is on antirejection medication. Which single organism is the most likely cause of his symptoms?**

A. Candida
B. Cryptococcus
C. Tinea Capitis
D. Tinea Corporis
E. Tinea Pedis

28. **A three-year-old child has had fever, conjunctivitis and spasms of severe coughing followed by a 'whoop' for eight days. The provisional diagnosis is whooping cough. Which single statement is the most accurate?**

    A. Symptom resolution occurs with approximately two weeks
    B. The incubation period is one to two days
    C. There is no vaccination against whooping cough
    D. Whooping cough is caused by *Bordatella pertusis*
    E. Whooping cough is caused by a Gram-positive anaerobic rod

29. **A 78-year-old female is brought from her care home with a fever, worsened confusion, and purple urine in her catheter bag. Her HR is 126 bpm, BP 135/86 mmHg, RR 20 breaths/min, SaO$_2$ 96% on room air and temperature 38.5°C. Which single organism is the most likely cause of her symptoms?**

    A. *Candida albicans*
    B. *Klebsiella pneumoniae*
    C. *Salmonella Enterica*
    D. *Staphylococcus aureus*
    E. *Streptococcus pyogenes*

30. **A 55-year-old female has had a fever, bloody diarrhoea, and abdominal pain. She attributes her symptoms to undercooked chicken at a restaurant. Cultures reveal a Gram-negative spiral-shaped bacteria. Which single organism is the most likely to have caused the symptoms?**

    A. *Campylobacter jejuni*
    B. *Clostridium perfringens*
    C. *Escherichia coli O157:H7*
    D. *Salmonella typhimurium*
    E. *Shigella dysenteriae*

31. **A 29-year-old man has had fevers, rigors, stomach pains, and bloody diarrhoea. He also has a painless ulcer with a black centre on his right forearm. He has recently returned from Central Africa where he was working as a farm hand. Which single organism is most likely in this case?**

    A. *Bacillus anthracis*
    B. *Entamoeba histolytica*
    C. *Francisella tularensis*
    D. *Rickettsia rickettsii*
    E. *Treponema pallidum*

32. **A 68-year-old sewer worker has had a high fever, jaundice, severe headaches, and a rash, which was preceded by several days of cough, mild fever, and muscle pains. Which single combination of diagnosis and treatment is most likely in this patient?**
    A. Legionella—IV amoxicillin
    B. Legionella—*Per os*, by mouth (PO) doxycycline
    C. Leptospirosis—IV doxycyline
    D. Leptospirosis—PO flucloxacillin
    E. Yellow Fever—IV aciclovir

33. **A 27-year-old female with a previous history of sexual transmitted infection presents with abdominal pain, intermenstrual bleeding, and vaginal discharge. A diagnosis of pelvic inflammatory disease (PID) is suspected. Which single statement regarding PID is most accurate?**
    A. Antibiotics should only be started once the causative organism is identified
    B. Chlamydia infection maybe associated with perihepatitis
    C. It usually results from haematogenous spread of organisms
    D. The most common causative organism is gonorrhoea
    E. The risk of tubular infertility is 50%.

34. **A seven-year-old boy with sickle cell disease has had a high fever and right thigh pain. His parents are concerned as he was recently treated for osteomyelitis. Which is the most likely causative organism in this patient?**
    A. *Enterobacter aerogenes*
    B. Group A Streptococcus
    C. *Haemophilus influenzae*
    D. *Salmonella enterica*
    E. *Staphylococcus aureus*

35. **A 73-year-old woman with a diagnosis of small cell lung cancer presents with a high fever at home. She completed her second cycle of chemotherapy 11 days ago. You decide that this patient is at risk of neutropenic sepsis and decide to start empiric antibiotic therapy. She has no known drug allergies. Which single antibiotic is most appropriate for this patient?**
    A. Clarithromycin
    B. Co-amoxiclav
    C. Colomycin
    D. Piperacillin with tazobactam (Tazocin)
    E. Vancomycin

1. B. ~~Endemic to Northern Africa.~~

A. Dengue is only spread by the Aedes Mosquito.
B. Correct answer: Dengue fever is endemic to countries in Central Africa, Central and South America, the Caribbean, the Eastern Mediterranean, South and Southeast Asia.
C. The mortality rate is between 1 to 5% if left untreated by less than 1% with adequate treatment. Treatment is supportive with IV fluids, antipyretics, and supportive care.
D. Dengue is spread by several species of mosquito of the Aedes type, principally *A. aegypti.*
E. The Dengue virus is a single-stranded RNA virus with five distinct serotypes.

Goering R, Dockrell H (2012). *Mims' Medical Microbiology*, 5th edition. London, UK: Elsevier.

Harrison M (2017). *Revision Notes for the FRCEM Primary*, 2nd edition. Oxford, UK: Oxford University Press.

2. D. Ceftriaxone and amoxicillin.

A. Amoxicillin should not be used in isolation to treat neonatal sepsis.
B. This child has suspected neonatal sepsis. The child has both risk factors for sepsis and 'red flag' findings for neonatal sepsis. As such the child requires treatment with broad spectrum antibiotics such as benzylpenicillin and gentamicin.
C. Ceftriaxone should not be used in children younger than three months.
D. Correct answer: Cefotaxime can be used in neonates to treat suspected meningitis but only in combination with amoxicillin.
E. Clindamycin is not used to treat neonatal infection but is the drug of choice for penicillin allergic mothers with GBS infection in labour.

Risk factors for neonatal sepsis include:

- Invasive group B streptococcal infection in a previous baby
- Maternal group B streptococcal colonization
- Bacteriuria or infection in the current pregnancy
- Prelabour rupture of membranes
- Preterm birth following spontaneous labour (before 37 weeks' gestation)
- Suspected or confirmed rupture of membranes for more than 18 hours in a preterm birth
- Intrapartum fever higher than 38°C, or confirmed or suspected chorioamnionitis
- Parenteral antibiotic treatment given to the woman for confirmed or suspected invasive bacterial infection (such as septicaemia) at any time during labour, or in the 24-hour periods before and after the birth
- Suspected or confirmed infection in another baby in the case of a multiple pregnancy

'Red flag' findings for neonatal sepsis include:

- Altered behaviour or responsiveness
- Altered muscle tone (e.g. floppiness)
- Feeding difficulties (e.g. feed refusal)
- Feed intolerance, including vomiting, excessive gastric aspirates, and abdominal distension
- Abnormal heart rate (bradycardia or tachycardia)
- Signs of respiratory distress
- Respiratory distress starting more than four hours after birth
- Hypoxia (e.g. central cyanosis or reduced oxygen saturation level)
- Jaundice within 24 hours of birth
- Apnoea
- Signs of neonatal encephalopathy
- Seizures
- Need for cardiopulmonary resuscitation
- Need for mechanical ventilation in a preterm baby
- Need for mechanical ventilation in a term baby
- Persistent fetal circulation (persistent pulmonary hypertension)
- Temperature abnormality (lower than 36°C or higher than 38°C) unexplained by environmental factors
- Signs of shock
- Unexplained excessive bleeding, thrombocytopenia, or abnormal coagulation
- Oliguria persisting beyond 24 hours after birth
- Altered glucose homeostasis (hypoglycaemia or hyperglycaemia)
- Metabolic acidosis (base deficit of 10 mmol/litre or greater)
- Local signs of infection (e.g. affecting the skin or eye)

The National Institute for Health and Care Excellence (2015). Neonatal infection: Antibiotics for prevention and treatment. Available at: https://www.nice.org.uk/guidance/cg149/chapter/1-Guidance

3. D. *Staphylococcus aureus.*

A. *Bacillus anthracis* is the pathogen responsible for anthrax and exposure would seem unlikely in this patient however it has been reported to cause cavitating pneumonia.

B. Haemophilus influenza is a less common cause of pneumonia and rarely causes cavitation.

C. *Klebsiella pneumoniae* is the most common cause of cavitating pneumonia and is more frequent in older, institutionalized patients, or those with a history of aspiration.

D. Correct answer: *Staphylococcus aureus* is an emerging cause of pneumonia and can cause cavitation however it is more common in immunocompromised patients.

E. *Streptococcus pneumoniae* is the most common cause of pneumonia in all age groups except neonates but very rarely causes cavitation.

A useful pneumonic for remembering the causes of cavitating pneumonia is TANKS:

T—Tuberculosis

A—Aspergillus

N—Nocardia

K—Klebsiella

S—Staphylococcus

Harrison M (2017). *Revision Notes for the FRCEM Primary*, 2nd edition. Oxford, UK: Oxford University Press.

Llewelyn H (2011). *Oxford Handbook of Clinical Diagnosis*, 2nd edition. Oxford, UK: Oxford University Press.

4. A. *Chlamydia trachomatis.*

A. Correct answer: Chlamydia trachomatis is a brown ovoid shaped non-mobile bacterium responsible for causing Chlamydia.

B. *Escherichia coli* is a Gram-negative, facultatively anaerobic, rod-shaped bacterium, which can be responsible for numerous infections.

C. Neisseria gonorrhoeae is a Gram-negative coffee bean-shaped diplococci responsible for causing Gonorrhoea.

D. Treponema pallidum is a spirochaete bacterium, which causes Syphilis.

E. Trichomonas vaginalis is an anaerobic, flagellated protozoan parasite and the causative agent of trichomoniasis.

Goering R, Dockrell H (2012). *Mims' Medical Microbiology*, 5th edition. London, UK: Elsevier.

Harrison M (2017). *Revision Notes for the FRCEM Primary*, 2nd edition. Oxford, UK: Oxford University Press.

5. E. Trimethoprim 200 mg twice a day orally.

A. Cefalexin 500 mg twice daily for seven days is used in the treatment of uncomplicated lower urinary tract infections in pregnant women.

B. Ciprofloxacin 500 mg twice daily for seven days is used in the treatment of acute uncomplicated pyelonephritis with no risk factors for the development of complications.

C. Co-amoxiclav 500/125 mg three times a day for 14 days is an alternative to ciprofloxacin for the treatment of pyelonephritis.

D. Gentamicin 5 mg/kg as a single intravenous dose is not recommended for the treatment of UTI.

E. Correct answer: This patient appears to be suffering with an uncomplicated lower urinary tract infection. The treatment of choice is Trimethoprim 200 mg twice a day for three days or Nitrofurantoin 50 mg four times a day for three days.

The National Institute for Health and Care Excellence (2015). Urinary tract infections in adults. Available at: https://www.nice.org.uk/guidance/qs90

6. B. *Staphylococcus aureus.*

A. *Clostridium perfringens* is responsible for gas gangrene and necrotizing fasciitis.

B. Correct answer: *Staphylococcus aureus* is the second most common cause of cellulitis.

C. *Streptococcus pyogenes* is a group A β-haemolytic streptococci responsible for up to two-thirds of the cases of cellulitis.

D. *Pasteurella multocida* is usually found in cellulitis related to cat bites.

E. *Pseudomonas aeruginosa* is more commonly seen in older hospitalized patients or the immunocompromised.

Goering R, Dockrell H (2012). *Mims' Medical Microbiology*, 5th edition. London, UK: Elsevier.

7. C. Clarithromycin.

A. Co-amoxiclav is a combination of amoxicillin and clavulanic acid and therefore not suitable for penicillin allergic patients.

B. Ciprofloxacin is effective against *Mycoplasma pneumoniae* but is not the first line agent of choice.

C. Correct answer: Clarithromycin is safe in penicillin allergic patients and effective against *Mycoplasma pneumoniae*.

D. Meropenem should be avoided in penicillin allergic patients if possible as should all cephalosporins, carbapenems, and beta-lactam antibiotics due to a theoretical risk of cross reactivity causing anaphylaxis.

E. Tazocin is a combination of Piperacillin + Tazobactam and therefore not suitable for this patient.

Harrison M (2017). *Revision Notes for the FRCEM Primary*, 2nd edition. Oxford, UK: Oxford University Press.

8. A. Coxsackievirus.

This child has clinical features suggestive of meningitis. The Lumbar puncture results show typical findings for viral meningitis. Table 3.1 compares CSF findings in viral and bacterial meningitis.

Table 3.1 Cerebrospinal fluid (CSF) findings

	WCC	**Protein**	**Glucose**
Viral	Lymphocytosis	Normal or mildly raised	Normal
Bacterial	Neutrophilia	Raised	Low or normal

A. Correct answer: Coxsackievirus as well as echovirus is an enterovirus. Enteroviruses are the most common cause of viral meningitis. Other causes of viral meningitis include mumps, measles, and arboviruses (such as West Nile virus).

B. Group B streptococci is the most common cause of bacterial meningitis in children less than three months of age.

C. *Haemophilus influenzae* type B was previously the most common cause of bacterial meningitis but has declined in the developed world due to widespread vaccination.

D. HSV-1 typically causes encephalitis. HSV-2 can cause meningitis.

E. *Neisseria meningitides* is the most common cause of bacterial meningitis in older children and adults.

Harrison M (2017). *Revision Notes for the FRCEM Primary*, 2nd edition. Oxford, UK: Oxford University Press.

9. D. Treatment of choice is acyclovir.

A. It is diagnosed by PCR on CSF.

B. It has an untreated mortality of up to 70% and a treated mortality rate of 15–20%.

C. HSV predominantly affects the temporal lobes.

D. Correct answer: The treatment of choice is high dose intravenous acyclovir.

E. It is usually caused by HSV -1 with less than 10% of cases caused by HSV-2.

Harrison M (2017). *Revision Notes for the FRCEM Primary*, 2nd edition. Oxford, UK: Oxford University Press.

10. C. Haemolytic uraemic syndrome.

Below is a list of all current Notifiable Diseases in the United Kingdom:

- Acute encephalitis
- Acute infectious hepatitis
- Acute meningitis
- Acute poliomyelitis
- Anthrax
- Botulism
- Brucellosis
- Cholera
- Diphtheria
- Enteric fever
- Food poisoning
- Haemolytic uraemic syndrome (HUS)
- Infectious bloody diarrhoea
- Invasive group A streptococcal disease
- Legionnaires' disease
- Leprosy
- Malaria
- Measles
- Meningococcal septicaemia
- Mumps
- Plague
- Rabies
- Rubella
- Severe acute respiratory syndrome (SARS)
- Scarlet fever
- Smallpox
- Tetanus
- TB
- Typhus
- Viral haemorrhagic fever
- Whooping cough
- Yellow fever

Note that there is a separate list of notifiable organisms which laboratories need to report. Knowledge of this list is not required but be aware that it includes all rickettsia species, coronavirus species, and even varicella species.

Public Health England (2010). Notifiable diseases and causative organisms. Available at: https://www.gov.uk/guidance/notifiable-diseases-and-causative-organisms-how-to-report

11. D. *Staphylococcus aureus.*

A. *Candida albicans* is also more prevalent in the intravenous drug using population but is unlikely to show on routine blood culture.

B. *Cardiobacterium hominis* is a member of the slow growing HACEK group of organisms. It is more common in the intravenous drug using population (particularly those who lick their needles prior to use) but is slow-growing, and often difficult to detect on routine blood culture.

C. *Coxiella burnetii* is uncommon and results in 'culture negative' endocarditis.

D. Correct answer: *Staphylococcus aureus* is the most common causative organism of infective endocarditis in the intravenous drug using population.

E. *Streptococcus viridans* is the most common cause in patients with native valves.

Goering R, Dockrell H (2012). *Mims' Medical Microbiology*, 5th edition. London, UK: Elsevier.

12. D. Respiratory syncytial virus.

A. *Bordetella pertussis* is the causative bacteria in Whooping Cough.

B. *Haemophilus influenza* does not cause bronchiolitis and infection is uncommon due to widespread vaccination.

C. Parainfluenza virus can cause bronchiolitis, but it is uncommon compared to other viruses such as metapneumovirus or Rhinovirus

D. Respiratory syncytial virus is the most common cause of bronchiolitis in the United Kingdom.

E. *Streptococcus pneumoniae* is among the leading causes of community acquired pneumonia in adults and meningitis in children. It does not cause bronchiolitis.

Harrison M (2017). *Revision Notes for the FRCEM Primary*, 2nd edition. Oxford, UK: Oxford University Press.

13. C. *Clostridium perfringens.*

The patient has highly lethal gas gangrene infection, which is caused by exotoxin produced by Gram-positive anaerobic clostridia. *C perfringens* causes such infections in 80 to 90% situations. *C. septicum* and *C histolyticum* causes only 10–20% cases.

Clostridium tetani causes tetanus and *C. botulinum* causes botulism by producing toxins in the food.

Wyatt J, Illingworth RN, Graham CA, et al. (2012). *Oxford Handbook of Emergency Medicine*, 4th edition. Oxford, UK: Oxford University Press.

14. B. *Plasmodium knowlesi.*

Malaria is a protozoal disease caused by plasmodium species. Transmission is via female anopheles mosquitoes. Symptoms include cyclical fevers, headaches, myalgia, arthralgia, rigors, sweats, and malaise. Treatment is with primaquinine, chloroquinine, quinine, mefloquinine, or purimethamine.

A. *Plasmodium falciparum* is the most dangerous plasmodial species and can prove fatal. It is most common in sub-Saharan Africa.

B. Correct answer: *Plasmodium knowlesi* is most common in Southeast Asia.

C. *Plasmodium malariae* is commonly found in sub-Saharan Africa, the western Pacific islands, and South America.

D. *Plasmodium ovale* is now classified into two separate species. It is commonly found in West Africa, Thailand, Bangladesh, Vietnam, and the Philippines.

E. *Plasmodium vivax* is most common in certain parts of North America and Latin America. It commonly causes splenomegaly.

Harrison M (2017). *Revision Notes for the FRCEM Primary*, 2nd edition. Oxford, UK: Oxford University Press.

15. A. *Ascaris lumbricoides.*

A. Correct answer: *Ascaris lumbricoides* is roundworm and causes Ascariasis. Transmission is by soil containing eggs. Symptoms include pneumonitis, conjunctivitis, abdominal pain, weight loss, diarrhoea, anorexia, and anal itching as well as liver abscesses, gastrointestinal (GI) obstruction and seizures.

B. *Enterobius vernicularis* is threadworm. Symptoms include anal itching and visible eggs and worms in stool.

C. *Necator Americanus* is hookworm. Patients are often asymptomatic but may have abdominal pain, weight loss, and chronic GI blood loss.

D. *Taenia Saginata* is beef tapeworm.

E. Taenia Solium is pork tapeworm.

Goering R, Dockrell H (2012). *Mims' Medical Microbiology*, 5th edition. London, UK: Elsevier.

Harrison M (2017). *Revision Notes for the FRCEM Primary*, 2nd edition. Oxford, UK: Oxford University Press.

16. C. Intranasal influenza vaccine.

Live attenuated vaccines are contraindicated in any patient who is immunosuppressed including HIV patients with inadequate CD4 cell counts, patients on chemotherapy or radiotherapy, patients with bone marrow transplant in the last 12 months, and patients on immunosuppressive drugs such as methotrexate.

The following are live attenuated vaccines:

- Measles, mumps, and rubella (MMR)
- BCG
- Poliomyelitis—oral Sabin vaccine
- Yellow fever
- Oral typhoid (not available in the United Kingdom)
- Herpes zoster (shingles) vaccine
- Intranasal influenza vaccine—Fluenz

The National Health Service (2013). Contraindications and Special considerations. Available at: https://www.gov.uk/government/publications/contraindications-and-special-considerations-the-green-book-chapter-6

17. B. EBV.

A. Most healthy children and adults infected with CMV have no symptoms and may not have known that they have been infected. Some may develop mild illness. In adults, infections may be severe in immunocompromised or elderly patients. CMV is a member of the Herpesvirus family along with EBV, HSV-1 & -2, varicella zoster virus and human herpesviruses (HHV)-6, -7 & -8. They share properties. They have a genome of double-stranded linear DNA with a viral envelope.

B. Correct answer: The patient has glandular fever caused by EBV or human herpes virus-4. It affects teenagers and young adults. The infection spreads via droplets via kissing. EBV is a member of the gamma herpesvirus family and, *in vitro*, replicate in lymphoid tissue. There are two types: EBV-1 and EBV-2.

C. Gram-positive coccus, frequently colonizes the human genitalia and gastrointestinal tracts. It may infect neonates, pregnant women, and other adults resulting in sepsis. In the laboratory,

GBS is identified by its zone of beta haemolysis around grey-white colonies in blood agar media.

D. Please see the discussion on option A. Though both HSV-1 and -2, both can cause genital infections, in young women and men, the HSV-1 has been associated with the increasing proportions of infections in genitalia. It may cause extragenital complications, which could be meningitis and proctitis.

E. *T. gondii* is an obligate intracellular protozoan parasite causes toxoplasmosis. The infection in humans occurs through ingestion of raw or undercooked meat, drinking contaminated water, or transplacental transmission. Besides the mild flu-like symptoms in the early stages, the adults are asymptomatic following the infection. The occasional symptomatic patients have fevers, chill, and sweats with cervical lymph node enlargements. It persists as latent infection for the rest of the life and can recur if the person becomes immunocompromised.

Gupta P (2011). *Oxford Assess and Progress: Emergency Medicine.* Oxford, UK: Oxford University Press.

UpToDate (2017). Acquired cytomegalovirus infection in children. Available at: https://www.uptodate.com/contents/acquired-cytomegalovirus-infection-in-children?source=search_result&search=virology%20of%20CMV&selectedTitle=1~150

18. B. Ceftriaxone.

This patient has signs and symptoms of gonorrhoea, which is confirmed by the microscopy results.

Primary syphilis presents as small painless genital ulcers and lymphadenopathy ten days to three months after infection.

Secondary syphilis causes a pruritic rash, myalgia, arthralgia, patchy hair loss, and weight loss several months after infection.

Tertiary syphilis presents years to decades after infection and symptoms vary widely depending on body system involvement.

A. Benzylpenicillin is the treatment of choice for suspected syphilis.

B. Correct answer: Ceftriaxone or any third-generation cephalosporin is appropriate for the treatment of gonorrhoea.

C. Co-amoxiclav has no role in the treatment of any sexually transmitted infection.

D. Doxycycline is used in the treatment of chlamydia. Chlamydia is often asymptomatic but can cause vaginal, urethral, or rectal mucoid discharge, post-coital or intermenstrual bleeding, abdominal pain, fever, and scrotal swelling. Complications include endometritis, PID, salpingitis, prostatitis, and epididymitis. Patients are usually treated for gonorrhoea at the same time as chlamydia due to the high rate of co-infection.

E. Metronidazole is used in conjunction with other antibiotics for the treatment of PID.

Harrison M (2017). *Revision Notes for the FRCEM Primary,* 2nd edition. Oxford, UK: Oxford University Press.

19. C. Mycoplasma TB is a Gram-negative acid-fast bacilli.

A. Culture using Lowenstein–Jensen Agar is highly sensitive, but the mycobacteria are very slow-growing, and results can take between two to eight weeks.

B. Ziehl–Neelsen staining can detect acid-fast bacilli but cannot differentiate between mycobacteria species. A false negative is also possible.

C. Correct answer: Mycoplasma TB is a Gram-negative acid-fast bacilli. It is an obligate aerobe. Symptoms of TB are varied depending the body system affected.

Primary TB is usually pulmonary and often asymptomatic.

Post-primary TB often results in fevers, night sweats, weight loss, and lethargy.

Pulmonary TB results in cough, haemoptysis, pleural effusion, and cavitating lesions on CXR.

Miliary TB presents as disseminated infection.

Genitourinary TB results in hydronephrosis, haematuria, dysuria, orchitis, prostatitis, and epididymitis.

Gastrointestinal TB leads to fevers, nausea, weight loss, constipation, perforation, and obstruction

Tuberculoma, Potts disease, meningitis, and cerebral abscess are also possible.

D. According to nice guidance only patients with drug resistant TB or those undergoing droplet prone procedures require respiratory precautions and barrier nursing.

E. Treatment is with combination therapy of rifampicin, isoniazid, pyrazinamide, ethambutol, or streptomycin depending on local policy due to the high rates of drug resistance.

Goering R, Dockrell H (2012). *Mims' Medical Microbiology*, 5th edition. London, UK: Elsevier.

Harrison M (2017). *Revision Notes for the FRCEM Primary*, 2nd edition. Oxford, UK: Oxford University Press.

The National Institute for Health and Care Excellence (2011). Tuberculosis: Clinical diagnosis and management of tuberculosis, and measures for its prevention and control. Available at: http://www.nice.org.uk/guidance/cg117/chapter/guidance#management-of-respiratory-tb

20. A. Human tetanus immunoglobulin.

Human tetanus immunoglobulin should be administered regardless of tetanus immunization status to all patients with a tetanus-prone wound.

A tetanus-prone wound is either a wound that has extensive devitalization, or a wound that has heavy contamination with material likely to contain tetanus spores (e.g. soil or manure) and:

- Requires surgical intervention that has been delayed by six hours or more.
- Has significant devitalization or is a puncture-type injury.
- Has a foreign body.

With regards to tetanus vaccination a fully immunized person will have had a primary course of three vaccines followed by two boosters spaced 10 years apart. Patients from the United Kingdom aged less than 65 are usually fully vaccinated. Patients who are not fully vaccinated require a booster vaccination in the following circumstances.

- Fully immunized—booster not required.
- Primary immunization complete, boosters incomplete but up to date—booster not required but administer if the next dose is due soon and it is convenient to do so.
- Primary immunization incomplete or boosters not up to date—administer a reinforcing dose and continue with the recommended schedule.
- Not immunized or immunization status unknown or uncertain—give an immediate dose of vaccine and continue with the full five-dose schedule.

The National Institute for Health and Care Excellence (2012). Lacerations. Available at: http://cks.nice.org.uk/lacerations#!scenariorecommendation:11

21. B. Rabies symptoms in humans include hydrophobia, aerophobia, confusion, paranoia, delirium, and fever.

A. Once symptoms develop rabies is fatal and there is no benefit to further treatment. Because of this the focus in rabies treatment is prevention and early post-exposure treatment to prevent symptom development.

B. Correct answer: Rabies symptoms include hydrophobia, aerophobia, confusion, paranoia, delirium, and fever, flu-like illness, seizures, and itching/tingling in the wound.

C. Rabies is caused by lyssaviruses, of which the two most common are rabies virus and Australian bat lyssavirus.

D. According to Public Health England even fully immunized individuals require post-exposure treatment with at least two doses of rabies vaccine.

E. Only patients who are unimmunized or partially immunized require human rabies immunoglobulin treatment following exposure. This patient is considered fully immunized and has a low risk exposure; as such he requires treatment with two doses of rabies vaccine.

Harrison M (2017). *Revision Notes for the FRCEM Primary*, 2nd edition. Oxford, UK: Oxford University Press.

Public Health England (2015). PHE guidelines on rabies post-exposure treatment (January 2015). Available at: https://www.gov.uk/government/uploads/system/uploads/attachment_data/file/402386/Rabies_PHE_guidelines_on_postexposure_treatment_January_2015.pdf

22. C. Measles.

A. Chickenpox is caused by the varicella zoster virus. In younger children the earliest feature is characteristic small itchy blisters. Older children may have a prodrome of malaise, headache, fever, and oral sores before the rash develops. It is a self-limiting condition but complications such as pneumonia and meningitis can develop. Children are usually treated conservatively with supportive measures although there is some evidence for the use of acyclovir to reduce symptom duration. Adults usually suffer with more severe symptoms and treatment with oral acyclovir is advised. A varicella vaccine is available.

B. Erythema infectiosum is also known as Slap Cheek or fifth disease. It is caused by parovirus B19 infection. Symptoms include low-grade fever, headache, malaise, coryza and rash (typically bright red across the cheeks with a lacy red rash across the body). It is a self-limiting condition that does not require specific treatment. There is no available vaccine.

C. Correct answer: Measles is caused by the measles virus. Symptoms include high-grade fever, coryza, conjunctivitis, rash which typically starts behind the ears and Koplik spots in the mouth. Complications include pneumonia, subacute sclerosing panencephalitis, and corneal ulceration. There is no specific treatment beyond supportive measures. A vaccine is available for prevention.

D. Mumps is also known as epidemic parotitis. It is caused by the mumps virus. Symptoms include low-grade fever, headache, malaise, and then painful parotid swelling. Serious complications include testicular swelling leading to infertility, meningitis, pancreatitis, ovarian inflammation, and sensorineural hearing loss. Treatment is supportive. A vaccination is available.

E. Rubella is also known as German measles. It is caused by a togavirus called the rubella virus. Symptoms include low-grade fever, rash starting on the face and spreading to the rest of the body, cervical lymphadenopathy, and flu-like symptoms. There is no specific treatment although vaccination is available via the MMR vaccine or a separate rubella vaccination.

Harrison M (2017). *Revision Notes for the FRCEM Primary*, 2nd edition. Oxford, UK: Oxford University Press.

23. C. Semen.

HIV has been isolated from variety of body fluids: blood and blood products, serum, semen, vaginal secretions, urine, CSF, tears, breast milk, alveolar fluid, synovial fluid, bone marrow, and saliva. Only a few modes of transmission have been established unscreened blood/ blood products (blood transfusion before 1985 in the United Kingdom), semen, vaginal secretions, breast milk, and transplacental.

Gupta P (2011). *Oxford Assess and Progress: Emergency Medicine*. Oxford, UK: Oxford University Press.

House of Parliament (2014). Post Note. HIV prevention in the UK. Available at: http://researchbriefings.parliament.uk/ResearchBriefing/Summary/POST-PN-463#fullreport

Wyatt J, Illingworth RN, Graham CA, et al. (2012). *Oxford Handbook of Emergency Medicine*, 4th edition. Oxford, UK: Oxford University Press.

24. B. HIV is a single-stranded RNA retrovirus.

A. HIV transmission can be via three routes: sexual intercourse (most common in men who have sex with men), infected blood or blood products (intravenous drug users, or blood transfusions pre-1985) or vertical transmission (transplacental, vaginal birth, or breastfeeding). Vertical transmission is the least common route of transmission in the United Kingdom.

B. Correct answer: HIV is a single-stranded RNA retrovirus, which contains reverse transcriptase.

C. In the United Kingdom, AIDS is defined as a CD4 cell count of less than 200 and a serious opportunistic infection or AIDS-defining illness.

AIDS-defining illnesses include:

- Candidiasis of the bronchi, trachea, lungs, and oesophagus
- Mycobacterium TB
- Cerebral toxoplasmosis
- Cytomegalovirus disease
- Kaposi sarcoma
- Lymphoma
- HIV wasting syndrome
- HIV-related encephalopathy

D. All patients with a low CD4 count should receive prophylactic treatment to prevent against serious opportunistic infection.

E. Treatment is aimed at preventing viral replication, but this is achieved almost exclusively through polypharmacy with a combination of nucleoside reverse transcriptase inhibitors, non-nucleoside reverse transcriptase inhibitors, and protease inhibitors.

Goering R, Dockrell H (2012). *Mims' Medical Microbiology*, 5th edition. London, UK: Elsevier.

25. E. Transmission is via respiratory droplets.

- A. Antigenic drift occurs in all type of influenza. Antigenic shift occurs only in influenza Type A.
- B. Antigenic drift causes yearly minor changes in surface antigen expression due to random mutations in the viral RNA. Antigenic Drift is a re-assortment of RNA segments which causes more profound changes in antigen expression.
- C. Ribavarin is an antiviral, which is used to treat respiratory syncytial virus and only in very severe cases. Antivirals are available for the treatment of influenza, but they only reduce symptom duration by 48 hours and may lead to resistance so are not routinely used.
- D. The incubation period of influenza is 18–72 hours. Peak illness is after four to five days with gradual recovery.
- E. Correct answer: Transmission is via respiratory droplets and viral shedding occurs within 24 hours and lasts for up to 10 days.

Goering R, Dockrell H (2012). *Mims' Medical Microbiology*, 5th edition. London, UK: Elsevier.

Harrison M (2017). *Revision Notes for the FRCEM Primary*, 2nd edition. Oxford, UK: Oxford University Press.

26. C. The risk of HIV infection is approximately 0.3%.

- A. The risk of hepatitis B infection is approximately 30% from a confirmed hepatitis B positive donor.
- B. The risk of hepatitis C infection is approximately 3% from a confirmed Hepatitis C positive donor.
- C. Correct answer: The risk of HIV infection is approximately 0.3% from a confirmed HIV positive donor.
- D. The risk of infection is greater with a hollow bore needle than a solid needle. Visible contamination of the needle with blood also increases the risk of possible infection.
- E. A full risk assessment needs to be performed for both the recipient and donor of the needle stick but in all likelihood post-exposure prophylaxis will need to be offered to this patient.

Harrison M (2017). *Revision Notes for the FRCEM Primary*, 2nd edition. Oxford, UK: Oxford University Press.

27. B. Cryptococcus.

- A. Candida is part of the normal flora found in the mouth, skin, vagina, and GI tract. It frequently presents as an opportunistic infection in the immunocompromised or following antibiotic use. It causes both localized and generalized infections.
- B. Correct answer: Cryptococcus is an opportunistic mycosis, which typically affects those who come into contact with soil containing bird faeces. It is also referred to as pigeon fancier's lung. Typical pulmonary features include cough, dyspnoea, fever, malaise, and pleuritic pain. It can also cause extrapulmonary infections especially in the immunocompromised. Treatment is with antifungal agents.
- C. Tinea Capitis is also known as scalp ringworm.
- D. Tinea Corporis is also known as ringworm.
- E. Tinea Pedis is also known as athletes' foot.

Goering R, Dockrell H (2012). *Mims' Medical Microbiology*, 5th edition. London, UK: Elsevier.

28. D. Whooping cough is caused by *Bordatella Pertusis.*

A. The catarrhal phase of the disease lasts one to two weeks. This is followed by the paroxysmal phase in which the characteristic 'whoop' develops which lasts up to four weeks. There is then a three- to four-week convalescent stage. Erythromycin in the catarrhal stage can reduce duration and severity of symptoms but has no role once coughing has developed.

B. The incubation period is 5 to 14 days.

C. Routine vaccination against whooping cough occurs in the United Kingdom at two, three, and four months of age with a booster at pre-school age.

D. Correct answer: Whooping cough is caused by *Bordatella Pertusis*, which is a Gram-negative aerobic rod.

E. Whooping cough is caused by *Bordatella Pertusis.*

Harrison M (2017). *Revision Notes for the FRCEM Primary*, 2nd edition. Oxford, UK: Oxford University Press.

29. B. *Klebsiella pneumoniae.*

This patient has purple urine bag syndrome, which occurs in patients with urinary catheters and co-existent urinary tract infections. It is most common in elderly females from care home settings. Tryptophan in the diet is metabolized to indole, which is converted to indoxyl sulphate and excreted in urine. In patients with a urinary tract infection the indoxyl sulphate is metabolized to indirubin and indigo by the colonizing bacteria. Treatment depends on the causative organism. The most common organisms involved are:

- *Providencia stuartii*
- *Providencia rettgeri*
- *Klebsiella pneumoniae*
- *Proteus mirabilis*
- *Escherichia coli*
- *Morganella morganii*
- *Pseudomonas aeruginosa*

Goering R, Dockrell H (2012). *Mims' Medical Microbiology*, 5th edition. London, UK: Elsevier.

30. A. *Campylobacter jejuni.*

A. Correct answer: *Campylobacter jejuni* is a Gram-negative, microaerophilic, oxidase-positive, catalase-positive bacteria. It is responsible for of 75% of UK food poisoning cases. It commonly causes bloody diarrhoea and abdominal pains. It is typically treated with azithromycin.

B. *Clostridium perfringens* is a Gram-positive, rod-shaped, anaerobic, spore-forming pathogenic bacterium. It is the third most common cause of UK food poisoning.

C. *Escherichia coli O157:H7* is an enterohemorrhagic serotype of the bacteria *Escherichia coli*. It can cause bloody diarrhoea, fevers, and can progress to HUS and renal failure. It accounts for almost 2% of UK food poisoning cases.

D. *Salmonella typhimurium* is a rod-shaped Gram-negative bacteria responsible for approximately 20% of cases of food poisoning in the United Kingdom. Typical features include abdominal pain, vomiting, and diarrhoea (not typically bloody)

E. *Shigella dysenteriae* is a Gram-negative, facultative anaerobic, non-spore-forming, rod-shaped bacteria which is closely related to Salmonella. Typical symptoms include diarrhoea (containing blood, mucous or pus), fever, nausea, vomiting, stomach cramps, and flatulence. It can lead to HUS.

Goering R, Dockrell H (2012). *Mims' Medical Microbiology*, 5th edition. London, UK: Elsevier.

Harrison M (2017). *Revision Notes for the FRCEM Primary*, 2nd edition. Oxford, UK: Oxford University Press.

31. A. *Bacillus anthracis.*

This patient has features of both intestinal and cutaneous anthrax as well as a potential high-risk exposure history.

A. Correct answer: *Bacillus anthracis* is a Gram-positive, endospore-forming, rod-shaped bacterium responsible for anthrax. Anthrax is most common in Africa, Central and Southern Asia. Infection is through spore exposure and is most common in those who work with contaminated animal or contaminated animal products.

B. *Entamoeba histolytica* is the primary causative organism in amoebic dysentery. Symptoms include violent diarrhoea (with blood or mucous) flatulence abdominal bloating and signs of dehydration. Skin manifestations are not a feature. It is most prevalent in tropical climates.

C. *Francisella tularensis* is the causative organism of Tularemia. Symptoms include fever, lethargy, loss of appetite, signs of sepsis, and lymphadenopathy. Skin lesions are not a typical feature. It is endemic in North America and parts of Asia and spread by contact with contaminated animals or tick bites.

D. *Rickettsia rickettsia* is the organism responsible for Rocky Mountain spotted fever, which is found throughout North, Central, and South America. It is spread by tick bites and has not been reported in other parts of the world. Symptoms include fever, nausea, and vomiting, headaches, myalgia, maculopapular and petechial rashes, and abdominal pain.

E. *Treponema pallidum* is the causative organism of syphilis. The chancre in primary syphilis can often be confused with the ulceration seen in anthrax. However, syphilis would not account for these patients' other features. More information on syphilis is available in other parts of this chapter.

Anthrax symptoms are divided into four categories:

Inhalational

- Fever
- Chest discomfort
- Shortness of breath
- Confusion
- Cough
- Nausea
- Vomiting
- Headache
- Sweats (often drenching)
- Extreme tiredness
- Body aches
- Abdominal pain

Gastrointestinal

- Fever
- Swelling of neck
- Sore throat
- Painful swallowing
- Hoarseness

- Nausea
- Bloody vomiting
- Bloody diarrhoea
- Headache
- Abdominal pain
- Fainting
- Abdominal distension

Injection

- Fever
- Blisters at injection site
- A painless skin sore with a black centre
- Swelling around the sore
- Abscesses deep under the

Cutaneous

- A group of small blisters that may itch
- Swelling can occur around the sore
- A painless ulcer with a black centre
- Ulcer are usually on the face, neck, arms, or hands

Centre for Disease Control and Prevention (2016). Anthrax. Available at: https://www.cdc.gov/anthrax/index.html

Goering R, Dockrell H (2012). *Mims' Medical Microbiology*, 5th edition. London, UK: Elsevier.

32. C. Leptospirosis—IV doxycyline.

This patient has risk factors for as well as signs and symptoms of Weil's disease (the most severe form of leptospirosis). Leptospirosis is caused by spirochaete bacteria belonging to the genus Leptospira.

Symptoms include fever, headaches, nausea, vomiting, myalgia, rashes, and conjunctivitis, and can progress to jaundice, signs of meningitis, peripheral oedema, and haemoptysis in severe cases of Weils disease.

Risk factors for the disease include occupational exposures such as farmers, sewer works, and fishermen, recreational exposures such as sailors and divers and foreign travel.

- A. Amoxicillin is not effective against Legionella.
- B. Legionella is caused by Legionella pneumophila is a thin, aerobic, pleomorphic, flagellated, non-spore-forming, Gram-negative bacterium. It typically presents as an atypical pneumonia. Treatment is with either PO or IV macrolide antibiotics.
- C. Correct answer: Leptospirosis is treated with oral or IV tetracycline depending on severity.
- D. Some penicillins such as amoxicillin or ampicillin can be used in the treatment of leptospirosis but flucloxacillin is not effective and given the severity of this patient's symptoms intravenous therapy would be preferred.
- E. Yellow Fever is a viral illness, which causes fever, chills, loss of appetite, nausea, muscle pains, and headaches which can cause jaundice in severe cases. It is spread by mosquito bites and found in subtropical areas. Treatment is supportive. There is no role for antivirals.

Harrison M (2017). *Revision Notes for the FRCEM Primary*, 2nd edition. Oxford, UK: Oxford University Press.

33. B. Chlamydia infection maybe associated with perihepatitis.

PID refers to an infection of the upper genital tract. It is typically caused by sexually transmitted infections and results in symptoms of abdominal or pelvic pain, fevers, deep dyspareunia, abnormal vaginal bleeding, abnormal vaginal or cervical discharge, and right upper quadrant pain.

A. Antibiotics should be started immediately based on clinical suspicion to reduce the risk of complications. The choice of antibiotic depends on the patient's risk for gonorrhoea infection. Up to date guidelines can be found on the National Institute for Health and Care Excellence (NICE) website.
B. Correct answer; Chlamydia infection can lead to Curtis-Fitz-Hugh syndrome (perihepatitis) where scar tissue forms on Glisson's capsule causing right upper quadrant pain.
C. The most common route of spread is via ascending infection from the lower genital tract.
D. In the United Kingdom, over 50% of cases are caused by chlamydia infection and approximately 20% by gonorrhoea.
E. The risk of tubular infertility can be as high as 20% in severe PID but is often much lower. Other potential complications include an increased risk of ectopic pregnancy and chronic abdominal or pelvic pain.

Harrison M (2017). *Revision Notes for the FRCEM Primary*, 2nd edition. Oxford, UK: Oxford University Press.

National Institute for Health and Care Excellence (2016). Pelvic inflammatory disease. Available at: http://cks.nice.org.uk/pelvic-inflammatory-disease#!topicsummary

34. D. *Salmonella enterica.*

Osteomyeltitis is a severe infection of the bone and bone marrow. Acute osteomyelitis almost invariably occurs in children, usually as the result of haematogenous spread. It typically affects the long bones such as the femur (35%) or tibia (30%) in children and is more common in the vertebrae and pelvis in adults. Treatment is with prolonged antibiotic therapy.

Table 3.2 shows the most common organisms by age.

Table 3.2 Common organisms

Age group	Most common organisms
Newborns (<4 months)	*Staphylococcus aureus*
	Enterobacter species
	Group A and B *Streptococcus species*
Children (<18 years)	*Staphylococcus aureus*
	Group A *Streptococcus species*
	Haemophilus influenzae
	Enterobacter species
Adult	*Staphylococcus aureus*
	Occasionally *Enterobacter* or *Streptococcus species*
Sickle cell anaemia patients	Salmonella species

Goering R, Dockrell H (2012). *Mims' Medical Microbiology*, 5th edition. London, UK: Elsevier.

Harrison M (2017). *Revision Notes for the FRCEM Primary*, 2nd edition. Oxford, UK: Oxford University Press.

35. D. Piperacillin with tazobactam (Tazocin).

A neutrophil count 0.5×10^9 per litre or lower is defined as neutropenia. Patients with signs of sepsis who are at risk of neutropenia (acute leukaemia's, stem cell transplants or solid tumours receiving chemotherapy) should be treated empirically with Tazocin 4.5 g IV. Treatment should not be delayed for blood results. More targeted antibiotics may be started once a causative organism has been identified.

National Institute for Health and Care Excellence (2016). Neutropenic sepsis: Prevention and management in people with cancer. Available at: https://www.nice.org.uk/guidance/cg151

1. **A 75-year-old has had a fever and tachycardia having been discharged two days ago following treatment for urosepsis. His most recent blood cultures showed *E. Coli* only sensitive to aminoglycosides. He has no known drug allergies. Which single antibiotic is most appropriate for this patient?**
   A. Cefalexin
   B. Co-Amoxiclav
   C. Doxycycline
   D. Gentamicin
   E. Trimethoprim

2. **A 28-year-old man is treated with oral amoxicillin for a presumed lower respiratory tract infection and discharged from the emergency department (ED). Which single statement regarding amoxicillin is most accurate?**
   A. Amoxicillin is baceteriostatic
   B. Amoxicillin is mostly effective against Gram negative organisms
   C. Amoxicillin is safe in patients with a known allergy to co-amoxiclav
   D. Ampicillin is a derivative of amoxicillin
   E. Resistance to amoxicillin is mostly due to beta-lactamase production

3. **A 56-year-old female has had palpitations for six days. She is haemodynamically stable. The electrocardiogram shows atrial fibrillation with ventricular rate of 145 beats per minute. The treatment plan is to use metoprolol. Which class of drug does metoprolol fall into according to the Vaughan Williams Classification?**
   A. Ia
   B. II
   C. III
   D. IV
   E. V

4. **A 24-year-old has had signs and symptoms of acute severe asthma. He has had a poor response to initial nebulized salbutamol given by the ambulance crew. Which single statement regarding salbutamol is the most accurate?**

A. Can only be given via the nebulized route

B. Has the same mechanism of action as ipratropium

C. Is long acting

D. Primarily acts at beta-1 receptors

E. Side effects include tachycardia and headache

5. **An eight-year-old boy with known anaphylaxis to bee stings presents to the ED 20 minutes after being stung. He has shortness of breath, stridor, and a widespread urticarial rash. He weighs 25 kg. Which single medication is the most appropriate first line management of this patient?**

A. Adrenaline 1:1,000 0.25 mL intramuscular (IM)

B. Adrenaline 1:1,000 0.25 mL intravenous (IV)

C. Adrenaline 1:10,000 0.25 mL IM

D. Adrenaline 1: 10,000 0.25 mL IV

E. Adrenaline 1:1,000 2.5 mL IM

6. **A 62-year-old man presents with a non-infectious exacerbation of his chronic obstructive pulmonary disease (COPD): He is treated with intravenous hydrocortisone and nebulized bronchodilators. He improves significantly and is discharged home on a course of oral prednisolone. Which single statement regarding steroid medications in this circumstance is the most accurate?**

A. Dexamethasone has a very short duration of action

B. Hydrocortisone has a longer duration of action than prednisolone

C. Hydrocortisone has greater anti-inflammatory potency than prednisolone

D. Prednisolone has a half-life of approximately ~~200 minutes~~ 60 minutes

✓E. Prednisolone has peak effect within three hours

7. **A seven-year-old girl is brought to the ED with a fracture of distal forearm, which is grossly deformed requiring manipulation under ketamine sedation. Which single statement regarding ketamine is the most accurate?**

A. Emergence phenomena is more common in children

B. Ketamine is a non-competitive N-methyl-D-aspartate receptor (NMDA) receptor antagonist

C. It is safe for use in patients with cardiac disease

D. It has an onset of action of five minutes when given intravenously

E. The most common side effect is respiratory depression

8. **A 22-year-old rugby player presents with an anterior dislocation of his right shoulder joint. You have decided to use propofol for reduction of his shoulder. Which single statement regarding propofol is the most accurate?**

   A. Causes respiratory depression rarely
   B. Contraindicated in patients with a soya bean allergy
   C. Has duration of action of up to 30 minutes
   D. Hypertension is a common side effect
   E. Predominantly acts on NMDA receptors

9. **A 48-year-old man with a large frontal intracranial haemorrhage is awaiting transfer to a neurosurgical centre. He is intubated and ventilated in the resuscitation room when he becomes increasingly hypertensive and bradycardic. He has a dilated right pupil on examination. His approximate body weight is 80 kg. Which single medication is the most appropriate to treat this patient at this stage?**

   A. 400 mL 10% mannitol IV
   B. 400 mL 20% mannitol IV
   C. 500 mL 3% sodium chloride IV
   D. 1,000 mL 20% mannitol IV
   E. 1,000 mL 3% sodium chloride IV

10. **A 78-year-old man presents with malaise, weakness, and palpitations. His electrocardiogram (ECG) shows peaked T waves with flattened P waves globally. His has a serum potassium level of 7.1 mmol/l. Which statement regarding the treatment is the most accurate?**

    A. 10 mL of 10% calcium gluconate IV
    B. 50 mL of 50% dextrose with 50 IU of actrapid insulin
    C. Benefit of nebulized salbutamol is doubtful
    D. IV fluids should be restricted
    E. Sodium bicarbonate administration is contraindicated

11. **A 41-year-old female has had an open distal tibia fracture. She is screaming in pain and opiate analgesia has been prescribed. She has no known drug allergies. Which statement regarding opiate analgesia is the most accurate?**

    A. Alfenatnil has an onset time of less than 60 seconds
    B. Codeine is safe to be given intravenously
    C. Fentanyl has a longer duration of action compared to morphine
    D. Morphine predominantly acts on κ receptors
    E. Tramadol should be avoided because it has more side effects than codeine

12. **A seven-year-old boy has had a painful right arm following an injury while playing football. He has no known drug allergies and weighs 25 kg. Which is the most appropriate analgesia for this patient?**

A. Ibuprofen 300 mg PO
B. Paracetamol 400 mg IV
C. Paracetamol 600 mg PO
D. Paracetamol 400 mg IV + codeine 30 mg PO
E. Paracetamol 400 mg PO + ibuprofen 150 mg PO

13. **A 55-year-old man has had worsening symptoms of angina. He has been recently started on diltiazem after having a drug reaction to a beta-blocker. Which statement regarding diltiazem is the most accurate?**

A. All calcium channel blockers act the same site to cause negative inotropy and chronotropy
B. Diltiazem is a dihydropyridimine
C. Nimodipine does not cross the blood brain barrier
D. Use Diltiazem with caution in patients also taking beta-blockers
E. Verapamil is the least cardioselective agent

14. **A 22-year-old woman is agitated following the use of cocaine. She has heart rate (HR) of 130 beats per minute and BP115/ 75 mmHg. You decide to treat her with benzodiazepines to decrease the agitation. Which statement regarding benzodiazepines is the most accurate?**

A. All benzodiazepines work by potentiating the action of gamma-aminobutyric acid (GABA) receptors
B. Diazepam is the preferred agent because of its predictable absorption
C. Lorazepam cannot be given orally
D. Midazolam has the longest half-life
E. Midazolam has the shortest onset time when given intravenously

15. **A 38-year-old female with bipolar disorder has had a manic episode after stopping her lithium several weeks ago. Which statement regarding lithium therapy is the most accurate?**

A. Lithium is safe due to its wide therapeutic window
B. Lithium toxicity should be treated with the specific reversal agent
C. Patients on lithium do not require routine blood tests
D. Toxicity rarely causes cardiovascular manifestations
E. Tremor is among the most common side effects

16. **A 55-year-old female has had an out of hospital cardiac arrest. She is intubated and ventilated without sedation. She has a normal sinus rhythm on her ECG but has required several boluses of adrenaline to maintain her blood pressure. Which statement regarding adrenaline is the most accurate?**

    A. Can cause lactic acidosis as a side effect
    B. Has an identical mechanism of action to Noradrenaline
    C. Must never be given through a peripheral cannula
    D. Primarily effects alpha receptors
    E. Raises blood pressure primarily through vasoconstriction

17. **A 47-year-old man has been treated in the ED for profound septic shock. Despite adequate intravenous fluid resuscitation, he remains hypotensive with a persistently raised lactate. You decide to start vasopressors. Which statement regarding vasoactive medication is the most accurate?**

    A. Dobutamine has a longer half-life than other vasopressors.
    B. Dobutamine has a negative inotropic effect.
    C. Noradrenaline at high doses may cause peripheral ischaemia.
    D. Vasopressin actions on vassopressin-3 receptors are responsible for its vasoconstrictive properties.
    E. Vasopressin is an endogenous catecholamine.

18. **A 38-year-old female has had an open fracture of his left tibia following a fall from a horse. He has no other injuries. He is allergic (anaphylaxis) to penicillin. Which is the single most appropriate antibiotic in this patient?**

    A. Cefuroxime 1.5 g within six hours of injury
    B. Clindamycin 600 mg IV within three hours of injury
    C. Clindamycin 600 mg IV within six hours of injury
    D. Co-amoxiclav 1.2 g IV within three hours of injury
    E. Flucloxacillin 1 g within three hours of injury

19. **A 65-year-old male presents to the ED with signs and symptoms of gout in his right first metatarso-phalangeal joint. After investigating him you decide to discharge him home with non-steroidal anti-inflammatory drugs (NSAIDs) and a proton pump inhibitor. Which statement regarding proton pump inhibitors is the most accurate?**

    A. Cause inhibition of cytochrome P450
    B. Have fewer side effects than H_2 receptor antagonists
    C. Lansoprazole is considered less effective than omeprazole
    D. Less effective than H_2 receptor antagonists
    E. Ranitidine is a proton pump inhibitor

20. **A 33-year-old female is brought to the ED with lower abdominal pain and ongoing vomiting. The symptomatic management with analgesia and antiemetics have been initiated. Which statement regarding antiemetics is the most accurate?**
    A. Cyclizine acts only at the chemoreceptor trigger zone in the Central nervous system
    B. Cyclizine can cause oculogyric crisis as a side effect
    C. Metoclopramide cannot be given orally
    D. Metoclopramide has both D2 receptor and 5-HT3 receptor activity
    E. Ondansetron is a D2 receptor antagonist

21. **A 73-year-old female presents to the ED with gradually worsening shortness of breath and decreasing exercise tolerance. She is diagnosed with worsening of her congestive cardiac failure and diuretics are started. Which statement regarding diuretics is the most accurate?**
    A. Acetazolamide is a potent diuretic
    B. Furosemide is a loop diuretic
    C. Spironolactone can cause hypokalaemia as a side effect
    D. Thiazide diuretics can cause deafness at high doses
    E. Thiazide diuretics act as an aldosterone antagonist

22. **A 58-year-old male is brought to the resuscitation room with dense right-sided hemiparesis, which started 60 minutes ago. His computed tomography (CT) scan of the head is normal. The treatment by thrombolysis for an acute stroke has been considered. Which statement regarding thrombolytic is the most accurate?**
    A. History of recent haemorrhage is not a contraindication to thrombolysis
    B. Streptokinase is the recommended thrombolytic of choice
    C. Symptom onset longer than 3.5 hours is a contraindication
    D. Thrombolytic drugs must never be administered to patients in cardiac arrest
    E. Thrombolytic drugs work by activating plasminogen to plasmin

23. **A 92-year-old female is brought to the ED from her nursing home with palpitations and feeling generally unwell for several days having been started on digoxin for atrial fibrillation (AF) by her general practitioner. Which statement regarding digoxin is the most accurate?**
    A. Arrhythmias are uncommon in patients taking digoxin
    B. It acts by inhibiting Na/K pump activity in myocyte cell membranes
    C. Its toxicity is precipitated by hyperkalaemia
    D. It decreases central vagal activity
    E. The toxicity is uncommon due to the wide therapeutic range

24. **A 55-year-old male presents to the ED complaining of palpitations intermittently for the last few weeks. His ECG shows that he is in AF with a ventricular rate of 160 beats per minute. The rate control strategy with beta-blockers has been planned. Which statement regarding beta-blockers is the most accurate?**

    A. Bisoprolol is a non-cardioselective beta-blocker
    B. Cardioselective beta-blockers have primarily Beta-2 receptor effects
    C. Esmolol is a long acting beta-blocker with a half-life of more than 9 hours
    D. Metoprolol has hepatic elimination
    E. Metoprolol has positive inotropic and chronotropic effects

25. **A 33-year-old female has had generalized tonic clonic seizure, which resolved within a few seconds. This is her third seizure in six months. She is back to baseline and keen to go home. The neurologist has advised to start an antiepileptic medication for her prior to discharge. Which statement regarding antiepileptics is the most accurate?**

    A. Carbamazepine is a hepatic enzyme inducer and should be used cautiously in patients taking other medications
    B. Phenytoin is considered safe in pregnancy
    C. Phenytoin is generally safe due to its wide therapeutic window
    D. Sodium valproate binds inactivated sodium channels in the central nervous system (CNS) preventing them returning to the resting state thus preventing further firing of these neurons
    E. Sodium valproate generally causes the most side effects of the antiepileptic medications

26. **A 24-year-old female has been feeling unwell. She is type 1 diabetic and has been on insulin for many years. She has started vomiting and has vague abdominal pain. Diabetic ketoacidosis is suspected. She has been given intravenous fluids and insulin and monitored closely. Regarding treatment with insulin, which statement is correct?**

    A. Absorption of insulin is same irrespective of the site of injection in the subcutaneous tissue in the body
    B. Can be given in the dialysate fluid infused into peritoneal cavity for patients on peritoneal dialysis
    C. Can be given orally, but has delayed onset of action in this patient's situation
    D. Fat and protein synthesis are decreased by insulin
    E. Insulin corrects the polydipsia and polyuria by its antidiuretic action

27. **An 84-year-old male has had episode of sweating and altered consciousness. He has type 2 diabetes. He is on combinations of medications including antibiotics started recently. The ambulance crew recorded his bedside capillary blood glucose level of 1.9 mmol/L. Which combination of medications might have contributed to the symptoms?**

    A. Metformin with alcohol
    B. Metformin with nifedepine
    C. Sulfonylureas with vancomycin
    D. Sulfonylureas with ranitidine
    E. Sulfonylureas with bendroflumethazide

28. **A 34-year-old female has been on levothyroxine for some time. She has started feeling unwell for the last week or so. Which single symptom might be because of the adverse reaction of the drug?**

    A. Abdominal cramps
    B. Constipation
    C. Heat tolerance
    D. Hypotension
    E. Weight gain

29. **An 88-year-old female has had a fall while trying to go to toilet at home. She could not get up on her own. She is on several medications for her high blood pressure, constipation, osteoporosis, heart failure, and arthritis. Her serum potassium level is 2.5 mmol/L, sodium 136 mmol/L, urea 5.0 mmol/L, and creatinine 95 micromol/L. Which single factor is the most likely cause of her blood results?**

    A. Constipation
    B. Chronic kidney disease
    C. Laxative abuse
    D. Non-steroidal anti-inflammatory drug
    E. Spironolactone

30. **A 38-year-old female has had a fall while trying to run to board a bus. She could not get up on her own because of severe pain and deformity to her right ankle. She was given morphine intravenously by the ambulance crew following which she feels severe nausea. Cyclizine has been prescribed. Which statement is the most accurate about the drug?**

    A. A member of antihistamine group
    B. Absorption through oral route is unreliable
    C. Acts by blocking the dopaminergic receptors
    D. Antagonist to H1 receptor
    E. Mechanism of action of the antiemetic effect is unclear

31. **A 28-year-old female has had a severe acute asthma. She has been given nebulized salbutamol and ipratropium through oxygen, and intravenous steroids. She has been prescribed intravenous magnesium as well. Which statement is correct regarding magnesium use in this situation?**

    A. Acts possibly by inhibiting Ca+ influx into airway smooth muscles
    B. Equally effective if given through nebulization and intravenously
    C. Serum magnesium level monitoring may be useful to determine its efficacy
    D. There is no contraindication and has excellent safety profile
    E. Infusion of 4 g over 20 minutes is the usual dose

32. **A 48-year-old female has been feeling unwell for the past week or so. She has type 2 diabetes, for which she has been recently started metformin. Her heart rate is 70 bpm, blood pressure 145/88mmHg and temperature of 36.8°C with capillary blood sugar level of 10.8 mmol/L. Which statement is correct about metformin?**

    A. Contraindicated in active alcohol abuse
    B. Decreases insulin-mediated glucose utilization in peripheral tissues
    C. Has lipolytic affect that increases the serum free fatty acid concentration
    D. It typically lowers fasting blood glucose concentrations by about 40%
    E. Side effects include adverse cardiovascular events

33. **An 88-year-old female has had red painful area on her left leg following a scratch received by striking to furniture at home. She lives alone and mobilizes with a walking stick. She is not allergic to any medication. Her heart rate is 75 bpm, blood pressure 165/92mmHg and temperature of 36.8°C: Which is the most appropriate antibiotic regime?**

    A. Amoxycillin 500 mg three time a day for 14 days
    B. Amoxycillin and flucloxacillin in combination for seven days
    C. Clarithromycin 500 mg twice a day for five days
    D. Co-amoxiclav 200/125 mg three times a day for five days
    E. Flucloxacillin 500 mg four times a day for seven days

34. **A 62-year-old male has been feeling unwell for a week. He has cough with yellow expectoration and been on cyclosporine for kidney transplant 10 months ago. He has vomited today a couple of times. He has high cholesterol. He is allergic to penicillin. His HR is 90 bpm, BP145/90mmHg and T of 36.8°C: Which single most interaction is correct in between the medications?**

    A. Cyclosporine can be given safely with ibuprofen
    B. Cyclosporine levels may increase if given with clarythromycin
    C. Metoclopramide can be combined safely with cyclosporine
    D. No added toxicity to kidneys if cyclosporine is given with aminoglycosides
    E. Statins can be given safely with cyclosporines

35. **A 42-year-old man has had pain in his right ankle following a sprain. He is not on any medication or allergic to any drug. An advice has been given to start ibuprofen tablets as an analgesic. Which single most appropriate statement is correct?**

    A. If ibuprofen does not work, other type of NSAID may not work

    B. It is safer to give another NSAID if patient develops toxicity with ibuprofen

    C. NSAIDs increase nitric oxide synthetase, which help in reducing the inflammation

    D. NSAIDs in general stimulate cyclooxygenase enzyme, which helps in formation of prostaglandins

    E. NSAIDs interfere in the migration of granulocytes to sites of inflammation

36. **A 32-year-old man has had injury to his right shoulder joint. He has anterior subluxation of the joint, which has happened four times in the past. He is not on any medication or allergic to any drug. He has been given a mixture of 50% oxygen and 50% nitrous oxide to inhale for pain relief. Which statement about nitrous oxide is correct?**

    A. Can safely be given to intoxicated patients

    B. Contraindicated in third trimester of pregnancy as it crosses the placenta in high concentrations

    C. Decreases cerebral blood flow and intracranial pressure

    D. May act on opiate receptors to cause mild analgesia

    E. Onset of action is usually in 10 minutes

37. **A 32-year-old man has had a large amount of alcohol consumption. He has reduced conscious level. He has been drinking a significant amount for many years. Which statement about alcohol (ethanol) is correct?**

    A. Acute excess alcohol consumption can safely be treated with disulphiram

    B. Alcohol is the most widely abused addictive drug

    C. Ethanol is chemically very active substance in physiological condition

    D. Intoxication actions of alcohol are specifically mediated

    E. Unpleasant side effects after excessive alcohol consumption are because of the metabolite, acetaldehyde

38. **A 32-year-old man has had a laceration of 3 cm on his right foot by trading on a broken glass in his garden three hours ago. He has a small glass piece inside his foot on X-ray. He is on cyclosporine for renal transplant done two years ago. He is Caribbean in origin and came to the United Kingdom 10 years ago and unable to remember his tetanus status. Which is the most appropriate management?**

    A. Co-amoxiclav in enough to prevent tetanus infection

    B. Immediate dose of vaccine followed by a five-dose course

    C. No need of immediate immunoglobulin

    D. Tetanus vaccine is a live vaccine, so should be avoided

    E. There is risk of rejection of the transplanted organ by the vaccine

39. **A 30-year-old man has had a fall from a roof on the concrete ground. He is suspected to have pelvic injuries. He has no long-term disease and he is not on any medications. His heart rate is 116 beats per minute; blood pressure is 95/68mmHg and respiratory rate 24 breaths per minute. Intravenous fluid has been started. Which is the most appropriate statement about fluids?**

A. Hartmann's solution has osmolality of 303–347 mOsm/L

B. Hartmann's solution has maximum intravascular volume expansion of 35% of the administered volume

C. Normal saline has maximum intravascular volume expansion of 35% of the administered volume

D. Normal saline has osmolality of 285–308 mOsm/L

E. Plasmatic half-life of normal saline is two hours

40. **A 90-year-old man has not opened bowel for a week. He is having abdominal pain and mild distension. The colon and rectum are loaded with stool on abdominal X-ray. The plan is to insert a suppository and discharge with a laxative. Which is the single most appropriate statement about laxatives?**

A. Glycerol suppositories act as a rectal stimulant

B. Lactulose is a stimulant diuretic useful in hepatic encephalothy

C. Liquid paraffin is an osmotic laxative

D. Movicol is a bulk-forming laxative

E. Phosphate enemas are contraindicated for bowel preparations in surgical conditions

41. **A 72-year-old woman has had shortness of breath over the past few days. There is no cough. But has pain in the left side of the chest, which is worse on inspiration. She has been treated for breast cancer. The chest is clear on auscultation. Her heart rate is 100 bpm, respiratory rate 32 breaths per minute, blood pressure 132/79mmHg, and oxygen saturation of 86% on air. A diagnosis of pulmonary embolism has been confirmed. Which is the most accurate statement about warfarin?**

A. Adult targeted international normalized ratio (INR) range is 3–4 in this condition

B. Chronic daily alcohol use increases INR

C. Cranberry juice may decrease the warfarin effect

D. Onset of action of warfarin is 72–96 hours

E. Warfarin works by reducing the synthesis of active clotting factors

42. **A 42-year-old woman has had shortness of breath and pleuritic chest pain over the past few days. She has been treated for ovarian cancer. The chest is clear on auscultation. Her heart rate is 110 bpm, respiratory rate 34 breaths per minute, blood pressure 130/70 mmHg, and oxygen saturation of 88% on air. A diagnosis of pulmonary embolism has been confirmed and anticoagulation initiated with low molecular weight heparin (LMWH). Which is the most accurate statement about LMWH?**

   A. Average molecular weight of LMWH is 15,000 Daltons
   B. Has shorter half-life than unfractionated heparin
   C. Is a polysaccharide with approximately 45 saccharide units
   D. It acts indirectly by binding to antithrombin
   E. Monitoring by blood tests is not required

43. **A 46-year-old woman has had pain in the right upper abdomen for the last couple of days. Her heart rate is 110 bpm, respiratory rate 20 breaths per minute, blood pressure 130/70mmHg, and temperature 38.6°C: A diagnosis of acute cholecystitis has been suspected and antibiotics prescribed. Which is the most accurate statement about antibiotics in such situation?**

   A. All patients with penicillin allergies will have cross-sensitivity
   B. Cephalosporins inhibit cell wall synthesis by binding to the bacterial enzymes
   C. Cefuroxime is first generation cephalosporin
   D. Cefuroxime is inactivated by bacterial beta-lactamases
   E. No interaction occurs with concurrent alcohol intake

44. **A 66-year-old woman has had post-herpetic pain on the right eighth thoracic dermatome following shingles a few weeks ago. Gabapentin has been started. Which is the most accurate statement about the medication?**

   A. Agitation is one of the common side effects
   B. Gabapentin and alcohol are safe combination
   C. Gabapentin binds to $GABA_A$/ $GABA_B$ receptors to produce its action
   D. Gabapentin has half-life of five to seven hours
   E. It is safe to withdraw the drug abruptly

45. **A 66-year-old woman has dislocated her right prosthetic hip joint while falling on the floor. The reduction is planned to be done with procedural sedation and analgesia (PSA). Which is the most accurate statement about the PSA?**

   A. Common side effect of ketamine is hypotension and dry mouth
   B. Duration of ketamine's effect following intravenous injection is 30 minutes
   C. Ketamine can safely be given to elderly patients with co-morbidities
   D. Ketamine is a phencyclidine derivative that acts as a dissociative sedative
   E. Propofol is safer in patients with cardiac disease

46. **A 45-year-old man has had painful and swollen right ankle joint. He has had this before. He is on antihypertensive. The provisional diagnosis is acute gouty arthritis. He has been prescribed colchicine. Which statement is the most accurate regarding colchicine?**

    A. Biological effects are directly related to plasma concentrations
    B. Elimination half-life is 10–15 hours
    C. Inhibits migration of white blood cells to the inflamed joint
    D. Most effective when given for acute attacks of more than 72–96 hours
    E. Safe in patients with renal and hepatic impairment

47. **A 28-year-old medical professional has had a needle stick injury while taking a blood sample from a patient. He is worried about transmission of hepatitis B virus as he has not taken the booster dose of the vaccine for many years. Which statement is the most accurate regarding hepatitis B vaccine?**

    A. A titre or >10 IU/mL of anti-HBs is defined as positive immune response
    B. Contraindicated in chronic liver disease patients
    C. Efficacy is around 80% against all hepatitis B virus (HBV) infection
    D. Past HBV infected patients does not require the vaccine
    E. The second and third dose should be separated by an interval of at least one month

48. **A 92-year-old male has had a fall while trying to go to toilet at home. He could not get up on his own. He feels weak and lethargic. He is on several medications for high blood pressure, constipation, osteoporosis, heart failure, and arthritis. He has been also treated for metastatic prostate cancer. His serum potassium level is 4.0 mmol/L, sodium 136 mmol/L, urea 5.0 mmol/L, creatinine 95 micromol/L and calcium 3.6 mmol/L. Which statement is the most accurate?**

    A. Absorption of calcium through gastrointestinal tract is around 50% of the amount ingested
    B. In plasma, only 45% of the total calcium exists as physiologically important ionized form
    C. Only 50% of the filtered calcium is absorbed through renal tubules
    D. Parathyroid hormone directly influences the absorption of calcium from gastrointestinal tract
    E. Renal reabsorption of calcium is not influenced by parathyroid hormone

49. **A 15-year-old boy has had cough, lethargy, and fever. He has not had his school-aged vaccinations. Which single set of vaccines listed would this child be due?**

    A. Diphtheria, tetanus, pertussis, and polio (DTaP/IPV or dTaP/IPV)
    B. Diphtheria, tetanus, pertussis, polio, and Hib (DTaP/IPV/Hib), Meningococcal C conjugate (MenC), Rotavirus
    C. Diphtheria, tetanus, pertussis, polio, and Hib (DTaP/IPV/Hib), pneumococcal conjugate (PCV), rotavirus
    D. Hib/MenC conjugate, PCV, measles, mumps, and rubella (MMR)
    E. Tetanus, diphtheria, and polio (Td/IPV), MenC

50. **A 45-year-old man has had pain in the joints for the last week. He has been well in the past. There is no known allergy to drugs. Which statement about aspirin is correct?**
    A. Aspirin also acts as prostaglandin independent neutrophil activation
    B. At low dosage (75 mg/day), primarily inhibits COX-2
    C. Gastrointestinal side effects are primarily caused by COX-1 inhibition
    D. Inhibits COX-2 more than the COX-1 enzymes in all doses
    E. Inhibits only COX-1 when used as doses between 4 to 8 grams per day

51. **A 55-year-old man has had cardiac arrest. The cardiopulmonary resuscitation (CPR) has been started. His rhythm is pulseless electrical activity (PEA): he has been given adrenaline. Which statement about adrenaline is correct in this situation?**
    A. Cerebral blood flow in increased by its beta-adrenergic action
    B. Cerebral perfusion pressure is increased by its beta-adrenergic effect
    C. Coronary blood flow is increased by its alpha-adrenergic effects
    D. Coronary perfusion pressure is increased through its beta-adrenergic effect
    E. Systemic vasoconstriction is mediated by beta-adrenergic action

52. **A 60-year-old man has had cardiac arrest. The CPR has been started. His rhythm is ventricular fibrillation (VF). He has been given amiodarone intravenously after the delivery of three shocks. Which statement about amiodarone is correct in this situation?**
    A. It causes peripheral vasodilation through beta-blocking affects
    B. It decreases the refractory period
    C. It has mild positive chronotropic action
    D. It increases the atrioventricular conduction
    E. It increases the duration of action potential

53. **A 32-year-old man has attended the ED with sudden onset of palpitation. His ECG is shown in Figure 4.1. He has been given adenosine intravenously. Which statement about adenosine is correct in this situation?**
    A. It blocks conduction through conduction pathways
    B. It delays conduction through myocardial cells
    C. It facilitates transmission through atrioventricular (AV) node
    D. Its half-life is 10–15 minutes
    E. It is a naturally occurring purine nucleotide

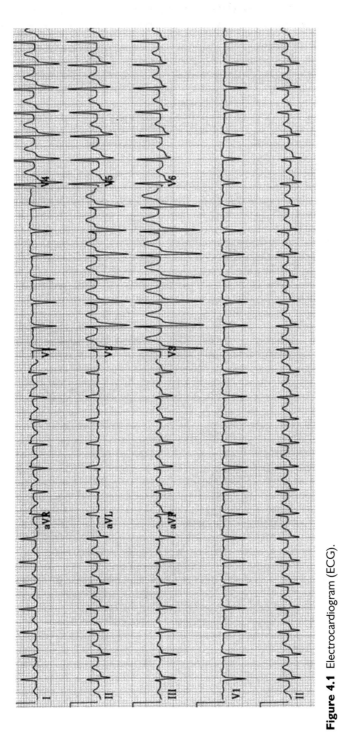

Figure 4.1 Electrocardiogram (ECG).

Reproduced with permission from Ali Khavandi (eds), *Essential Revision Notes for the Cardiology KBA*, Figure 7.5 Copyright © 2014 with permission from Oxford University.

1. D. Gentamicin.

Gentamicin is the only aminoglycoside antibiotic.

Table 4.1 shows the different antibiotic classes, mechanism of action, and some examples of each. Familiarization of various classes of antibiotics is essential.

Table 4.1 Different antibiotic classes

Class	Examples	Mechanism
Aminoglycosides	Gentamicin Neomycin Tobramycin	Inhibits the translocation of the peptidyl-tRNA inhibiting protein synthesis
Carbapenems	Meropenem Ertapenem	Inhibition of cell wall synthesis
Cephalosporins	Cefalexin (first generation) Cefuroxime (second generation) Cefotaxime (third generation) Ceftriaxone (third generation)	Disrupts the synthesis of the peptidoglycan layer of bacterial cell walls
Glycopeptides	Teicoplanin Vancomycin	Inhibits peptoglycan synthesis
Lincosamides	Clindamycin	Inhibits protein synthesis by binding to 50S subunit of bacterial ribosomal RNA
Macrolides	Clarithromycin Erythromycin	Inhibition of bacterial protein biosynthesis thereby inhibiting translocation of peptidyl-tRNA
Penicillins	Amoxicillin Penicillin V Flucloxacillin	Disrupt the synthesis of the peptidoglycan layer of bacterial cell walls
Quinolones	Ciprofloxacin	Inhibits the bacterial DNA gyrase inhibiting DNA replication and transcription
Tetracyclines	DoxycyclineTetracycline	Inhibits the binding of aminoacyl-tRNA to the mRNA-ribosome complex

Source data from The routine immunisation schedule, Public Health England 2016.

Harrison M (2017). *Revision Notes for the FRCEM Primary*, 2nd edition. Oxford, UK: Oxford University Press.

2. E. Resistance to amoxicillin is mostly due to beta-lactamase production.

A. Amoxicillin is bactericidal.

B. Amoxicillin is predominantly effective against gram positive organisms.

C. Co-amoxiclav contains clavulanic acid and amoxicillin and as such amoxicillin should be avoided in patients with a documented allergy.

D. Amoxicillin is a derivative of ampicillin and is better absorbed orally than ampicillin.

E. Correct answer: Beta-lactamase production by bacteria leads to resistance against penicillin including amoxicillin.

Harrison M (2017). *Revision Notes for the FRCEM Primary*, 2nd edition. Oxford, UK: Oxford University Press.

Joint Formulary Committee (2015). *British National Formulary*, 69th edition. London, UK: BMJ Group and Pharmaceutical Press.

3. B. II.

Table 4.2 shows the Vaughan Williams classification of drugs, complete with mechanisms of action and examples.

Table 4.2 Vaughan Williams classification of drugs

Class	Examples	Mechanism
Ia	Procainamide	Sodium channel blockade (intermediate association/dissociation)
Ib	Lidocaine	Sodium channel blockade (fast association/dissociation)
Ic	Flecianide Propafenone	Sodium channel blockade (slow association/dissociation)
II	Esmolol Bisoprolol Metoprolol	Beta blockade
III	Amiodarone	Potassium channel blockade
IV	Verapamil Diltiazem	Calcium channel blockade
V	Adenosin Magnesium Digoxin	Unknown mechanism (direct nodal blockade)

Source data from Vaughan Williams, EM, Classification of antiarrhythmic drugs. In: *Symposium on Cardiac Arrhythmias*, Sandoe E, Flensted-Jensen E, Olsen KH (eds), 1970.

Joint Formulary Committee (2015). *British National Formulary*, 69th edition. London, UK: BMJ Group and Pharmaceutical Press.

4. E. The most common side effects of salbutamol use include tachycardia, palpitations, hypotension, hypokalaemia, tremor, and headache.

A. Salbutamol can be given via the inhaled, nebulized, intravenous or oral route (there is no clinical indication for oral administration).

B. Ipratropium is an antimuscarinic that blocks vagally mediated bronchoconstriction.

C. Salbutamol is short acting. Salmeterol is long acting.

D. Salbutamol primarily acts on Beta-2 receptors but does have some Beta-1 effects at high doses. Beta-2 receptors are found throughout smooth and striated muscle as well as blood vessels and motor nerve terminals. Beta-1 receptors are predominantly found in cardiac tissues.

E. Correct answer: The most common side effects of salbutamol use include tachycardia, palpitations, hypotension, hypokalaemia, tremor, and headache.

Knowledge of the most up to date BTS/SIGN guidelines on the classification and treatment of asthma is essential.

Table 4.3 outlines the current classification of asthma severity.

Table 4.3 Asthma severity classification

Acute moderate asthma	Increasing symptoms PEF >50–75% best or predicted No features of acute severe asthma
Acute severe asthma	Any one of: - PEF 33–50% best or predicted - respiratory rate ≥25/min - heart rate ≥110/min - inability to complete sentences in one breath
Life-threatening asthma	Any one of the following in a patient with severe asthma: PEF <33% best or predicted SpO_2 <92% PaO_2 <8 kPa 'Normal' $PaCO_2$ (4.6–6.0 kPa) Altered conscious level Exhaustion Arrhythmia Hypotension Cyanosis Silent chest Poor respiratory effort
Near fatal asthma	Raised $PaCO_2$ and/or requiring mechanical ventilation with raised inflation pressures

Source data from *SIGN 153*, British guideline on the management of asthma: A national clinical guideline September 2016.

Harrison M (2017). *Revision Notes for the FRCEM Primary*, 2nd edition. Oxford, UK: Oxford University Press.

The British Thoracic Society (2016). British Guidelines on the Management of Asthma. Available at: https://www.brit-thoracic.org.uk/document-library/clinical-information/asthma/btssign-asthma-guideline-2016

5. A. Adrenaline 1:1,000 0.25 mL IM.

Anaphylaxis is an acute life-threatening emergency. Initial treatment should be with immediate IM adrenaline. The intramuscular route is preferred due to difficulties in obtaining access, complications of IV adrenaline, and the longer lasting effect of IM dosing.

The correct dose of IM adrenaline is 10 mcg/kg (equivalent to 0.01 mL/kg of 1:1,000 adrenaline). For a 25 kg child, the dose would be 250 mcg or 0.25 mL of 1:1,000 adrenaline.

Adrenaline for anaphylaxis can also be dosed based on age:

<6 years old: 150 mcg

6–12 years old: 300 mcg

>12 years old: 500 mcg

Note that adrenaline can be given IV for anaphylaxis at a dose of 1 mcg/kg (0.01 mL of 1:10,000 adrenaline) but this should only be used by people familiar with the drug and not used as first line treatment.

Additional medications used in the treatment of anaphylaxis are:

> Hydrocortisone IV 2–4 mg/kg
> Chlorphenamine IV 2.5 mg to 10 mg total dose depending on age
> Oxygen
> Normal saline fluid boluses at 20 mL/kg
> H_2 antagonists such as ranitidine are sometimes also used but their efficacy is unclear

Advanced Life Support Group (2014). *Advanced Paediatric Life Support*, 5th edition. Oxford, UK: Blackwell Publishing Limited

6. D. Prednisolone has a half-life of approximately 200 minutes. [handwritten: 60] [handwritten: Actual Answer is Ⓔ]

Table 4.4 compares the three most common corticosteroids used in clinical practice in the ED.

Table 4.4 Comparison of common corticosteroids

	Hydrocortisone	**Prednisolone**	**Dexamethasone**
Routes	PO, IV, IM	PO	PO, IV, IM
Dose	100–500 mg IV	10–60 mg	1–24 mg IV
	20–30 mg PO		1–10 mg PO
Relative potency	1	4	30
Onset of action	Variable	<1 hour	1 hour
Peak effect	1–2 hours	1–2 hours	1 hour
Half-life	90 mins	60 mins [handwritten: 60]	200 mins
Duration of action	8–12 hours	12–36 hours	36–54 hours

Harrison M (2017). *Revision Notes for the FRCEM Primary*, 2nd edition. Oxford, UK: Oxford University Press.

Joint Formulary Committee (2015). *British National Formulary*, 69th edition. London, UK: BMJ Group and Pharmaceutical Press.

7. B. Ketamine is a non-competitive NMDA receptor antagonist.

A. Emergence phenomena is one of several possible side effects to ketamine but is far more common in adults. Other side effects include: hallucinations, tachycardia, hypertension, increased secretions, anxiety, raised intraocular and intracranial pressure, and arrhythmias.

B. Correct answer: Ketamine acts as a non-competitive antagonist of NMDA receptor calcium channel pores causing a dissociative anaesthetic effect.

C. Contraindications including acute porphyria, stroke, recent head trauma, known raised intracranial pressure (ICP), hypertension, cardiac disease, psychiatric history or psychosis, laryngospasm or airway instability, and adverse reactions to ketamine. It is worth noting that there is some controversy regarding the use of ketamine in patients with head injury and psychiatric disease as there is emerging evidence for its safety. However, the Royal College of Emergency Medicine (RCEM) guidance has not yet changed to reflect this.

D. Ketamine has a rapid onset of less than 60 seconds when given intravenously and up to five minutes when given intramuscularly.

E. Ketamine is the preferred sedation agent in children because it has very low rates of respiratory depression when given at appropriate doses. Standard doses are 2.5 mg/kg IM or 1 mg/kg IV.

Harrison M (2017). *Revision Notes for the FRCEM Primary*, 2nd edition. Oxford, UK: Oxford University Press.

The Royal College of Emergency Medicine (2012). *Paediatric Procedural Sedation with Ketamine in the Emergency Department*. Available at: http://secure.rcem.ac.uk/code/document.asp?id=4880

8. B. Contraindicated in patients with a soya bean allergy.

A. Respiratory depression and hypotension are the most common side effects of propofol sedation.

B. Correct answer: Propofol is contraindicated in egg and soya allergy, porphyria, stroke, raised ICP, and young children for prolonged infusions or large doses. It is worth noting that the use of propofol in children is a contentious point as the previously described increased risk of propofol infusion syndrome may no longer be valid. However, other safer alternatives exist for the sedation of children (such as ketamine and benzodiazepines) and it is best avoided.

C. Propofol has a rapid onset of 30–90 seconds and a rapid off set of between 5 to 10 minutes (offset time is dose dependent).

D. Side effects include flushing, painful injection, bradycardia, hypotension, apnoea, respiratory depression, and anaphylaxis.

E. The exact mechanism of action for propofol is unknown. It is phenol derivative and is thought to act predominantly on GABA-A receptors.

Harrison M (2017). *Revision Notes for the FRCEM Primary*, 2nd edition. Oxford, UK: Oxford University Press.

9. B. 400 mL 20% mannitol IV.

This patient appears to be suffering from an acute rise in his intracranial pressure and as such a medication to reduce his ICP is warranted. There is no evidence for the superiority of either hypertonic saline (3% sodium chloride) or Mannitol and the treatments appear to have comparable efficacy.

The dose of mannitol is 1–2 g/kg intravenously over 20–30 minutes. In an 80 kg patient the dose would be 80–160 g, giving a dose of 400–800 mLs of 20% mannitol or 800–1,600mLs of 10% mannitol.

The dose of 3% sodium chloride is 3–5 mL/kg over 10–20 minutes intravenously. In an 80 kg patient, the dose would be 240–400 mLs.

Joint Formulary Committee (2015). *British National Formulary*, 69th edition. London, UK: BMJ Group and Pharmaceutical Press.

10. A. 10 mL of 10% calcium gluconate IV.

This patient is suffering from acute severe hyperkalaemia (defined as a serum potassium concentration above 6.5 mmol/l or potassium concentration above 5.5 mmol/l in the presence of ECG changes) and requires urgent treatment.

A. Correct answer: 10% calcium gluconate or 10% calcium chloride should be administered by slow intravenous injection to stabilize the myocardium and reduce the risk of arrhythmias. This dose may need to be repeated and should be titrated against improvement in the ECG.

B. 10–15 IU of fast acting insulin such as actrapid is used to decrease extracellular potassium. This is co-administered with 50 mL of 50% dextrose over 15–30 minutes to decrease the risk of hypoglycaemia.

C. Nebulized salbutamol at a dose of 20 mg can be used to reduce serum potassium levels. Intravenous salbutamol may also be considered.

D. Most patients suffering from hyperkalaemia are also suffering from Acute Kidney injury or are volume deplete. As such administration of intravenous fluids may improve their serum potassium levels through dilution and improved renal function. Potassium containing fluids such as Hartman's solution should be avoided.

E. The use of sodium bicarbonate may be considered to reverse acidosis and decrease extracellular potassium, particularly in refractory cases or patients who are peri-arrest or in cardiac arrest.

Joint Formulary Committee (2015). *British National Formulary*, 69th edition. London, UK: BMJ Group and Pharmaceutical Press.

11. A. Alfenatnil has an onset time of less than 60 seconds.

A. Correct answer: Morphine primarily acts on μ receptors.

B. Tramadol has fewer side effects compared to codeine particularly with regards to respiratory depression and constipation.

C. Fentanyl has duration of action of up to 60 minutes compared to morphine, which can last more than three times as long.

D. Alfentanil has a very rapid onset and offset limiting its use in the ED.

E. Codeine should be avoided in the intravenous form because of histamine release.

Table 4.5 shows comparisons between common opiate analgesics.

Table 4.5 Comparison of common opiate analgesics

	Codeine	Tramadol	Morphine	Fentanyl	Alfentanil
Routes	PO	PO	IV, PO	IV, Transdermal	IV
Dose	30–60 mg	50–100 mg	10 mg	100 mcg	500 mcg
Onset of action	30–60 mins	30–60 mins	5–10 mins	3 mins	<1 min
Duration of action	4–6 hours	4–6 hours	3–4 hours	30 mins	<10 mins

Harrison M (2017). *Revision Notes for the FRCEM Primary*, 2nd edition. Oxford, UK: Oxford University Press.

Joint Formulary Committee (2015). *British National Formulary*, 69th edition. London, UK: BMJ Group and Pharmaceutical Press.

12. E. Paracetamol 400 mg PO + ibuprofen 150 mg PO.

A. The ibuprofen dose for a child is 5–10 mg/kg.

B. 400 mg would be an appropriate dose for this child but starting an intravenous line on a child takes time and as such other routes are preferred.

C. The standard dose for paracetamol in a child is 15–20 mg/kg.

D. Codeine is contraindicated in children under 12 due to the risk of respiratory depression.

E. Correct answer: 400 mg would be a reasonable dose of paracetamol for this child and an appropriate first line analgesic. The combination with ibuprofen also provides a synergistic benefit in decreasing pain.

Joint Formulary Committee (2015). *British National Formulary*, 69th edition. London, UK: BMJ Group and Pharmaceutical Press.

13. D. Use diltiazem with caution in patients also taking beta-blockers.

A. Calcium channel blockers all effect L-type voltage sensitive calcium channels but their site of action varies.

B. Diltiazem is a benzothiazepine. Verapamil is a phenylalkylamine. Amlodipine is a dihydropyridimine.

C. Nimodipine crosses the blood brain barrier and affects the cerebral arteries making it useful in the treatment of aneurysmal subarachnoid haemorrhage.

D. Correct answer: Both verapamil and diltiazem affect conduction through the AV node and can cause asystole when used in conjunction with beta-blockers. As such caution is advised when using these drugs in combination.

E. Verpamil is the most relatively cardioselective calcium channel blocker, acting to decrease myocardial contractility and decreased heart rate.

Harrison M (2017). *Revision Notes for the FRCEM Primary*, 2nd edition. Oxford, UK: Oxford University Press.

14. A. All benzodiazepines work by potentiating the action of GABA receptors.

All benzodiazepines work by facilitating the action of GABA-A within the CNS leading to CNS depression.

Table 4.6 shows the three most commonly used benzodiazepines.

Table 4.6 Comparison of common benzodiazepines

	Midazolam	**Diazepam**	**Lorazepam**
Routes	PO, IM, IV	PO, PR, IM, IV	IV, IM, PO
Onset	3–5 mins (IV)	5–90 mins (PR)	1–3 mins (IV)
	15–20 mins (IM/PO)	variable (PO)	15–30 mins (IM)
Peak effect	Variable	5–90 mins depending on route and dose	<3 hours (IM)
			<10 mins (IV)
Duration of action	20–40 mins (IV)	Up to 60 mins (IV)	Up to 12 hours
	1–6 hours (PO/IM)	Up to 24 hours (PO/PR)	
Half-life	1–4 hours	20–40 hours	8–12 hours

Harrison M (2017). *Revision Notes for the FRCEM Primary*, 2nd edition. Oxford, UK: Oxford University Press.

Joint Formulary Committee (2015). *British National Formulary*, 69th edition. London, UK: BMJ Group and Pharmaceutical Press.

15. E. Tremor is among the most common side effects.

A. Lithium has a very narrow therapeutic range and as such require careful monitoring and prompt treatment of toxicity.
B. There is no specific reversal agent for lithium. Treatment of toxicity is with supportive measures and hemofiltration if required.
C. All patients require routine lithium levels, renal function, and liver function tests while on treatment.
D. Toxicity can cause nausea, vomiting, ataxia, dysarthria, weakness, renal failure, come, seizures, renal failure, ECG changes, arrhythmias, circulatory failure, and death.
E. Correct answer: Common side effects include fine tremor, gastrointestinal (GI) disturbance, thyroid problems, and weight gain.

Harrison M (2017). *Revision Notes for the FRCEM Primary*, 2nd edition. Oxford, UK: Oxford University Press.

16. A. Can cause lactic acidosis as a side effect.

A. Correct answer: Adrenaline can cause hypokalaemia, lactic acidosis, and tachyarrhythmia as some of the more frequent side effects of its use.
B. Noradrenaline is another endogenous catecholamine but unlike adrenaline it has primarily alpha-1 effects causing it to act as a vasoconstrictor and inotrope with little chronotropic effect.
C. Adrenaline can be given through a peripheral IV line during cardiac arrest and in emergencies such as post-cardiac arrest or refractory anaphylaxis, but central administration is preferred due to the risks associated with extravasations.
D. Adrenaline has both alpha and beta-receptor effects but primarily acts on beta-receptors with beta-1 receptors more strongly affected than beta-2.
E. Due to its actions on beta-adrenreceptors, its primary action is as an inotrope and chronotrope, not as a vasoconstrictor although its alpha effects do cause some vasoconstriction.

Table 4.7 compares the receptor activity of various catecholamine medications.

Table 4.7 Inotropes, vasopressors, and other vasoactive agents

	Alpha—1	Alpha—2	Beta—1	Beta-2
	Vasoconstriction Inotropy		Inotropy Chronotropy	Inotropy Vasodilation Bronchodilation
Adrenaline	++	+	++++	+++
Noradrenaline	++++	+	++	+
Metaraminol	++++	+		
Ephedrine			++++	
Dobutamine	+		++++	++

Adapted from *Emergency Medicine Australasia*, Senz, A. and Nunnink, L., Review article: Inotrope and vasopressor use in the emergency department, pp. 342–51. © 2009 The Authors. Journal compilation © 2009 Australasian College for Emergency Medicine and Australasian Society for Emergency Medicine.

Harrison M (2017). *Revision Notes for the FRCEM Primary*, 2nd edition. Oxford, UK: Oxford University Press.

Life in the Fast Lane (2016). Inotropes, vasopressors and other vasoactive agents. Available at: http://lifeinthefastlane.com/ccc/inotropes-vasopressors-and-other-vasoactive-agents (accessed 6 October 2016).

17. C. Noradrenaline at high doses may cause peripheral ischaemia.

A. Dobutamine has a similar half-life compared to other vasoactive medications of approximately 3 minutes.

B. Dobutamine has positive inotropic effects by action on beta-1 and beta-2 receptors.

C. Noradrenaline can cause reflex bradycardia, peripheral ischaemia, and hypertension as common side effects.

D. Vasopressin acts on vasopressin-1 receptors in vascular smooth muscle to cause vasoconstriction. Vasopressin 2 receptors are also found in the vascular endothelium as well as the kidneys. Vasopressin-3 is found in the pituitary and is responsible for prolactin and adrenocorticotropic hormone (ACTH) release.

E. Vasopressin is an endogenous peptide. Both adrenaline and noradrenaline are endogenous catecholamine and dobutamine is a synthetic catecholamine.

Table 4.8 compares the effects of common vasoactive medications.

Table 4.8 Comparison of effects of common vasoactive medications

	Adrenaline	Noradrenaline	Dobutamine	Vasopressin
Class	endogenous catecholamine	endogenous catecholamine	synthetic catecholamine	endogenous peptide
Mechanism	Beta > Aplha	Alpha > Beta	Beta-1 + Beta-2	V1R = vasoconstriction
				V2R = renal + endothelium
				V3R = pituitary
Effects	HR +	SVR +	inotropy +	Antidiuresis
	inotropy +		myocardial work +	SVR +
	CO +		HR +	platelet aggregation +
	vasodilation + bronchodilation +		coronary perfusion +	
Uses	cardiac arrest	septic shock	low CO state	septic shock
	low CO state			
Side effects	lactic acidosis	reflex bradycardia	myocardial ischaemia	pulmonary hypertension
	low K	hypertension	tachyarrhythmia	splanchnic ischaemia
	low PO4	peripheral ischaemia		uterine contraction

Courtesy of lifeinthefastlane.com. Copyright © 2007–2017.

Harrison M (2017). *Revision Notes for the FRCEM Primary*, 2nd edition. Oxford, UK: Oxford University Press.

Life in the Fast Lane (2016). Inotropes, vasopressors and other vasoactive agents. Available at: http://lifeinthefastlane.com/ccc/inotropes-vasopressors-and-other-vasoactive-agents (accessed 6 October 2016).

18. B. Clindamycin 600 mg IV within three hours of injury.

The local guidelines on antibiotics may vary, but most orthopaedic guidelines for management of open fractures are based on the British Orthopaedic Association Standards for Trauma (BOAST) guidelines, which state that antibiotics should be administered within 3 hours of the time of injury. IV co-amoxiclav or iv cefuroxime are the recommended first line treatments however both are contraindicated in this patient due to penicillin allergy. In this circumstance, the BOAST guideline recommends 600 mg IV clindamycin.

British Orthopaedic Association and British Association of Plastic, Reconstructive and Aesthetic Surgeons Standard for Trauma (2009). The management of severe open lower limb fractures. Available at: https://www.boa.ac.uk/wp-content/uploads/2014/05/BOAST-4-The-Management-of-Sever-Open-Lower-Limb-Fractures.pdf (accessed 6 October 2016).

19. A. Cause inhibition of cytochrome P450.

A. Correct answer: Proton pump inhibitors (PPIs) can potentiate drug effects due to inhibition of cytochrome P450. A complete list of drugs that effect cytochrome P450 can be found earlier in this chapter.

B. H_2 receptor antagonists are generally considered to have fewer side effects than PPIs. Common side effects of PPIs include nausea, vomiting, abdominal pain, constipation, rashes, and headaches.

C. Most studies suggest that omeprazole is less effective that lansoprazole but the use of antacids can reduce the action of lansoprazole limiting its usefulness in patients also using medications such as Gaviscon.

D. PPIs are almost 100% effective at suppression of acid whereas H_2 receptor antagonists are less than 90% effective. Omeprazole and lansoprazole are the two most commonly utilized PPIs.

E. Ranitidine is an example of an H_2 receptor antagonist.

Harrison M (2017). *Revision Notes for the FRCEM Primary*, 2nd edition. Oxford, UK: Oxford University Press.

Joint Formulary Committee (2015). *British National Formulary*, 69th edition. London, UK: BMJ Group and Pharmaceutical Press.

20. D. Metoclopramide has both D2 receptor and 5-HT3 receptor activity.

A. Cyclizine acts on H1 receptors found in the chemoreceptor trigger zone (CTZ) but also has some action on the vestibular system directly.

B. Cyclizine is an H1 receptor antagonist. As such side effects include anticholinergic effects such as dry mouth, sedation, urinary retention, and blurred vision. Oculogyric crisis is a side effect of D2 receptor antagonist and is commonly seen in young females taking metoclopramide. Other side effects of D2 receptor antagonists include tachycardia, akathisia, and dystonia.

C. Metoclopramide like most antiemetics can be given by multiple routes including orally.

D. Correct answer: Metoclopramide primarily acts on D2 receptors but also has activity at 5-HT3 receptors.

E. Ondansetron is a 5-HT3-receptor antagonist. It acts both centrally at the CTZ of the CNS and has some limited effects directly on the GI tract. Common side effects include headache, flushing, and bradycardia.

Harrison M (2017). *Revision Notes for the FRCEM Primary*, 2nd edition. Oxford, UK: Oxford University Press.

Joint Formulary Committee (2015). *British National Formulary*, 69th edition. London, UK: BMJ Group and Pharmaceutical Press.

21. B. Furosemide is a loop diuretic.

A. Acetazolamide is a carbonic anhydrase inhibitor that has weak diuretic action. It is used to treat mountain sickness and acute glaucoma.

B. Correct answer: Furosemide is an example of a loop diuretic. Loop diuretics act by inhibiting the Na/K/2Cl co-transporter in the thick ascending loop of Henle.

C. Spironolactone is a potassium sparing diuretic. It acts as an aldosterone antagonist increasing sodium and water excretion but reducing potassium excretion. As such it can cause hyperkalaemia as a side effect of use.

D. The risk of deafness at high doses is associated with loop diuretics. Side effects of loop diuretics include hypokalaemia, hyponatraemia, hypocalcaemia, hypomagnesaemia, and hypovolaemia among others. The side effects of thiazide diuretics include hyponatraemia, hypomagnesaemia, hypercalcaemia, weakness, and impotence.

E. Thiazide diuretics work by inhibiting Na/Cl co-transport in the proximal part of the distal tubule.

Harrison M (2017). *Revision Notes for the FRCEM Primary*, 2nd edition. Oxford, UK: Oxford University Press.

22. E. Thrombolytic drugs work by activating plasminogen to plasmin.

A. There are absolute contraindications to thrombolysis including, evidence of haemorrhage on CT, active bleeding, aortic dissection, recent major surgery, recent GI haemorrhage, and cerebral neoplasm. There are also numerous relative contraindications such as severe hypertension, liver disease, traumatic CPR, and pregnancy. Side effects of thrombolytic include nausea, haemorrhage, hypotension, bradycardia, and reperfusion injury.

B. Alteplase is the recommended thrombolytic for use in cerebrovascular accident (CVA) according to current National Institute for Health and Care Excellence (NICE) guidance.

C. Nice guidance states that thrombolysis for acute stroke can be administered up to 4.5 hours after confirmed symptom onset.

D. Thrombolytic drugs are indicated in peri-arrest or cardiac arrest patients with a confirmed or suspected large pulmonary embolus.

E. Correct answer: Thrombolytic drugs activate plasminogen to plasmin, which lyses fibrin and leads to clot breakdown.

National Institute for Health and Care Excellence (2016). Acute stroke. Available at: https://pathways.nice.org.uk/pathways/stroke (accessed 9 October 2016).

23. B. It acts by inhibiting Na/K pump activity in myocyte cell membranes.

A. Common side effects of digoxin include arrhythmias, nausea, vomiting, rashes, confusion, and visual changes.

B. Correct answer: Digoxin acts by inhibiting Na/K pump activity in myocyte cell membranes, increasing intracellular sodium, reducing calcium extrusion via Na/Ca exchange transporters, increasing available calcium in sarcoplasmic reticulum leading to more forceful cardiac contraction.

C. Hypokalaemia, hypocalcaemia, acidosis, and renal failure can all precipitate digoxin toxicity. Hyperkalaemia is caused by digoxin toxicity.

D. Digoxin increases central vagal activity and facilitates muscarinic transmission in the heart. This slows the heart rate, slows the atrioventricular conductance, and prolongs the refractory period of the atrioventricular node.

E. Digoxin has a very narrow therapeutic range and as such toxicity is relatively common. Symptoms of digoxin toxicity include confusion, malaise, palpitations/arrhythmias, tachycardia, visual changes, and multiple ECG abnormalities.

Neal MJ (2005). *Medical Pharmacology at a Glance*, 5th edition. Oxford, UK: Blackwell Publishing.

24. D. Metoprolol has hepatic elimination.

A. Bisoprolol, metoprolol, atenolol, and esmolol are all cardioselective drugs.

B. Cardioselective beta-blockers preferentially act on Beta-1 receptors to reduce the cardiac output, lower blood pressure, and reduce intraocular pressure. No beta-blocker is truly cardio-specific and all cause some degree of Beta-2 effects usually at higher doses.

C. Esmolol is an incredibly short acting beta-blocker with a half-life of six to nine minutes, which is usually given as intravenous boluses or as an IV infusion. Bisoprolol is the longest cardioselective beta-blocker with a half-life of 9–12 hours.

D. Correct answer: Metoprolol has primarily hepatic elimination. Atenolol is eliminated by the kidneys. Bisoprolol has both renal and hepatic elimination.

E. Like all beta-blockers, metoprolol has negative inotropic and chronotropic effects due to their Beta-1 receptor activity.

Harrison M (2017). *Revision Notes for the FRCEM Primary*, 2nd edition. Oxford, UK: Oxford University Press.

Joint Formulary Committee (2015). *British National Formulary*, 69th edition. London, UK: BMJ Group and Pharmaceutical Press.

25. A. Carbamazepine is a hepatic enzyme inducer and should be used cautiously in patients taking other medications.

A. Correct answer: Carbamzepine is a cytochrome P450 inducer and as such has various interactions with other medications. See question 3 for further information on these medications.

B. Phenytoin has numerous side effects including aplastic anaemia, leucopoenia, gum hypertrophy, and teratogenicity. As such it is not considered safe in pregnancy. Carbamzepine and sodium valproate have similar side effect profiles.

C. Phenytoin has a very narrow therapeutic window, which can be difficult to maintain and requires careful blood level monitoring.

D. Sodium valproate works by reducing GABA inactivation thereby increasing GABA mediated inhibition. Phenytoin works by binding inactivated Na channels in the CNS preventing them returning to the resting state, as these channels are more prevalent in rapidly firing neurones (i.e. those involved in seizure activity). They are preferentially blocked thus preventing further firing of these neurons and further seizures. Carbamazepine has an almost identical mechanism of action to phenytoin.

E. Sodium valproate is usually the best tolerated of the common antiepileptic medications with the least side effects.

Harrison M (2017). *Revision Notes for the FRCEM Primary*, 2nd edition. Oxford, UK: Oxford University Press.

Joint Formulary Committee (2015). *British National Formulary*, 69th edition. London, UK: BMJ Group and Pharmaceutical Press.

26. B. Can be given in the dialysate fluid infused into peritoneal cavity for patients on peritoneal dialysis.

A. Absorption of subcutaneous insulin varies according to the injection site, the blood supply, and degree of tissue hypertrophy at the injection site.

B. Correct answer: Insulin can be given in dialysate fluid infused into the peritoneal cavity for patients on peritoneal dialysis therapy.

C. Insulin is not effective when taken orally because the GI tract breaks down the protein molecule before it reaches the bloodstream.

D. Insulin is an anabolic, or building, hormone that helps:

i. promote storage of glucose as glycogen

ii. increase protein and fat synthesis

iii. low the breakdown of glycogen, protein, and fat

iv. balance fluids and electrolytes.

E. Insulin does not have any antidiuretic action. It corrects the polydipsia and polyuria associated with osmotic diuresis by decreasing the blood glucose level.

Eckman M, Labus D (Eds.) (2009). *Clinical Pharmacology Made Incredibly Easy* (eBook from OVID), 3rd edition. Philadelphia, PA: Lippincott Williams & Wilkins.

27. B. Metformin with nifedepine.

Hypoglycaemia may occur when sulfonylureas are combined with alcohol, anabolic steroids, chloramphenicol, cimetidine, clofibrate, coumadin, fluconazole, gemfibrozil, MAOIs, phenylbutazone, ranitidine, salicylates, or sulphonamides.

It may also occur when metformin is combined with cimetidine, nifedipine, procainamide, ranitidine, or vancomycin.

Hypoglycaemia is less likely to occur when metformin is used as a single agent.

Hyperglycaemia may occur when sulfonylureas are taken with corticosteroids, dextrothyroxine, rifampin, sympathomimetics, and thiazide diuretics.

Eckman M, Labus D (Eds.) (2009). *Clinical Pharmacology Made Incredibly Easy* (eBook from OVID), 3rd edition. Philadelphia, PA: Lippincott Williams & Wilkins.

28. A. Abdominal cramps.

Adverse reactions to thyroid drugs.

Most adverse reactions to thyroid drugs result from toxicity.

GI system:

- Diarrhoea
- Abdominal cramps
- Weight loss
- Increased appetite

CVS:

- Palpitations
- Sweating
- Tachycardia
- Hypertension
- Angina
- Arrhythmias

General:

- Headache
- Tremor
- Insomnia
- Nervousness
- Fever
- Heat intolerance
- Menstrual irregularities

Eckman M, Labus D (Eds.) (2009). *Clinical Pharmacology Made Incredibly Easy* (eBook from OVID), 3rd edition. Philadelphia, PA: Lippincott Williams & Wilkins.

29. C.   Laxative abuse.

- Long-term laxative ingestion causes increased and unregulated losses of K^+. The body store of K^+ is depleted if there is no concomitant increase in dietary K^+ intake.
- The patient does not have any evidence of chronic kidney disease (CKD), hence this is not a contributory factor in this case.
- Spironolactone is a K^+ sparing diuretic, hence it may cause hyperkalaemia.
- NSAIDs may promote development of hyperkalaemia by lowering renal rennin secretion and impairing the angiotensin II-induced aldosterone release. The fall of aldosterone as a result may reduce urinary K^+ excretion raising the serum K+ concentration.

Potassium is necessary for proper functioning of all nerve and muscle cells and for nerve impulse transmission. It is also essential for tissue growth and repair and for maintenance of acid-base balance.

Eckman M, Labus D (Eds.) (2009). *Clinical Pharmacology Made Incredibly Easy* (eBook from OVID), 3rd edition. Philadelphia, PA: Lippincott Williams & Wilkins.

Gennary FJ, Wiese WJ (2008). Acid-base disturbances in gastrointestinal disease. *Clin J Am Soc Nephrol*, **3**(6), 1861–8.

UpToDate (2017). NSAIDs: Electrolyte complications. Available at: http://www.upToDate.com/contents/nsaids-electrolyte-complications

30. D.   Antagonist to H1 receptor.

A. Cyclizine has properties of histamines. It also exerts a central anticholinergic action.

B. It is absorbed well from GI tract and metabolized in the liver.

C. Phenothiazines produce their antiemetic effects by blocking the dopaminergic receptors in the CTZ in the brain. It may also directly depress the vomiting centre. But cyclizine does not act through dopaminergic receptors.

D. Correct answer; but also see answers above. Cyclizine is a histamine H1-receptor antagonist. It is used to treat nausea, vomiting, and dizziness due to motion sickness or vertigo. It also works in opioid induced nausea or vomiting.

E. The action in motion sickness is not clear, but it is thought that the drug may have a direct effect on labyrinth. Please see A also.

Eckman M, Labus D (Eds.) (2009). *Clinical Pharmacology Made Incredibly Easy* (eBook from OVID), 3rd edition. Philadelphia, PA: Lippincott Williams & Wilkins.

31. A. Acts possibly by inhibiting Ca+ influx into airway smooth muscles.

A. Correct answer: Magnesium can induce bronchial smooth muscle relaxation in a dose-dependent manner by inhibiting calcium influx into the cytosol, histamine release from mast cells, or acetylcholine release from cholinergic nerve endings.

B. The efficacy of magnesium through nebulization is controversial. Larger trials are needed to establish this.

C. Magnesium is predominantly an intracellular ion. Therefore, serum level does not represent the degree of cellular deficit. So, it would not be useful to monitor serum magnesium level for enhancing the efficacy of $MgSO_4$ therapy.

D. Though it has excellent safety profile, higher dose may cause hypermagnesaemia resulting in muscle weaknesses. It is contraindicated in presence of renal insufficiency.

E. The usual dose is 2 g over 20 minutes intravenously, which has a minimal risk of major toxicity in patients with normal renal function. Higher dose may produce toxicity. There is no published report which has examined the efficacy of 4 g.

Song W, Chang Y (2012). Magnesium sulfate for acute asthma in adults: a systematic literature review. *Asia Pacific Allergy*, **2**(1), 76–85.

UpToDate (2017). Management of acute exacerbations of asthma in adults. Available at: https://www.uptodate.com/contents/treatment-of-acute-exacerbations-of-asthma-in-adults

32. A. Contraindicated in active alcohol abuse.

A. Correct answer: Metformin is contraindicated in patients with factors predisposing to lactic acidosis. Active alcohol abuse is one of the predisposing factors.

B. It increases insulin-mediated glucose utilization in peripheral tissue (muscle and liver), particularly after meals. It works by inhibiting gluconeogenesis decreasing the hepatic glucose output.

C. Metformin has antilipolytic action that lowers the free fatty acid concentration in the blood.

D. It typically lowers the concentration of fasting blood sugar by about 20%.

E. Metformin does not have adverse cardiovascular effects. It appears to lower long-term cardiovascular mortality compared to sulfonylurea monotherapy.

UpToDate (2017). Metformin in the treatment of adults with type 2 diabetes. Available at: https://www.uptodate.com/contents/metformin-in-the-treatment-of-adults-with-type-2-diabetes-mellitus

33. E. Flucloxacillin 500 mg four times a day for seven days.

A. Antibiotic of choice in patients with known lymphoedema.

B. This combination is used when there is evidence of infection with *staphylococcus aureus* (folliculitis or pus formation) until the infection is clear.

C. Clarithromycin is the drug of choice in patients with allergic to penicillin.

D. Co-amoxiclav is prescribed in mild facial/ orbital cellulitis in the dosage of 500/125 mg three times a day for seven days.

E. Correct answer: In adults with uncomplicated cellulitis (Eron Class I), this is the drug of choice.

Clinica Knowledge Summaries (2015). Cellulitis—acute. Available at: http://cks.nice.org.uk/cellulitis-acute#!topicsummary

34. B. Cyclosporine levels may increase if given with clarythromycin.

A. There is increased risk of nephrotoxicity and hypertension if ibuprofen is used with cyclosporine.

B. Correct answer: The level of cyclosporine may increase if used with macrolides.

C. Metoclopramide increases the concentration of cyclosporines.

D. There is elevated risk of nephrotoxicity if the drugs are used together.

E. Muscle toxicity and rarely acute renal failure may occur if given concurrently with statins.

Spicer ST, Liddle C, Chapman JR, et al. (1997). The mechanism of cyclosporine toxicity induced by clarithromycin. *Br J Clin Pharmacol*, **43f**(2), 194–6.

UpToDate. Cyclosporine. Available at: https://www.uptodate.com/contents/cyclosporine

35. E. NSAIDs interfere in the migration of granulocytes to sites of inflammation.

A. If a patient does not respond to an NSAID of one class, the different class of NSAID should be tried.

B. It is not safe to give another NSAID if patient develops toxicity with one. Some toxicity is unique to particular classes of NSAIDs, while others are related to the general mode of action of inhibition of prostaglandin synthesis.

C. NSAIDs may decrease available nitric oxide synthetase, which produces nitric oxide in large amounts causing inflammatory reaction such as vasodilation, increased vascular permeability, and so on.

D. NSAIDs in general inhibit the cyclooxygenase enzyme, which ultimately reduces the formation of prostaglandins.

E. Correct answer: NSAIDs interfere with neutrophil-endothelial cell adherence by decreasing the availability of L-selectins, thereby removing a critical step in the migration of granulocytes to sites of inflammation.

UpToDate (2017). NSAIDS therapeutic use and variability of response in adults. Available at: https://www.uptodate.com/contents/nsaids-therapeutic-use-and-variability-of-response-in-adults

36. D. May act on opiate receptors to cause mild analgesia.

A. CNS depressant effect of ethyl alcohol may be enhanced by the CNS depressant effect of N_2O (nitrous oxide).

B. Avoid using N_2O in first and second trimesters of pregnancy. Use during labour is considered acceptable.

C. N_2O increases the cerebral blood flow and intracranial pressure.

D. Correct answer: It has analgesic action similar to morphine.

E. The onset of action by inhalation is two to five minutes. It is absorbed through lungs and excreted through exhaled gases.

UpToDate. Nitrous oxide drug information. Available at: https://www.uptodate.com/contents/nitrous-oxide-drug-information

37. E. Unpleasant side effects after excessive alcohol consumption are because of the metabolite, acetaldehyde.

A. Disulphiram, which blocks the mitochondrial aldehyde dehydrogenase 2 (ALDH2) leads to accumulation of acetaldehyde resulting in facial flushing, tachycardia, palpitations, dizziness, nausea, vomiting, and even death if heavy drinking continues. aldehyde dehydrogenase (ALDH) helps in conversion of acetaldehyde to acetate.

B. Tobacco is the most widely used addictive drug.

C. Ethanol is chemically an inert substance under physiological condition.

D. Alcohol is a non-specific drug and intoxicating actions of alcohol are due to summation of effects on numerous molecular targets.

E. Correct answer: The ethanol metabolite acetaldehyde mediates much of the unpleasant side effects and the hangover experienced after excessive alcohol consumption. Acetaldehyde is formed in the liver after the oxidation of alcohol in the liver.

Wallner M, Olsen RW (2008). Physiology and pharmacology of alcohol: the imidazobenzodiazepine alcohol antagonist site on subtypes of $GABA_A$ receptors as an opportunity for drug development? *Br J Pharmacol*, **154**(2), 288–98.

38. B. Immediate dose of vaccine followed by a five-dose course.

The patient has a tetanus-prone wound.

A. The antibiotics are administered to patients with clinical tetanus. Penicillin G was long considered the treatment of choice, but now metronidazole is considered as the choice of antimicrobial.

B. Correct answer: The full dose of vaccine should be provided as is done in normal circumstances. Please see the green book for reference no. 1.

C. The wound is tetanus prone. Hence the patient should receive the immunoglobulin immediately at a separate site by intramuscular injection (250 IU).

D. Tetanus vaccine is not a live vaccine. It is made from a cell-free purified toxin extracted from a strain of *C. tetani*.

E. There is no evidence of rejection of the graft by using the vaccine.

Gov.uk (2016). The routine immunisation schedule. Available at: https://www.gov.uk/government/uploads/system/uploads/attachment_data/file/523050/PHE_Complete_Immunisation_Schedule_SPRING16.pdf

Medscape (2017). Tetanus Medication. Available at: http://emedicine.medscape.com/article/229594-medication

Rubin LG, Levin MJ, Liungman P, et al. (2013). IDSA clinical practice guideline for vaccination of the immunocompromised host. *Clin Infect Dis*, 58(3), e44–e100.

UpToDate (2017). Immunizations in solid organ transplant candidates and recipients. Available at: https://www.uptodate.com/contents/immunizations-in-solid-organ-transplant-candidates-and-recipients

39. D. Normal saline has osmolality of 285–308 mOsm/L.

A. The osmolality of Hartmann's solution is 250–273 mOsm/L.

B. The maximum volume expansion (as a percentage of administered volume) is 20–25%, in case of Hartmann's solution which is similar to normal saline.

C. The sodium concentration is similar to extracellular fluid (ECF) (extracellular fluid). Within the ECF, the fluid is distributed between the interstitial fluid (ISF) and intravascular fluid by three-quarters and one-quarter, respectively. Ringers and Hartmann's both contain lactate in addition to salt and electrolytes.

D. Correct answer: Normal saline has 9 gm of NaCl/L water, 154 mmol/L sodium, 154 mmol/L chloride, pH 5.0, and osmolality of 308 mosm/L.

E. Plasmatic half-life of normal saline and Hartmann's solution are the same: 0.5 hours.

Anaesthesia UK (2004). Crystalloids. Available at: http://www.frca.co.uk/article.aspx?articleid=291

40. A. Glycerol suppositories act as a rectal stimulant.

A. Correct answer: Glycerol suppositories act as rectal stimulant by virtue of the mildly irritant action of glycerol.

B. Lactulose is a semi-synthetic disaccharide, which is not absorbed from the gastrointestinal tract. It produces an osmotic diarrhoea of low faecal pH and discourages the proliferation of ammonia-producing organisms. It is therefore useful in the treatment of hepatic encephalopathy.

C. Liquid paraffin is a faecal softener.

D. Macrogols are inert polymers of ethylene glycol, which sequester fluid in the bowel; giving fluid with macrogols may reduce the dehydrating effect sometimes seen with osmotic laxatives.

E. Phosphate enemas are useful in bowel clearance before radiology, endoscopy, and surgery.

National Institute for Health and Care Excellence (n.d.). Constipation. Available at: https://bnf.nice.org.uk/treatment-summary/constipation.html

41. E. Warfarin works by reducing the synthesis of active clotting factors.

A. The target range of INR for treatment of venous thromboembolism is 2–3.

B. Chronic daily ethanol use increases the metabolism of oral anticoagulants and decreases PT/INR. Hence, avoid taking alcohol during treatment.

C. Cranberry juice may increase the warfarin effect.

D. The onset of action following oral anticoagulation is 24–72 hours. Full therapeutic effect is reached in 5–7 days. The INR may increase in 36–72 hours.

E. Correct answer: The coagulation factors II, VII, IX, X, Protein C and S requires vitamin K for its synthesis in liver. Warfarin competitively inhibits the enzyme (VKORC1), which reactivates vitamin K resulting in depleting the reserve of functional vitamin K, which in turn reduces the formation of active clotting factors.

UpToDate, Warfarin drug information. Available at: https://www.uptodate.com/contents/warfarin-drug-information?source=search_result&search=warfarin&selectedTitle=1~150

42. D. It acts indirectly by binding to antithrombin.

A. Average molecular weight of LMWH is 4,000 to 5,000 Daltons. The molecular weight of unfractionated heparin is 15,000 Daltons.

B. The half-life of unfractionated heparin is 45 minutes to one hour, but the half-life of LMWH is about two hours.

C. Unfractionated heparin has 45 saccharide units. The LMWH has approximately 15 saccharide units on average.

D. Correct answer: It acts indirectly by binding to antithrombin (heparin cofactor 1), which induces a conformational chage in antithrombin, which inactivates the coagulation factors (factor IIa and factor Xa).

E. An aPTT (or antifactor Xa activity) of 1.5 to 2.5 times the mean of the control value or upper limit of the normal range is widely accepted for maintenance therapy. This should be checked four to six hours of initiation of heparin.

UpToDate (2017). Heparin and lmw heparin dosing and adverse effects. Available at: https://www.uptodate.com/contents/heparin-and-lmw-heparin-dosing-and-adverse-effects?source=machineLearning&search=mechanism%20of%20action%20of%20heparin&selectedTitle=3~150&sectionRank=1&anchor=H3#H3

43. B. Cephalosporins inhibit cell wall synthesis by binding to the bacterial enzymes.

A. Because penicillins and cephalosporins are chemically similar (beta-lactam molecular structure), cross-sensitivity occurs in 10 to 15% of patients.

B. Correct answer: Cephalosporins penetrate the bacterial cell wall and bind with proteins on the cytoplasmic membrane. Following this destruction of cell wall, body's defence mechanisms destroy the bacteria.

C. There are four generations of cephalosporins. Cefuroxime is a second-generation cephalosporin.

D. Cefuroxime cannot be inactivated by bacterial beta-lactamases.

E. Acute alcohol intolerance develops if patients receiving cephalosporins drinks alcohol with or up to 72 hours after taking a dose. The signs and symptoms are headache, flushing, nausea, vomiting, or abdominal cramps within 30 minutes of alcohol ingestion.

Weil J, Miramonti J, Ladisch MR (1995). Cephalosporin C: Mode of action and biosynthetic pathway. *Enzyme and Microbial Technology*, **17**(1), 85–7.

44. D. Gabapentin has half-life of five to seven hours.

A. Gabapentin causes CNS depression and dizziness, drowsiness, ataxia, and fatigue as adverse reaction.

B. CNS depressant effect may be enhanced if used concomitantly with alcohol.

C. Gabapentin is structurally related to GABA, but it does not bind to the GABAA/ GABAB receptors. High affinity gabapentin binding sites are located throughout the brain. Gabapentin may work through these sites to modulate the release of excitatory neurotransmitters.

D. Correct answer: The half-life is increased with decreasing renal function.

E. Abrupt withdrawal of the drug may precipitate seizure activity. So, the therapy should be withdrawn gradually.

UpToDate, Gabapentin drug information. Available at: https://www.uptodate.com/contents/gabapentin-drug-information

45. D. Ketamine is a phencyclidine derivative that acts as a dissociative sedative.

A. The reported side effects of ketamine include tachycardia, hypertension, laryngospasm, nausea, vomiting, hypersalivation, and so on.

B. Following an intravenous injection, the onset of action is immediate. The duration of its effect is 10–20 minutes.

C. Gabapentin is structurally related to GABA, but it does not bind to the GABAA/ GABAB receptors. High affinity gabapentin binding sites are located throughout the brain. Gabapentin may work through these sites to modulate the release of excitatory neurotransmitters.

D. Correct answer: It produces a trance-like state and provides sedation, analgesia, and amnesia, while preserving upper airway muscle tone, airway protective reflexes, and spontaneous breathing.

E. In elderly patients with major co-morbidities, surgery is best performed in the operation theatre. Patients without major co-morbidities may be safer with an ultra-short-acting sedative, such as propofol.

UpToDate (2017). Procedural sedation in adults outside the operating room. Available at: https://www.uptodate.com/contents/procedural-sedation-in-adults-outside-the-operating-room

46. C. Inhibits migration of white blood cells to the inflamed joint.

A. The biological effects are not related to plasma concentrations but with intraleucocyte concentrations.

B. Colchicine elimination occurs via hepatic pathways and the elimination half-life ranged from 20 to 40 hours.

C. Correct answer: Colchicine is an extract of the plant Colchicum autumnale (automn crocus) used medically since ancient times. It binds to tubulin in leucocytes and prevents its polymerization into microtubules. This inhibits the phagocytic activity and migration of leucocytes to the areas of uric acid deposition, and hence reduces the inflammatory responses.

D. Colchicine is most effective if given within 12–24 hours of acute attack.

E. It should be avoided in severe renal and hepatic impairment.

Chappey O, Scherrmann JM (1995). Colchicine: recent data on pharmacokinetics and clinical pharmacology. *Rev Med Interne*, **16**(10), 782–9.

Neal MJ (2005). *Medical Pharmacology at a Glance*, 5th edition. Oxford, UK: Blackwell Publishing.

UpToDate (2017). Treatment of acute gout. Available at: http://www.uptodate.com/contents/treatment-of-acute-gout

47. D. Past HBV infected patients does not require the vaccine.

Development of hepatitis B surface antibody (anti-HBs) at a titre of >10 mIU/mL following vaccination is called a positive immune response.

Vaccination should be administered as early as possible because response rates to Hepatitis B (HepB) vaccine are low with decompensated cirrhosis (around 36%) and in liver transplant patients.

Currently available hepatitis B vaccines are extremely safe and have an efficacy of >90% against all HBV serotypes and genotypes.

Anti-HBc and antiHBs positive patients (marker of past infection with HBV) do not need the vaccine even if their titres are low.

There should be a gap of at least two months between the second and the third dose.

Chappey O, Scherrmann JM (1995). Colchicine: recent data on pharmacokinetics and clinical pharmacology. *Rev Med Interne*, **16**(10), 782–9.

Neal MJ (2005). *Medical Pharmacology at a Glance*, 5th edition. Oxford, UK: Blackwell Publishing.

UpToDate (2017). Treatment of acute gout. Available at: http://www.uptodate.com/contents/treatment-of-acute-gout

48. B. In plasma, only 45% of the total calcium exists as physiologically important ionized form.

A. The absorption of calcium through GI tract is incomplete. The net absorption is only 100 to 200 mg when 1,000 mg is ingested. This is because of requirement of activated vitamin D and formation of insoluble salts of calcium and other ions in the intestine, which are not absorbed.

B. Correct answer: In plasma, 40% of calcium is bound to albumin, 15% is in combination with citrate, sulphate, or phosphate and 45% is free, which is important physiologically.

C. Only ionized calcium is filtered through glomerulus. Between 97 to 99% of the filtered calcium is reabsorbed through subsequent segments of renal tubules. About 70% is absorbed passively in conjunction with sodium in the proximal tubules.

D. Parathyroid hormone (PTH) promotes renal formation of active vitamin D (1,25-dihydroxyvitamin D), which enhances intestinal calcium and phosphate absorption.

E. PTH through adenyl cyclase system in the distal tubules, rapidly reabsorbs the calcium.

UpToDate, Regulation of calcium and phosphate balance. Available at: https://www.uptodate.com/contents/regulation-of-calcium-and-phosphate-balance

49. E. Tetanus, diphtheria, and polio (Td/IPV), MenC.

Knowledge of the UK immunization schedule is required for the examination. Table 4.9 shows the immunization schedule as of 2015. Make sure to look at the most up to date list of immunizations prior to the examination.

Table 4.9 2015 immunization schedule

Age	Vaccines given
2 months	Diphtheria, tetanus, pertussis, polio, and Hib (DTaP/IPV/Hib), pneumococcal conjugate (PCV), rotavirus
3 months	Diphtheria, tetanus, pertussis, polio, and Hib (DTaP/IPV/Hib), meningococcal C conjugate (MenC), rotavirus
4 months	Diphtheria, tetanus, pertussis, polio, and Hib (DTaP/IPV/Hib), PCV
12 months	Hib/MenC conjugate, pneumococcal conjugate (PCV), measles, mumps, and rubella (MMR)
2–17 years (annually)	Influenza nasal spray
3 years 4 months	Diphtheria, tetanus, pertussis, and polio (DTaP/IPV or dTaP/IPV), measles, mumps, and rubella (MMR)
12–14 (girls only)	Human papillomavirus (HPV)
14 years	Tetanus, diphtheria, and polio (Td/IPV), MenC conjugate

The National Health Service (2014). The complete routine immunisation schedule from summer 2014. Available at: https://www.gov.uk/government/uploads/system/uploads/attachment_data/file/422787/8584_PHE_2015_Complete_Immunisation_Schedule_A4_13_accessible.pdf (accessed 10 May 2015).

50. C.   Gastrointestinal side effects are primarily caused by COX-1 inhibition.

A. COX (Cyclooxygenase) inhibition is the main mechanism of action of aspirin. However, it does not explain all the inflammatory effects of aspirin. Inhibition of neutrophil activation and responses is other PG-independent actions of aspirin.

B. At low dosage, it inhibits COX-1 resulting in inhibition of platelet aggregation.

C. Correct answer: The GI side effects of aspirin are mediated via COX-1 pathway. If used in conjunction with other COX-2 inhibitors, the side effects may continue to persist.

D. Aspirin reduces prostaglandin production by inhibiting both COX-1 and COX-2. In COX-2, the efficiency is 10-fold less than that of COX-1.

E. At higher dosages, aspirin acts by reducing COX-2 dependent prostaglandins and prostaglandin independent effects.

UpToDate (2016). Abramson SB et al.: Aspirin: Mechanism of action, major toxicities, and use in rheumatic diseases. Available at: https://www.uptodate.com/contents/aspirin-mechanism-of-action-major-toxicities-and-use-in-rheumatic-diseases

UpToDate (2017). Aspirin mechanism of action major toxicities and use in rheumatic diseases. Available at: https://www.uptodate.com/contents/aspirin-mechanism-of-action-major-toxicities-and-use-in-rheumatic-diseases

51. A.   Cerebral blood flow in increased by its beta-adrenergic action.

The systemic vasoconstriction is through alpha-adrenergic effects resulting in increase in coronary and cerebral perfusion pressures. The beta-adrenergic actions may increase coronary and cerebral blood flow (inotropic and chronotropic).

Nolan J, Soar J, Lockey A (2011). *Advanced Life Support Manual*, 6th edition. (Appendix A: Drugs used in the treatment of cardiac arrest). London, UK: Resuscitation Council.

52. E.   It increases the duration of action potential.

Amiodarone is a membrane-stabilizing class III anti-arrhythmic drug that increases the duration of action potential and refractory period in atrial and ventricular myocardium. The atrioventricular conduction is slowed with similar effects through the accessory pathways. It has mild negative inotropic action and results in peripheral vasodilation through alpha-blocking effects.

Nolan J, Soar J, Lockey A (2011). *Advanced Life Support Manual*, 6th edition. (Appendix A: Drugs used in the treatment of cardiac arrest). London, UK: Resuscitation Council.

53. E.   It is a naturally occurring purine nucleotide.

Adenosine blocks conduction through AV node but it does not have much effect on myocardial cells or conduction pathways. It is naturally occurring purine nucleotide. It has a very short half-left (10–15 seconds). It is contraindicated in asthma.

Nolan J, Soar J, Lockey A (2011). *Advanced Life Support Manual*, 6th edition. (Appendix A: Drugs used in the treatment of cardiac arrest). London, UK: Resuscitation Council.

1. **A paper has been published looking at the effectiveness of bystander cardiopulmonary resuscitation (CPR) in out of hospital cardiac arrest. The paper pooled together data from six different trials in order to achieve a sample size of over 3,000 patients over a 10-year period. That data was then analysed collectively. Which single type of study design best describes this type of trial?**
   A. Case–control study
   B. Meta-analysis
   C. Prospective cohort study
   D. Randomized control trial
   E. Retrospective cohort study

2. **The following results (Table 5.1) were obtained from a randomized control trial for a new diagnostic test, called DJW, for diagnosis of subarachnoid haemorrhage (SAH). Which is the single most appropriate description of the trial results?**
   A. DJW has a negative predictive value (NPV) of 75%
   B. DJW has a positive predictive value (PPV) of 50%
   C. DJW has a sensitivity of 20%
   D. DJW has a sensitivity of 75%
   E. DJW has a specificity of 20%

Table 5.1 Diagnosis of subarachnoid haemorrhage

	SAH	
	Present	**Absent**
DJW—Positive	8	10
DJW—Negative	32	30

SAH, subarachnoid haemorrhage.

3. **A recently published paper on catheter-directed thrombolysis for the treatment of pulmonary embolism (PE) showed a number needed to treat (NNT) of 28 and a number needed to harm (NNH) of 54. Which is the single most accurate outcome of this trial?**

A. An NNH of 54 would be considered too high

B. The absolute risk reduction (ARR) is 0.28

C. The ARR is 0.3   *0·03*

D. The NNT is too low

4. **A study looking at the use of bedside ultrasound for the diagnosis of small bowel obstruction quoted a sensitivity of 60% and a specificity of 85%. Which single statement best describes the outcome of this paper?**

A. The negative likelihood ratio is 4

B. The negative likelihood ratio is 40

C. The positive likelihood ratio is 0.4

D. The positive likelihood ratio is 4

E. The positive likelihood ratio is 40

5. **The following results in Table 5.2 were obtained from a randomized controlled trial (RCT) comparing the new drug, APW, with clonidine for sedation in intensive care. Success was determined as an improvement in Richmond Agitation-Sedation Scale (RASS) scores of more than 2 points. Which single statement most accurately describes the outcome of this trial?**

Table 5.2 Results comparison of APW with clonidine

	RASS score improvement	
	Present	**Absent**
APW	38	2
Clonidine	28	12

RASS, Richmond Agitation-Sedation Scale.

A. The ARR is 0.95

B. The ARR is 4

C. The event rate in the APW group is 0.7

D. The event rate in the control group is 0.7

E. The NNT for APW is 25

6. **A 44-year-old man is experiencing chest pain, which radiates to the left arm. The provisional diagnosis is acute myocardial infarction (AMI). In a recent publication, a group of authors concluded that detection of the enzyme 'MG420' in this patient's blood could be considered as definitive sign of AMI. To ascertain the accuracy of this test, which is the single most appropriate statement?**

   A. The blood test result and its correlation to AMI should be known to the researchers during the study

   B. The follow-ups of the patients should be long and complete

   C. There is no requirement for validation of this test in a second independent group of patients

   D. There should have been an independent and blind comparison with a 'gold' standard of diagnosis

   E. This test should have been applied only to the severe cardiac-sounding chest pain group of patients

7. **A 60-year-old man has had sudden severe central chest pain with radiation to back. A diagnosis of aortic dissection is suspected. There has been a meta-analysis published on role of D-dimer as a biomarker for acute aortic dissection. Which is the single most appropriate statement about meta-analysis?**

   A. Meta-analysis should exclusively include evidence from the RCTs

   B. Quality assessment protocols and data forms should be developed to reduce the bias on the estimate of the effect

   C. Separate selection criteria may not be necessary if more than one hypothesis is to be tested in a meta-analysis

   D. Statistical analysis should include only those patients who completed all stages of the study, rather than conducted on all subjects enrolled in the study

   E. Studies published in English language should only be included

8. **An 82-year-old female has sustained a fracture in the neck of the femur. She is in considerable pain. Recently, a randomized trial was published in the _Emergency Medicine Journal_ comparing the fascia iliaca block versus the '3-in-1' block for femoral neck fractures in the emergency department. The study has been discussed to ascertain which is the best method of analgesia for the patient. Which is the single most appropriate statement about appraising a RCT?**

   A. Allocation concealment allows a researcher to allocate a particular patient in a particular slot for a particular treatment

   B. _p_ values provide more useful information than confidence intervals (CIs) in such studies

   C. RCTs are at the top of the triangle of hierarchy of evidences

   D. Results from an RCT are still valid even if the selection bias could not be avoided

   E. The main purpose of randomization is to avoid selection bias

9. **A randomized controlled study has been planned involving three district general hospitals on the effectiveness of a medication on the cure of cystic fibrosis. Which statement is the single most appropriate to sources of bias in clinical trials?**

   A. Attrition bias includes when outcome data is available despite subject withdrawal from the study

   B. Blinding of the study participants and personnel after their enrolment may avoid performance bias

   C. Reporting bias refers to when the studies with insignificant results for the main outcome interest are more likely to be published than those with significant results

   D. The expectation bias refers to the absence of knowledge of the result of a test to the interpreters involved on the trial

   E. To determine the degree of pain in a trial, detection bias could not be avoided

10. **A critical appraisal has been planned on a paper published in the *Emergency Medicine Journal*, 'Lactate level, aetiology and mortality of adult patients in an emergency department: a cohort study'. Which statement is the single most appropriate regarding cohort studies?**

    A. Considered as the top level of evidences of hierarchy triangle

    B. Defines a set of people followed over a period of time

    C. Generally provides similar quality results as in RCTs

    D. Internal validity of the study is reduced if the loss of follow-up cases remain below 20%

    E. Is a type of case-based study

11. **A critical appraisal has been planned on a paper published in the *Emergency Medicine Journal*: 'Arterial lactate levels in an emergency department are associated with mortality: a prospective observational cohort study.' Which statement is the single most appropriate regarding the critical appraisal of this study?**

    A. Extraneous variables may be kept under control

    B. Relatively inexpensive to conduct such a study

    C. Sampling in such cases may not need to be explicit

    D. Takes a long time to complete the study

    E. The cases should be selected from a single hospital

12. **A study has been conducted in Canada to examine the relationship between the coping styles and burnout among 600 emergency medicine healthcare professionals in small, medium, and large emergency departments. The inclusion of the subjects is voluntary and confidential. The study has been approved by the local Ethics Board. Which statement is the single most appropriate to describe the study design?**

    A. Case–control study

    B. Cohort study

    C. Cross-sectional survey

    D. RCT

    E. Single-blinded control trial

1. E. Retrospective cohort study.

  A. Case–control studies are an example of observational studies which are particularly useful for looking for rare diseases.

  B. Meta-analysis involves pooling data from multiple studies, looking at the same intervention to increase the number of patients studied.

  C. Cohort studies are a type of observation study. Most cohort studies are prospective.

  D. RCTs are a type of experimental study for investigating the effect that different treatments have on patient groups.

  E. Correct answer: Cohort studies can also be retrospective and are sometimes known as 'historical cohort studies'.

Greenhalgh T (2014). *How to Read a Paper: The Basics of Evidence-Based Medicine*, 5th edition. Chichester, UK: Wiley-Blackwell.

2. C. DJW has a sensitivity of 20%.

See Table 5.3.

Table 5.3 DJW sensitivity

	SAH	
	Present	**Absent**
DJW—Positive	8 = a	10 = b
DJW—Negative	32 = c	30 = d

SAH, subarachnoid haemorrhage.

Sensitivity is the number of true positives correctly identified by a diagnostic test. This can be calculated as:

$$\text{Sensitivity} = \text{No. of True Positives} / (\text{No. True Positives} + \text{No. False Negatives})$$

$$\text{Sensitivity} = 8/40 \ (a/a+c) = 20\%$$

Specificity is the number of true negatives correctly identified by a diagnostic test. This can be calculated as:

$$\text{Specificity} = \text{No. True Negatives} / (\text{No. of True Negatives} + \text{No. False Positives})$$

$$\text{Specificity} = 30/40 \ (d/b+d) = 75\%$$

The NPV is the likelihood that a person who is tested negative for a disease does not have the disease. This can be calculated as:

$$NPV = \text{No. of True Negatives}/ \left(\text{No. of True Negatives} + \text{No. of False Negatives}\right)$$

$$NPV = 30/62 \; (d/c+d) = 48\%$$

The PPV is the likelihood that a person who tests positive for a disease actually has the disease. This can be calculated as:

$$PPV = \text{No. of True Positives}/ \left(\text{No. of True Positives} + \text{No. of False Positives}\right)$$

$$PPV = 8/18 \; (a/a+b) = 44\%$$

Greenhalgh T (2014). *How to Read a Paper: The Basics of Evidence-Based Medicine*, 5th edition. Chichester, UK: Wiley-Blackwell.

Harris M, Taylor G (2008). *Medical Statistics Made Easy*, 3rd edition. Bloxham, UK: Scion Publishing.

3. D. The ARR is 0.3.

The ARR can be calculated as the inverse of the number needed to treat or 1/NNT.

$$\text{Absolute Risk Reduction} \left(ARR\right) = 1/NNT$$

$$ARR = 1/28 = 0.03$$

The NNT is the number of patients who require a stated intervention in order for one patient to receive a benefit and is a useful method of describing the effectiveness of a treatment. The ideal NNT would be 1, but an NNT of 5–20 is more commonly used to represent a good therapeutic outcome. The closer the NNT is to 1, the better the intervention is considered to be. In this case the NNT is probably too high to be considered beneficial.

The NNH is defined as the number of patients who need to be exposed to a treatment or intervention to cause harm to one patient. Unlike NNT, the further the NNH is from 1 the better. An NNH of over 50 is acceptable in most circumstances.

Harris M, Taylor G (2008). *Medical Statistics Made Easy*, 3rd edition. Bloxham, UK: Scion Publishing.

4. D. The positive likelihood ratio is 4.

Likelihood ratios can be calculated as:

$$\text{A positive likelihood ratio} = \text{Sensitivity}/\left(1-\text{specificity}\right)$$

$$\text{A negative likelihood ratio} = \left(1-\text{sensitivity}\right)/\text{Specificity}$$

In this example a positive likelihood ratio is calculated as the Sensitivity/(1- specificity)

LR+ = Sensitivity/(1 – Specificity)

LR+ = 60%/(1 – 85%)

LR+ = 0.6/(1 – 0.85) = 4

In this example a negative likelihood ratio is calculated as (1 – sensitivity)/Specificity

LR– = (1 – sensitivity)/Specificity

LR– = (1 – 60%)/85%

LR– = (1 – 0.6)/0.85 = 0.47

A positive likelihood ratio of less than 5 or a negative likelihood ratio of more than 0.2 is rarely significant.

Greenhalgh T (2014). *How to Read a Paper: The Basics of Evidence-Based Medicine*, 5th edition. Chichester, UK: Wiley-Blackwell.

5. D. The event rate in the control group is 0.7

See Table 5.4.

Table 5.4 Control group event rate

	RASS score improvement	
	Present	**Absent**
APW	38 = a	2 = b
Clonidine	28 = c	12 = d

RASS, Richmond Agitation-Sedation Scale.

The event rate in the control group is calculated as:

$$CER = 28/40 \ (c/c+d) = 0.7 \ (70\%)$$

The event rate in the experimental group is calculated as:

$$EER = 38/40 \ (a/a+b) = 0.95 \ (95\%)$$

The ARR is calculated as:

$$ARR = EER - CER$$

$$ARR = 0.95 - 0.7 = 0.25 \ (25\%)$$

The NNT is calculated as:

$$NNT = 1/ARR$$

$$NNT = 1/0.25 = 4$$

Greenhalgh T (2014). *How to Read a Paper: The Basics of Evidence-Based Medicine*, 5th edition. Chichester, UK: Wiley-Blackwell.

Harris M, Taylor G (2008). *Medical Statistics Made Easy*, 3rd edition. Bloxham, UK: Scion Publishing.

6. D. There should have been an independent and blind comparison with a 'gold' standard of diagnosis.

A. The results of the diagnostic test in question (MG420) should not be known to those who are applying and interpreting the other, which would be compared with test. In this way, the investigators could avoid the conscious and unconscious bias towards the test results. Please see answer D.

B. The follow-ups are applicable when validating the accuracy of a therapeutic paper.

C. To be reassured of the accuracy of the new test, this should perform well if applied to a second independent set of patients (Was the test validated in a second, independent group of patients?).

D. Correct answer: The patients in this study should have undergone both the diagnostic test in question and the reference or 'gold' standard. Secondly, as mentioned in answer A, the results of one should not be known to those who are applying and interpreting the other.

E. The diagnostic test should be applied to all patients with mild, as well as severe chest pain. In this way, the diagnostic test could be evaluated in appropriate spectrum of patients.

Sackett DL, Starus SE, Richardson WS, Rosenberg W, Haynes RB (2000). *Evidence-Based Medicine: How to Practice and Teach EBM*, 2nd edition. London, UK: Churchill Livingstone.

7. B. Quality assessment protocols and data forms should be developed to reduce the bias on the estimate of the effect.

Meta-analysis is a quantitative, formal, epidemiological study design used to systematically assess the results of previous research to derive conclusions about that body of research.

A. Typically, but not necessarily, the study is based on randomized, controlled clinical trials. It is important to obtain all relevant studies, because loss of studies can lead to bias in the study. Database searches should be augmented with hand searches of library resources for relevant papers, books, abstracts, and conference proceedings. Cross-checking of references, citations in review papers, and communication with scientists who have been working in the relevant field are important methods used to provide a comprehensive search. If an analysis includes both randomized and non-randomized trials, it should separate these types of trials in its analysis.

B. Correct answer: Before assessing study quality, a quality assessment protocol and data forms should be developed. The goal of this process is to reduce the risk of bias in the estimate of effect.

C. If there is more than one hypothesis to be tested, separate selection criteria should be defined for each hypothesis. Inclusion criteria are ideally defined at the initial development stage of the study protocol.

D. It should be other way around. The statistical analysis should be conducted on all subjects that are enrolled in a study, rather than those that complete all stages of study considered desirable.

E. If the search is restricted to only one language, it may bias the conclusions. There have been examples of submission of trials with positive results to English language journals and those with negative results to a local language journal. It is important to overcome this difficulty, provided that the populations studied are relevant to the hypothesis being tested.

Haidich AB (2010). Meta-analysis in medical research. *Hippokratia*, **14**(Suppl 1), 29–37.

Sackett DL, Starus SE, Richardson WS, Rosenberg W, Haynes RB (2000). *Evidence-Based Medicine: How to Practice and Teach EBM*, 2nd edition. London, UK: Churchill Livingstone.

8. E. The main purpose of randomization is to avoid selection bias.

A. Allocation concealment is used to prevent selection bias. The allocation sequence is concealed from the researchers who are assigning a particular treatment to a particular patient. If this is not followed, the estimates of the treatment effect may be exaggerated by about 41%.

B. A CI conveys more useful information than a *p* value. It is able to provide an idea about how precise is the effect of a treatment. CI is the interval, which includes the true value in 95% of cases. The *p* value is the probability that any difference between two treatments would have risen by chance. A *p* value of <0.05 has been considered as 'statiscally significant'.

C. In the hierarchy of evidences triangle, the most rigorous methodology is systematic review with or without RCTs followed by RCTs.

D. Please see option (E).

E. Correct answer: The main aim of randomization is to remove, if possible, the selection bias. It also allows balancing various confounding factors between the control and treatment groups. Although an RCT should, in theory, eliminate selection bias, there are instances where bias can occur. Any selection bias in an RCT invalidates the study design and makes the results no more reliable than an observational study. As Torgesson and Roberts have suggested, the results of a supposed RCT which has had its randomization compromised by, say, poor allocation concealment may be more damaging than an explicitly unrandomized study, as bias in the latter is acknowledged and the statistical analysis and subsequent interpretation might have taken this into account.

Akonbeng AK (2005). Understanding randomised controlled trials. *Arch Dis Child*, **90**, 840–4.

Greenhalgh T (2006). *How to Read a Paper: The Basics of Evidence-Based Medicine*, 3rd edition. Oxford, UK: Blackwell Publishing.

Torgerson DJ, Torgerson CJ (2003). Avoiding bias in randomized controlled trials in educational research. *Br J Educ Stud*, **51**, 36–45.

9. B. Blinding of the study participants and personnel after their enrolment may avoid performance bias.

A. Attrition bias refers to systematic differences between groups in withdrawals from a study. Withdrawals from the study lead to incomplete outcome data. There are two reasons for withdrawals or incomplete outcome data in clinical trials. Exclusions refer to situations in which some participants are omitted from reports of analyses, despite outcome data being available. Attrition refers to situations in which outcome data are not available.

B. Correct answer: Performance bias refers to systematic differences between groups in the care that is provided, or in exposure to factors other than the interventions of interest. After enrolment into the study, blinding (or masking) of study participants and personnel may reduce the risk that the knowledge of which intervention was received, rather than the intervention itself, affects outcomes. Effective blinding can also ensure that the compared groups receive a similar amount of attention, ancillary treatment, and diagnostic investigations.

C. Reporting bias refers to systematic differences between reported and unreported findings. Within a published report those analyses with statistically significant differences between intervention groups are more likely to be reported than non-significant differences. This sort of 'within-study publication bias' is usually known as outcome reporting bias or selective reporting bias, and may be one of the most substantial biases affecting results from individual studies.

D. The expectation bias occurs when the interpreter is subconsciously influenced by the knowledge of the particular feature of the case; for example, the presence of chest pain when interpreting an electrocardiogram (ECG).

E. Detection bias refers to systematic differences between groups in how outcomes are determined. Blinding (or masking) of outcome assessors may reduce the risk that knowledge of which intervention was received, rather than the intervention itself, affects outcome measurement. Blinding of outcome assessors can be especially important for assessment of subjective outcomes, such as degree of postoperative pain.

Greenhalgh T (2006). *How to Read a Paper: The Basics of Evidence-based Medicine*, 3rd edition. Oxford, UK: Blackwell Publishing.

Higgins JPT, Green S (eds) (2011). *Cochrane Handbook for Systematic Reviews of Interventions* Version 5.1.0 [updated March 2011]. The Cochrane Collaboration. Available at: http://handbook.cochrane.org

10. E. Is a type of case-based study.

A. Cohort studies are placed at the third position, below the RCTs.

B. In epidemiology, the term cohort is used to define a set of people followed over a period of time. W. H. Frost, an epidemiologist from the early 1900s, was the first to use the word 'cohort' in his 1935 publication assessing age-specific mortality rates and tuberculosis. The modern epidemiological definition of the word now means a 'group of people with defined characteristics who are followed-up to determine incidence of, or mortality from, some specific disease, all causes of death, or some other outcome'.

C. Though RCTs remain more robust in methodology design, in certain specialties (e.g. surgery), well-designed cohort studies can play an important role in deriving evidences.

D. It is important to minimize loss to follow-up, as prospective cohort studies may require long follow-up periods. It may result in missing data. The internal validity of the study is compromised if too many patients are lost during the follow-up period. A general rule of thumb is that the loss to follow-up rate should not be more than 20% of the sample.

E. Correct answer: It is a type of observational study. Cohort studies and case–control studies are two primary types of observational study that help in exploring the association between a disease and its association to an agent the patient is exposed to. Cohort studies can be prospective or retrospective.

Morabia A (2004). *A History of Epidemiologic Methods and Concepts*. Basel, Switzerland: Birkhaeuser Verlag, pp. 1–405.

Song JW, Chung KC (2010). Observational studies: Cohort and case-controlled studies. *Plast Reconstr Surg*, **126**(6), 2234–42.

11. B. Relatively inexpensive to conduct such a study.

A. One of the disadvantages of such a study is that control over the extraneous variables may be inadequate.

B. Correct answer: It is relatively inexpensive to conduct such a study.

C. It is important to define the inclusion and exclusion criteria explicitly prior to the selection process.

D. Such studies are relatively quick to conduct.

E. Subjects may be sampled from a hospital, be members of a community, or from a doctor's individual practice. A subset of these subjects will be eligible for the study.

Song JW, Chung KC (2010). Observational studies: Cohort and case-controlled studies. *Plast Reconstr Surg*, **126**(6), 2234–42.

12. C. Cross-sectional survey.

A. In case–control studies, the patients undergo history and examination to find out any factors, which could have predisposed the disease/condition. The outcome status is identified at the outset of the project. The patients are then categorized as cases and controls. The controls are selected from the same population but without the condition.

B. Please see the answers in question 10.

C. Correct answer: In this type of observational study, the data is analysed and collected from a population at a specific point in time. A particular problem of such a study is the inability to obtain responses from the subjects, which may introduce bias in the outcome measure.

D. Both D and E are incorrect for obvious reasons. Please see other questions in the evidence-based medicine (EBM) sections for RCTs.

E. See answer D. Single-blinded control trials are randomized trials where the researchers, doctors, and patients in a clinical trial are prevented from knowing which study group each patient is in, so that the results could not be influenced.

Health Knowledge (2009). Cross-sectional Studies. Available at: http://www.healthknowledge.org.uk/public-health-textbook/research-methods/1a-epidemiology/cs-as-is/cross-sectional-studies

Song JW, Chung KC (2010). Observational studies: Cohort and case-controlled studies. *Plast Reconstr Surg*, **126**(6), 2234–42.

1. **A 32-year-old man has had malaise, headache, and myalgia for few days. He returned from a camping holiday in the woods with his family one week ago for the summer holidays. His BP is 125/84 mmHg, HR 82 bpm, RR 18 breaths/min, SaO$_2$ 98% in room air and temperature 38.1°C. He has flat discrete erythematous target lesions on the left calf, left buttock, and left thigh. Which is the single most appropriate statement?**

   A. Enzyme-linked immunosorbent assay (ELISA) is not useful in this case
   B. Immunoglobulins are only detectable in the first three months after the onset of symptoms
   C. Serological testing is the most practical and useful means of confirming clinical diagnosis
   D. Serum IgG levels are expected to be highest at this stage of illness
   E. Serum IgM levels are the highest six weeks after the onset of symptoms

2. **A 29-year-old female entertainer has just returned from a four-week tour in Tanzania. She became unwell on the flight back to the United Kingdom and arrives in the emergency department (ED) via ambulance, complaining of chills, headache, abdominal pains, lethargy, and difficulty breathing. Her BP is 115/76 mmHg, HR 101 bpm, RR 23 breaths/min, SaO$_2$ 97% in room air and temperature 39.8°C. She is diaphoretic and looks pale. She has palpable hepatosplenomegaly. Which is the single most appropriate statement with regards to parasitic spread?**

   A. Female psorophora mosquitoes serve as an animal vector
   B. *P. Falciparum* has a low risk of morbidity and mortality from end-organ damage
   C. *P. Falciparum*, if successfully treated, can still result in relapse
   D. *P. Malariae* exclusively offers an acute course of illness
   E. *P. Vivax* has a high risk of cerebral manifestations of disease including convulsions and coma

3. **A 21-year-old male student has just returned from India after six months. He has weight loss, a productive cough, night sweats, and difficulty in breathing. His BP is 125/68 mmHg, HR 111 bpm, RR 20 breaths/min, SaO$_2$ 95% in room air, temperature 38.5°C. He appears cachectic, pale, and sweaty. There is diffuse consolidation throughout his lung fields and significant hilar shadowing possibly lymphadenopathy on chest X-ray. Which one of the following statements is correct with regards to the mechanism of fever relating to this case?**

A. Lipopolysaccharide (LPS) is an example of an endogenous pyrogen and is not the cause of fever

B. Prostaglandin E$_2$ (PGE$_2$) lowers the set point temperature of the body

C. Pyrogens initiate the synthesis and release of cytokines, triggering the arachidonic acid pathway

D. Temperature is regulated by pituitary gland

E. The autonomic nervous system prevents heat loss by vasodilatation and sweating

4. **A 55-year-old gentleman has redness, swelling, and pain over his left knee joint for couple of days. He is known to have gout and alcohol excess. He is unable to fully weight bear on his left leg. His knee feels warm and his movement is restricted. The Hb is 134 g/dL, undifferentiated WCC 13.2 × 10^9/L, CRP 125 mg/L, creatinine 85 micromol/L, urea 6.5 mmol/L. Which is the single most appropriate statement with regards to inflammatory markers?**

A. CRP appears in the serum within days to weeks of inflammation or injury

B. CRP levels are unaffected by the presence of chronic liver disease (CLD)

C. Erythrocyte sedimentation rate (ESR) may be normal or elevated in this patient

D. Increase in serum ESR is detected earlier than CRP rise and correlates directly

E. Inflammatory markers in the acute-phase response are specific

5. **A seven-year-old boy has difficulty in breathing. His mother provides a history of mild asthma and mentions he had tried kiwi for the first time today. He has no known allergies and is otherwise well. His throat is inflamed, itchy, and has diffuse urticarial skin changes. How best can this patient's hypersensitivity reaction be classified?**

A. Acute: mediated by immunoglobulin E (IgE) antibody causing mast cell degranulation and release of inflammatory mediators

B. Antigen-antibody complex: complements C3a and C5a cause mast cells to degranulate

C. Cell-mediated: T-cell dependent recruitment of a range of white cell types such as macrophages and eosinophils

D. Cytotoxic: mediated by IgM or IgG and complement or phagocytic involvement

E. This is not an immunological hypersensitivity reaction and should be classified as 'food intolerance'

6. **A 35-year-old African female has fever and chest pain. She has had pain in the small joints of her hands for the last few months and been using paracetamol to control this. She is otherwise well. There is regular sinus rhythm with global ST-segment saddling on her electrocardiogram (ECG). Her BP is 118/84 mmHg, HR 98 bpm, RR 21 breaths/min, SaO$_2$ 96% in room air, temperature 37.9°C. A malar rash, which crosses the bridge of her nose with nasolabial sparing, is visible. Which is the single best statement with regards to diagnostic serum markers in this patient?**

A. C3 and C4 complement levels always correlate poorly with disease flare

B. CRP levels will be significantly elevated in this condition

C. Double-stranded DNA (dsDNA) antibodies are specific and their presence would be diagnostic

D. ESR is a specific marker for disease activity and its level would dictate prognosis and response to treatment

E. The absence of antinuclear antibodies (ANA) rules out the possibility of an autoimmune condition

7. **A 26-year-old policewoman has had complications from recent surgery on perianal fistulae. She is known to have Crohn's disease, and has had a previous right-sided hemicolectomy. She is on azathioprine, ciprofloxacin, and paracetamol for pain. She is concerned about pain and discharge of pus around one of her four fistulae. Which one of the following statements best describes the intended mechanism of immunosuppression of azathioprine?**

A. Asplenia

B. Bone marrow suppression

C. Complement deficiency

D. Lymphoma

E. Lymphopenia

8. **A 23-year-old male arrives with the police in the ED department. He is under the influence of alcohol and has been arrested for getting into an altercation. The police have bought him for assessment as he has sustained abrasions on his knuckles and knees. He is sporting a 4 cm jagged laceration on his forehead. On examination, it is determined that his forehead will need suturing. Which one statement is true with regards to wound healing?**

A. Alcohol consumption does not affect wound healing and increases the body's resistance against bacteria.

B. Capillary permeability increases to allow neutrophils and monocytes to scavenge debris.

C. Epithelialization via meiosis can be impeded in the presence of eschar or debris.

D. Fibroblasts synthesize and deposit highly disorganized collagen compounds two to four hours after injury.

E. Eosinophils release chemotactic agents to stimulate fibroblast proliferation and neovascularization.

9. **A 32-year-old female has had purulent vaginal discharge for the last five days. She started getting lower abdominal pains and dysuria two days ago. The abdominal pain has worsened. She noticed new dyspareunia on the previous night. She has a long-term partner with whom she has frequent unprotected sexual intercourse as she has long-term contraception in the form of the copper coil. Which one of the following statements is most correct in the diagnosis of pelvic inflammatory disease?**

A. In clinical practice, N. *Gonorrhoeae* and C. *Trachomatis* are distinguished by separate culture medium growths

B. N. *Gonorrhoeae* and C. *Trachomatis* are examples of anaerobic bacteria

C. Nucleic acid amplification testing (NAATs) has been estimated to have a sensitivity of approximately 90% and a specificity of approximately 99% for C. *Trachomatis*

D. The causative organisms for pelvic inflammatory disease in 22–28% of cases are N. *Gonorrhoeae* and C. *Trachomatis*

E. The growth of gram positive rods in agar culture medium is consistent with *Neisseria Gonorrhoeae* infection

10. **A 22-year-old nursery nurse has had acute onset diarrhoea and vomiting for seven days after eating a selection of food three hours prior to the start of her symptoms for a colleague's leaving party. She had cramping abdominal pain and feels dry and unable to tolerate any liquids or solids. Her BP is 98/60 mmHg, HR 102 bpm, RR 15 breaths/ minute, SaO$_2$ 99% in room air, temperature 37.6°C. The urine dip has ketones +++. Her capillary refill time is three seconds and she has mild generalized abdominal tenderness. Which of the following statements describes the most likely physiological mechanism for this patient's diarrhoea?**

A. Cellular damage to intestinal mucosa resulting in over-secretion of water, electrolytes, blood, mucus, and plasma proteins

B. Cytotoxins increase cellular permeability and cause over-secretion of water and electrolytes

C. Hypermotility of the bowel smooth muscle increases the interface of luminal contents and intestinal mucosa, increasing water, and electrolyte absorption

D. Osmotic movement of water into the intestinal lumen and its inability to reabsorb it

E. Osmotic effect of lipids due to malabsorption

11. **A 42-year-old female has had severe abdominal pain. She has taken** *X* **excess of alcohol in the past. She stopped drinking two years ago after a diagnosis of liver cirrhosis. She is due to go on holiday and has stopped her laxatives to reduce the frequency of her stools. Her abdomen is tense and tender due to ascites and she is noticeably jaundiced. Which one of the statements is correct with regards to the mechanism for jaundice in this patient?**

   A. Clinical jaundice is evident when serum bilirubin concentrations are lower than 2.0–3.0 mg/dL (34–51 μmol/L)

   B. The bilirubin has not undergone glucoronidation by the failing hepatocytes

   C. The hepatocyte has failed to excrete unconjugated bilirubin

   D. The overproduction of heme results in higher amounts of biliverdin

   E. There is a physical obstruction preventing bilirubin from being excreted into the intestine

12. **A 45-year-old father-of-two is generally feeling unwell with a fever for the last five days. In the last two days his voice has become uncharacteristically hoarse, and he is finding it painful to swallow. His pharynx is inflamed, tonsils are red and enlarged with white streaking, but not occluding the airway. He has tender cervical lymphadenopathy. His clinical observations and blood tests are normal. Which statement is correct with regards to the causative organism of tonsillopharyngitis in the case described?**

   A. 30% of cases are caused by viral infection

   B. Corynebacterium diptheriae is the most common pathogen for bacterial tonsillitis

   C. Group A β-haemolytic Streptococcus (GABHS) affects adults mostly aged 55 to 75

   D. Non-GABHS streptococcus species and GABHS can be clinically indistinguishable

   E. The pathogen is transmitted faeco-orally

13. **An 82-year-old woman has been brought in from her nursing home. She has reduced oral intake, worsening confusion, and drowsiness over the last week. She has a chesty cough but is unable to expectorate. Her BP is 111/62 mmHg, HR 95 bpm, RR 21 breaths/ min SaO$_2$ 92% in room air, temperature 35.6°C. There are crackles throughout in the chest but louder in the right mid-lower zone. Which one of the following statements is most appropriate with regards to risk factors for pneumonia?**

   A. Hospital-acquired pneumonias on the whole are caused by similar pathogens responsible for community acquired infections and therefore can be treated with the same antimicrobials

   B. Lungs are prone to infection due to the presence of potential pathogens within lung parenchyma

   C. Mucociliary clearance and elastic recoil decline with increasing age

   D. Obstructive respiratory disease such as chronic obstructive pulmonary disease (COPD) does not increase the likelihood of contracting pneumonia

   E. The flu vaccine prevents lower respiratory tract infections caused by streptococcus pneumoniae

14. **A 48-year-old business man has been feeling generally unwell for the last few weeks and short of breath with a new cough. He is on simvastatin, propranolol for anxiety, and Truvada. His BP is 152/89 mmHg, HR 98 bpm, RR 23 breaths/min, SaO$_2$ 86% in room air, temperature 38.3°C. One month ago, at his last hospital appointment, his CD4 count was 151 cells/µL. Which one of the following statements is not a sign or symptom of pneumocystis pneumonia?**

    A. Diffuse interstitial infiltrates on plain chest radiograph
    B. Elevated serum lactate dehydrogenase (LDH)
    C. Hypoxia
    D. Shortness of breath
    E. Productive cough

15. **A 48-year-old Caribbean man is found shaking and anxious in the middle of the road by paramedics. He stopped drinking alcohol 18 hours ago following an argument with his partner, after a 12-year history of alcohol excess. His observations are: BP 109/89 mmHg, HR 128 bpm, RR 20 breaths per minute, SaO$_2$ 95% in room air, temperature 36.1°C. While he is awaiting assessment, he vomits a significant amount of blood. His Hb is 112 g/dL, platelets 160 x 109 /L, MCV 102.6 femtoL. Which single option is the most likely cause for his anaemia?**

    A. Acute upper gastrointestinal bleed
    B. Alpha thalassaemia
    C. Bone marrow failure
    D. Folate deficiency
    E. Iron deficiency

16. **A six-year-old South Asian boy has had jaundice for 24 hours. He has yellow sclera and, palpable liver, and spleen. His father had jaundice as a child and since has avoided beans, aspirin, and antimalarial drugs. The child might have ingested beans in his chilli at a Mexican restaurant for a birthday party the day before. Which one of the following is NOT an expected laboratory finding for G6PD?**

    A. A positive direct antiglobulin test (Coomb's test)
    B. Decreased haptoglobin
    C. Elevated lactate dehydrogenase
    D. Heinz inclusion bodies in red cells on blood film
    E. Raised urinary haemoglobin

17. An 86-year-old gentleman has had slow bleeding from the tooth socket after the extraction of a molar tooth six days ago. The patient is on warfarin for a proximal deep vein thrombosis (DVT), which he has continued before and after the operation. Today his international normalized ratio (INR) is 2.3. Which single statement best describes the mechanism of impaired haemostasis by which this man is bleeding?

    A. Increased plasminogen to plasmin conversion
    B. Indirect inhibition of thrombin
    C. Inhibition of GpIIb/ IIIa complex
    D. Isolated deficiency of factor IX
    E. Reduced formation of active factors II, VII, IX, and X

18. A 55-year-old gentleman is referred from his GP urgently in light of recent blood test results. His bloods show: Hb 88 g/dL, platelets 122 x 10⁹/L, WCC 67.2 x 10⁹/L. His BP is 134/65 mmHg, HR 78 bpm, RR 15, SaO₂ 98% in room air and temperature 37.8°C. He has dropped two trouser sizes in the last six months and feels increasingly fatigued. He looks pale and has a markedly large palpable spleen. Which one of the following answers is false with regards to this patient's underlying condition?

    A. At higher white cell counts, the viscosity of blood can increase and lead to vaso-occlusive events
    B. If untreated, this disease could undergo blast transformation
    C. The blood film will show multiple small mature looking lymphocytes
    D. The bone marrow aspirate will be hypercellular with many myeloid progenitor cells
    E. The patient is likely to have a translocation involving chromosomes 9 and 22

19. A 24-year-old Nigerian woman is referred from outpatient radiology with a significantly widened mediastinum and hilar lymphadenopathy. She has been suffering with drenching night sweats, weight loss and fatigue for eight months, and she has noticed her neck seems bigger in size than it was previously. Which one of the following statements regarding lymphoma is appropriate?

    A. Epstein-Barr Virus is associated with Non-Hodgkin's lymphoma
    B. Involvement of lymph nodes on either side of the diaphragm is classed as stage II Hodgkin's
    C. Most likely diagnosis is Non-Hodgkin's lymphoma (NHL)
    D. Reed–Sternberg cells on histology distinguish Hodgkin's and Non-Hodgkin's
    E. Most lymphomas are T-cell in origin

20. **A 78-year-old lady has had a fall onto outstretched hands. Her forearm and wrist are swollen, painful, and deformed. There is volar displacement of a fractured distal radius on X-ray. Which is the single best statement regarding callus formation?**

   A. Callus consists of granulation tissue on fracture surfaces
   B. Callus formation begins within the trabecular space
   C. Callus formation is reduced in bones where periosteum is deficient
   D. Procallus is formed by deposition of calcium phosphate
   E. Remodelling of the callus is adversely affected by exercise

21. **A 34-year-old carpenter has accidentally sawn through the medial aspect of his left thumb. The wound is exposed down to the bone and bleeding. He has altered sensation on the medial side of the tip of his thumb. Which is the single best statement regarding peripheral neuronal injury?**

   A. Axonal skeleton is unaffected by injury
   B. Myelin sheath is reinforced by inflammatory markers post injury
   C. Repair and regeneration in central nervous system (CNS) injury is faster than the peripheral nervous system (PNS)
   D. Schwann cells help macrophages clear debris from degeneration
   E. The neurolemma degenerates post injury

1. C. Serological testing is the most practical and useful means of confirming clinical diagnosis.

A. Testing with ELISA is the gold standard for confirming a laboratory diagnosis of Lyme disease. In isolation, ELISA has sensitivity of 89% and a specificity of 72%. However, in patients with a low clinical probability, ELISA is likely to yield false positive results and can occur with the presence of other viral illnesses.

B. IgG antibodies, and, at times IgM antibodies, can persist for several years even after treatment and in the absence of symptoms. Presence of IgM/IgG is not diagnostic of current infection.

C. Correct answer: Although diagnosis of Lyme disease is primarily clinical, serology helps to confirm this. It is not without limitations however and need to be interpreted carefully, especially in the context of when the disease was contracted. The antibody response to *Borellia* develops slowly and can be blunted by the use of early antibiotic treatment.

D. IgG antibodies may be detectable two months after exposure and peaks at approximately 12 months.

E. Early in the infection, IgM levels may be undetectable. Serum IgM titres peak at three to six weeks after the onset of illness and return to pre-infection levels at four to six weeks.

Bolgiano EB, Sexton J (2010). Tick-borne illnesses. In: Marx JA, Hockberger RS, Wall RM (Eds.). *Rosen's Emergency Medicine*, 7th edition. Philadelphia, PA: Mosby Elsevier.

2. A. Female psorophora mosquitoes serve as an animal vector.

A. Correct answer: Species of the female Anopheles mosquito is the primary vector of malaria to humans. The *Psorophora* genus breeds in similar stagnant bodies of water, and tend to feed on larger mammals and, occasionally, humans.

B. Plasmodium Falciparum is a medical emergency as patients can deteriorate rapidly, progressing from acute fever to rigors and severe multiorgan failure and ultimately death. It is associated with typical features of cerebral malaria (oedema and encephalopathy), hypoglycaemia, and DIC.

C. Successfully treated P. Falciparum does not cause future relapse. However, *P. Vivax* and *P. Ovale*, although causing more benign illness, have a higher risk of resulting in relapses.

D. *P. Malariae* typically has a chronic course which can continue from months to years. Hepatosplenomegaly can develop over this time due to increased cellularity from the immune response; parasites can distend Kuppfer cells. Erythrocytes, which can also play host, reside in the sinusoidal system of the spleen.

E. *P. Vivax, P. Ovale*, and *P. Malariae* cause a milder form of malaria.

Bolgiano EB, Sexton J (2010). Tick-borne illnesses. In: Marx JA, Hockberger RS, Wall RM (Eds.). *Rosen's Emergency Medicine*, 7th edition. Philadelphia, PA: Mosby Elsevier.

3. C. Pyrogens initiate the synthesis and release of cytokines, triggering the arachidonic acid pathway.

A. Lipopolysaccaride (LPS) is an example of exogenous toxin found in the cell walls of gram-negative bacteria and mycobacterium. Lipopolysaccharide binding protein (LBP) binds to LPS forming a complex which triggers cytokine release following contact with macrophages. Exogenous pyrogens make use of endogenous factors to initiate a fever.

B. Prostaglandin E$_2$ (PGE$_2$) raises the set point by means of conserving heat such as peripheral vasoconstriction and increased muscle tone causing shivering. Fever is sustained until levels of pyrogens and PGE$_2$ decrease.

C. Correct answer: Endogenous pyrogens are produced by activated immune cells, being released into the circulation and binding with endothelial receptors and those on other leucocytes. PGE$_2$ is produced by the hypothalamus in response to cytokine release such as interleukin 1 (IL-1), IL-6, interferon, and tumour necrosis factor (TNF) and is a product of the arachidonic acid pathway. Cycloxogenase inhibitors block production of PGE$_2$.

D. Body temperature is controlled by the pre-optic area of the hypothalamus to maintain it between 36.0 to 37.8°C. Blood temperature is detected by neurons in the anterior hypothalamus which in turn uses mechanisms to rectify variations.

E. Vasodilatation and sweating occur in hyperthermic states in a bid to lower temperature by dissipating heat. Fever is not a hyperthermic state.

Blum FC (2010). Fever in the adult patient. In: Marx JA, Hockberger RS, Wall RM, (Eds.), *Rosen's Emergency Medicine*, 7th edition. Philadelphia, PA: Mosby Elsevier.

4. C. ESR may be normal or elevated in this patient.

A. CRP appears in the serum within hours of infection or tissue inflammation, peaking at 48 hours.

B. CRP is produced in the liver and its production is relatively unaffected by any other factors, however in CLD, CRP levels are often markedly elevated. This is thought to be due to damaged hepatocytes and increased macrophage activity within the liver.

C. Correct answer: ESR level is thought to be dependent on elevation of fibrinogen as an acute-phase protein, which has a half-life of approximately one week. It results in the ESR being raised for longer despite removal of the inflammatory stimulus.

D. Serum CRP levels rise more quickly than ESR and tends therefore to be the blood test of choice in an acute situation. ESR may therefore be normal while CRP is elevated. CRP returns to normal more quickly than ESR in response to therapy.

E. The acute-phase response is rapid and unspecific, with certain proteins including complement components and enzyme inhibitors rising rapidly in serum to deal with any type of damage.

Adam BA, Lowery III DW (2010). Arthritis. In: Marx JA, Hockberger RS, Wall RM, (Eds.), *Rosen's Emergency Medicine*, 7th edition. Philadelphia, PA: Mosby Elsevier.

Liu S, Ren J, Xia Q, et al. (2013). Preliminary case-control study to evaluate diagnostic values of C-reactive protein and erythrocyte sedimentation rate in differentiating active Crohn's disease from intestinal lymphoma, intestinal tuberculosis and Behcet's syndrome. *Am J Med Sci*, **346**(6), 467–72.

Playfair JHL, Chain BM (Eds.) (2009). Acute inflammation. In: *Immunology at a Glance*, 9th edition. Oxford, UK: Blackwell Publishing.

5. A.   Acute: mediated by IgE antibody causing mast cell degranulation and release of inflammatory mediators.

A. Correct answer: Type I—the most common form of hypersensitivity includes mild allergies such as hay fever through to anaphylaxis. IgE synthesis is induced by a particular antigen. This attaches to mast cells and causes a calcium influx into the cell and subsequent degranulation of the mast cell. Systemic release causes anaphylaxis, whereas localized release limits the reaction depending on the site of exposure. Atopic individuals have raised circulating IgE serum levels.

B. Type III—Type III is also IgM/IgG mediated and the antibody-antigen complexes circulate to the perivascular interstitial space, activating the complement pathway. Inflammatory response is largely due to complements C3a and C5a which are responsible for 'anaphylactoid' reactions and act on mast cells. This type is also responsible for transplant rejection.

C. Type IV—Also known as 'delayed' hypersensitivity reaction, helper T-cells recognize the antigen and activate B-cell and macrophage response. This has no relationship to the pathogenesis of anaphylaxis. An example of this is coeliac disease.

D. Type II—complement-fixing IgG or IgM engages a cell-bound antigen, activating the complement pathway and subsequent cell lysis. Complements C3a and C5a can also be involved.

E. Some food 'allergies' do not have an immune-based mechanism such as lactose intolerance. This is usually due to an impaired metabolism secondary to enzyme deficiency and does not result in systemic symptoms.

Playfair JHL, Chain BM (2009). Allergy and anaphylaxis. In: *Immunology at a Glance*, 9th edition. Oxford, UK: Blackwell Publishing.

Train TP, Meulleman RL (2010). Allergy, hypersensitivity and anaphylaxis. In: Marx JA, Hockberger RS, Wall RM (Eds.), *Rosen's Emergency Medicine*, 7th edition. Philadelphia, PA: Mosby Elsevier.

6. C.   Double-stranded DNA (dsDNA) antibodies are specific and their presence would be diagnostic.

A. Impaired clearance of dying cells is a pathway for the development of this systemic autoimmune disease. This includes deficient phagocytic activity and scant serum complement in addition to increased apoptosis. Thus, decreases in complement levels can correlate with disease flare in certain patients.

B. Monocytes are poorer at the uptake of apoptotic cells in systemic lupus erythematosus (SLE), thought to be due to reduced expression of CD44 surface molecules. Complement factors and CRP have a key role in organizing effective phagocytosis. As a result of impaired phagocytosis, CRP levels often remain low unless there is concurrent infection.

C. Correct answer: Antibodies against dsDNA and anti-Smith antibodies are the most specific for SLE and are subtypes of ANAs. dsDNA antibodies are present in 70% of cases and its absence has a strong negative predictive value with only 0.5% of the normal population testing positive for dsDNA antibodies.

D. ESR is non-specific and does not reflect disease activity. Those with ESR of 50–100 mm/hour often show minimal levels of disease activity.

E. When apoptotic material is not removed correctly by phagocytes, they are captured instead by antigen-presenting cells, which lead to development of ANA. Positive ANA occurs in more than 95% of patients with SLE and is positive in many connective tissue and autoimmune disorders. Higher titres correlate with positive predictive value of the disease. 5% of the normal population may also be positive for ANA.

Lisnevskaia L, Murphy G, Isenberg D (2014). Systemic lupus erythematosus. *Lancet*, **384**(9957), 1878–88.

Lehrmann JF, Sercombe CT (2010). Systemic lupus erythematosus and the vasculitidies. In: Marx JA, Hockberger RS, Wall RM (Eds.), *Rosen's Emergency Medicine*, 7th edition. Philadelphia, PA: Mosby Elsevier.

Playfair JHL, Chain BM (Eds.) (2009). Autoimmunity. In: *Immunology at a Glance*, 9th edition. Oxford, UK: Blackwell Publishing.

Rahman A, Isenberg DA (2008). Review article: Systemic lupus erythematosus. *N Engl J Med*, **358**(9), 929–39.

7. E. Lymphopenia.

A. The most common causes of asplenia are removal secondary to trauma, congenital aplasia, or haemoglobinopathies such as sickle cell anaemia. The patient discussed has a fully functioning spleen.

B. The most common side effect of azathioprine is bone marrow suppression, as it is a non-specific immunosuppressant. Severe pancytopaenia has been observed in approximately 1% of patients. But this is not the intended effect of the drug.

C. Complement deficiencies tend to be inherited through an autosomal recessive pattern and are classified as a primary cause for immunodeficiency. This patient has a secondary cause.

D. There is a hypothetical increased risk of lymphoma with azathioprine therapy. However, this is not an intended effect nor is it the cause for immunosuppression.

E. Correct answer: Azathioprine is a precursor of 6-mercaptopurine, which inhibits purine metabolism needed for DNA synthesis. This inhibits the production of B- and T-cells. Other antiproliferative drugs include cyclophosphamide and methotrexate.

Jones J, Bannister BA, Gillespie SH (2006). *Infection: Microbiology and Management* (Chapter 22). Chichester, UK: Wiley-Blackwell.

Playfair JHL, Chain BM (Eds.) (2009). Immunosuppression. In: *Immunology at a Glance*, 9th edition. Oxford, UK: Blackwell Publishing.

8. B. Capillary permeability increases to allow neutrophils and monocytes to scavenge debris.

A. While a serving of wine each day can be beneficial to blood flow, excessive alcohol consumption is detrimental to *wound healing*. It significantly increases the risk of *wound infection* by diminishing the body's resistance to bacteria and other harmful elements.

B. Correct answer: After tissue integrity is breached, platelet activating factors, and inflammatory cytokines are released from endothelial cells. This increases the capillary permeability to allow specialized leucocytes to migrate and clean the wound. Monocytes transform into phagocytic macrophages.

C. Meiosis occurs in specialized gamete cells in humans. Epithelialisation utilizes mitosis, similarly to most repairing tissues.

D. Collagen deposition occurs 48 hours after injury has occurred. Initially it is disorganized and of a gel-like consistency but with enzyme re-structuring, collagen is re-organized into characteristic cross-linked fibrils.

E. Macrophages following their transformation from monocytes are instrumental in development of new blood vessels and initiating fibroblast growth to start tissue repair.

Simon B, Hern Jr HG (2010). Wound management principles. In: Marx JA, Hockberger RS, Wall RM (Eds.), *Rosen's Emergency Medicine*, 7th edition. Philadelphia, PA: Mosby Elsevier.

9. C. NAATs has been estimated to have a sensitivity of approximately 90% and a specificity of approximately 99% for *C. Trachomatis*.

A. Clinically, gonorrhoea is diagnosed by growing *N. Gonorrhoeae* on agar culture medium. Culture for *C. Trachomatis* is useful in only a handful of non-genital specimens, but due to the development of more specific and sensitive testing through NAATs, culturing for chlamydia is infrequently performed. Culturing is often relatively insensitive, detecting only 60–80% of infections in asymptomatic women, and often giving falsely positive results.

B. Both pathogens are example of aerobic bacteria, although anaerobic bacteria can less frequently cause Pelvic inflammatory disease (PID). There can be up to 50% co-existing anaerobic infection in those suffering from chlamydia and/or gonorrhoea.

C. Correct answer: NAAT for chlamydia may be performed on genital or urinary specimens from men and women. Due to improved test accuracy, ease of specimen management, convenience in specimen management, and ease of screening sexually active men and women, the NAATs have largely replaced culture, the historic gold standard for chlamydia diagnosis.

D. *N. Gonorrhoeae* and *C. Trachomatis* are responsible for 75–90% of infections, 10% of which will continue onto PID often with other bacteria present.

E. *N. Gonorrhoeae* is characterized by growth of gram-negative diplococci in chocolate agar culture medium with CO_2. Although there are 11 species of *Neisseria* which colonize humans, only two are known to be pathogens.

Centers for Disease Control and Prevention (2014). Recommendations for the laboratory-based detection of *Chlamydia trachomatis* and *Neisseria gonorrhoeae*—2014. Available at: https://www.cdc.gov/mmwr/preview/mmwrhtml/rr6302a1.htm Retrieved 6 December 2016.

Centers for Disease Control and Prevention (2015). Pelvic inflammatory disease (PID). Clinical manifestations and sequelae. October 2014. Available at: https://www.cdc.gov/std/tg2015/pid.htm Retrieved 21 February, 2015.

Genco C, Wetzler L (Eds.) (2010). *Neisseria: Molecular Mechanisms of Pathogenesis*. Poole, UK: Caister Academic Press.

Haugland S, Thune T, Fosse B, et al. (2010). Comparing urine samples and cervical swabs for chlamydia testing in a female population by means of Strand Displacement Assay (SDA). *BMC Womens Health*, **10**(1), 9.

Sharma H, Tal R, Clark NA, Segars JH (2014). Microbiota and pelvic inflammatory disease. *Seminars in Reproductive Medicine*, **32**(1), 43–9.

10. B. Cytotoxins increase cellular permeability and cause over-secretion of water and electrolytes.

A. This describes inflammatory diarrhoea which encompasses dysentery. It is usually caused by invasive bacteria and parasites such as *Clostridium difficile* or *Entamoeba*. Non-infective causes include chemotherapy or inflammatory bowel disease.

B. Correct answer: This is the correct answer which describes secretory diarrhoea. Most acute cases fall in this category, with pathogens producing cytotoxins. Non-infective causes also include endocrine disorders or medications.

C. Abnormal motility of the bowel is always a component of acute diarrhoea and is also seen in chronic cases. Hypermotility decreases the contact time between luminal content and mucosa and therefore reduced the absorption of the contents.

D. Osmotic diarrhoea usually requires ingestion or malabsorption of osmotically active solutes. Osmotic laxatives are one such cause.

E. Steatorrhoea describes the malabsorption of fats and is another example of osmotic diarrhoea.

Collier RE, Gough JE, Clement PA (2010). Diarrhoea. In: Marx JA, Hockberger RS, Wall RM, (Eds.), *Rosen's Emergency Medicine*, 7th edition. Philadelphia, PA: Mosby Elsevier.

11. B. The bilirubin has not undergone glucoronidation by the failing hepatocytes.

A. Serum bilirubin manifests as visible jaundice when levels rise above the levels stated in (A). Clinical jaundice describes signs such as yellowing of the sclera or skin.

B. Correct answer: Decompensation of alcoholic liver disease is a common cause of hepatocellular jaundice. Bilirubin transport across the hepatocyte may be impaired at any point between the uptake of unconjugated bilirubin, conjugation, and excretion of conjugated bilirubin. Hence in hepatocellular jaundice, both unconjugated and conjugated bilirubin levels rise.

C. Hepatocytes release conjugated bilirubin. In hepatocellular disease, there is usually interference in all major steps of bilirubin metabolism, however, excretion is the rate-limiting step, and usually impaired to the greatest extent.

D. Overproduction of heme is a cause of pre-hepatic jaundice, usually due to increased haemolysis. The heme group is catabolized by heme oxygenase to biliverdin, which is in turn broken down further to bilirubin by biliverdin reductase. Although this is a cause of unconjugated hyperbilirubinaemia, it is not the cause for jaundice in the case described.

E. This describes post-hepatic or obstructive causes for conjugated hyperbilirubinaemia. A common cause of this is gallstones in the common bile duct and an interruption of flow of the bile pigments. This classically presents with dark urine and light stools in the patient with right upper quadrant pain.

Mathew KG (2008). *Medicine: Prep Manual for Undergraduates*, 3rd edition. Gurgaon, India: Elsevier India.

Wheatley MA, Heilpern KL (2010). Jaundice. In: Marx JA, Hockberger RS, Wall RM, (Eds.), *Rosen's Emergency Medicine*, 7th edition. Philadelphia, PA: Mosby Elsevier.

12. D. Non-GABHS streptococcus species and GABHS can be clinically indistinguishable.

A. Viruses are responsible for most cases of tonsillopharyngitis but occur in conjunction with coryzal symptoms and cough. Viral pharyngitis tends to be absent of cervical lymphadenopathy.

B. Diphtherial pharyngitis is a potentially lethal cause but is rare due to childhood vaccinations. It is often characterized by a grey-green pseudomembrane, which extends over the tonsils and soft palate, and can extend further into the larynx leading to airway obstruction.

C. GABHS mostly affects children aged between 5 and 15. 15% of cases affect those over the age of 15 and is rare in patients younger than three years of age, however, during epidemics, the incidence can double.

D. Correct answer: The presentation for 'strep throat' does not necessarily distinguish if the causative organism is Group A or non-group A. Generally, both present without a cough or coryzal symptoms. The Centor Criteria was developed to help decide if pharyngitis was being caused by GABHS and whether it should be treated: the presence of tonsillar exudates, tender lympadhenopathy, absence of cough, history of fever.

E. Most cases of tonsillopharyngitis are transmitted through respiratory secretions and aerosols, although transmission through food and fomite contact is possible.

Melio FR (2010). Upper respiratory tract infections. In: Marx JA, Hockberger RS, Wall RM, (Eds.), *Rosen's Emergency Medicine*, 7th edition. Philadelphia, PA: Mosby Elsevier.

13. C. Mucociliary clearance and elastic recoil decline with increasing age.

A. Patients coming from a healthcare setting (nursing homes, hospital, or extended care) are at higher risk of multidrug resistant pathogens such as pseudomonas aeruginosa or methicillin-resistant *Staphylococcus aureus* (MRSA) and the mortality associated is higher. They subsequently have a different treatment policy to community acquired infection.

B. Healthy lungs are a sterile environment. The upper respiratory tract and saliva is heavily colonized with both anaerobic and aerobic bacteria.

C. Correct answer: Older people are at greater risk of pneumonia due to decline of mucociliary clearance, poor elasticity, and reduced humoral and cellular immunity. With ageing, the quality of elastin produced deteriorates and therefore the recoil of alveoli is reduced. This increases the dead space due to smaller, less effect chest movement.

D. Cigarette smoking damaged mucociliary function as well as macrophage activity.

E. Both the flu and pneumococcal vaccines are offered in autumn and winter to elevated risk patient groups in the United Kingdom such as those above 65 years old, children, pregnant women, and those who are immunocompromised. *S. pneumoniae* is the most common organism responsible for community acquired pneumonias and the pneumococcal vaccine reduced the likelihood of serious infection. The annual flu vaccine is less specific, covering an umbrella of rapidly evolving influenza viruses (most commonly being caused by influenza type A).

Moran GJ, Talan DA (2010). Lower respiratory tract infections. In: Marx JA, Hockberger RS, Wall RM, (Eds.), *Rosen's Emergency Medicine*, 7th edition. Philadelphia, PA: Mosby Elsevier.

14. E. Productive cough.

A. The classic radiograph findings are bilateral interstitial infiltrates that begin in the perihilar region. Appearances can vary considerably, and other radiological signs include pleural effusion, hilar lymphadenopathy, cavitation, and lobar consolidation.

B. LDH is released during cell breakdown and can act as a surrogate marker for damage to alveoli in this case by pneumocystis jirovicii.

C. PCP damages the interstitial, fibrous tissue of the lungs, causing thickening of the alveolar septa leading to significant hypoxia due to impaired gas exchange.

D. Hypoxia, along with high arterial CO_2 levels, stimulates hyperventilatory effort, thereby causing dyspnoea.

E. Correct answer: Classically, PCP produces a non-productive cough as the viscosity of sputum is too thin for expectoration. This can be frustrating as gram staining of the sputum provides definitive histological diagnosis and therefore requires bronchoscopy and lavage for collection.

Hughes WT (1996). Pneumocystis carinii. In: Barron S (Ed.), *Barron's Medical Microbiology*, 4th edition. Galveston, Texas: University of Texas Medical Branch.

Moran GJ, Talan DA (2010). Lower respiratory tract infections. In: Marx JA, Hockberger RS, Wall RM, (Eds.), *Rosen's Emergency Medicine*, 7th edition. Philadelphia, PA: Mosby Elsevier.

15. D. Folate deficiency.

A. Anaemias which typically affect MCV are chronic in nature and caused by decreased red blood cell production. Although a singular acute upper gastrointestinal bleeding (UGI) bleed is a cause for a drop in haemoglobin and platelets, it does not affect the MCV.

B. Alpha Thalassaemia can range from asymptomatic carrier status to prenatal death and is seen in Asian and African American populations. It is characterized by microcytic, hypochromic anaemia where defective globin chains decrease haemoglobin synthesis and results in ineffective erythropoiesis.

C. Primary bone marrow involvement tends to result in normocytic anaemia and is a more challenging diagnosis to make where reticulocyte count is helpful which reflect red cell production.

D. Correct answer: Folic acid is absorbed in the duodenum and jejunum and is derived in the diet from green vegetables, cereal. Depletion in folate takes two to four months to affect haemoglobin and MCV. In conditions such as alcoholism or malabsorption syndromes result in macrocytic anaemias. Coenzyme derivatives of B12 and folate are responsible for DNA synthesis which results in larger red cells.

E. Iron deficiency is a common cause for microcytic anaemia, seen often in women of childbearing age and older patients with faecal occult blood loss. Bone marrow and cytochrome iron stores need to be deplete before a change in red blood cell (RBC) size is seen.

Janz TG, Hamilton GC (2010). Anemia, polycythemia, and white blood cell disorders. In: Marx JA, Hockberger RS, Wall RM, (Eds.), *Rosen's Emergency Medicine*, 7th edition. Philadelphia, PA: Mosby Elsevier.

16. A. A positive direct antiglobulin test (Coomb's test).

A. Correct answer: DAT/Coomb's test detects the presence of antibodies or complement on red cell membranes. The test uses rabbit IgG serum which reacts with IgG, IgM, or C3 proteins which can coat red cells, and results in agglutination of RBCs depending on the size of the immunoglobulin. G6PD is an example of an intrinsic haemolytic anaemia secondary to enzyme defect and therefore results in a negative DAT.

B. Haptoglobin binds with haemoglobin on a 1:1 ratio reflecting saturation and degradation of haemoglobin by the liver, and therefore absence of free plasma haptoglobin raises suspicion of an intravascular haemolysis.

C. LDH is released when the RBC is degraded peripherally or in marrow and is non-specific as to the cause of haemolysis.

D. Haemoglobin is irreversibly denatured by oxidants resulting in production of reactive oxygen species and early cell death. Heinz Bodies are clumps of damaged haemoglobin within red cells. These prematurely lysed cells are removed by macrophages in the spleen. The blood film often takes three weeks post the acute haemolytic episode to show this.

E. Haemoglobin which is unbound to haptoglobin is excreted by the kidneys and result in haemoglobinuria.

Ballinger A (2012). Haematological disease. In: Kumar P, Clark M (Eds.), *Essentials of Kumar and Clark's Clinical Medicine*, 5th edition. Philadelphia, PA: Saunders Elsevier.

Janz TG, Hamilton GC (2010). Anemia, polycythemia, and white blood cell disorders. In: Marx JA, Hockberger RS, Wall RM, (Eds.), *Rosen's Emergency Medicine*, 7th edition. Philadelphia, PA: Mosby Elsevier.

17. E. Reduced formation of active factors II, VII, IX, and X.

A. Fibrinolytic drugs such as streptokinase and alteplase hydrolyse peptide bonds in plasminogen to yield active enzyme plasmin which promotes clot lysis.

B. Heparins inactivate thrombin and factor Xa (which facilitates activation of factors Va, VIIIa, IXa, and XI, and converts fibrinogen to fibrin) via the activation of antithrombin.

C. Intimal injury exposes subendothelial collagen and von-Willebrand factor for platelet glycoproteins to bind to. The antiplatelet drug Clopidogrel in its biologically active form inhibits platelet aggregation.

D. Haemophilia Type B is an inherited deficiency of factor IX and effects 1 in 30,000 males.

E. Correct answer: Warfarin prevents the vitamin-K dependent γ-carboxylation of factors II, VII, IX, X to their biologically active forms, which affects both the intrinsic and extrinsic clotting pathway.

Ballinger A (2012). Haematological disease. In: Kumar P, Clark M (Eds.), *Essentials of Kumar and Clark's Clinical Medicine*, 5th edition. Philadelphia, PA: Saunders Elsevier.

18. C. The blood film will show multiple small mature looking lymphocytes.

A. Although it is relatively rare for hyperleukocytosis to occur, the condition does cause leukostasis and cause problems with pulmonary ventilation-perfusion mismatch, visual impairment, and deafness.

B. Blast crisis refers to transformation of chronic myeloid leukaemia (CML) into an acute (usually myeloid) leukaemia which results in an overproduction of premature blast cells by the bone marrow seen on biopsy. It is rare, aggressive, and has a high mortality.

C. Correct answer: CML is characterized by proliferation of the myeloid cell line which results in overproduction of mature and intermediate granulocytes. Lymphocytes are derived from lymphoid progenitor cells and form a distinct leukaemia.

D. The bone marrow aspirate shows a high quantity of myeloid progenitor cells.

E. The reciprocal translocation describes the Philadelphia chromosome which is associated with 95% of CML cases and results in a fusion gene, producing a protein with enhanced tyrosine kinase activity. It thereby alters cell growth and apoptosis.

Ballinger A (2012). Malignant disease. In: Kumar P, Clark M (Eds.), *Essentials of Kumar and Clark's Clinical Medicine*, 5th edition. Philadelphia, PA: Saunders Elsevier.

Janz TG, Hamilton GC (2010). Anemia, polycythemia, and white blood cell disorders. In: Marx J, Hockberger RS, Walls RM (Eds.), *Rosen's Emergency Medicine*, 8th edition (pp. 75–80). Philadelphia, PA: Saunders Elsevier.

19. D. Reed–Sternberg cells on histology distinguish Hodgkin's and Non-Hodgkin's.

A. EBV (or Human herpesvirus-4) is most commonly associated with infectious mononucleosis by transforming infected B-cells. It is also strongly associated with African Burkitt's Lymphoma and nasopharyngeal carcinoma. There is some association with Hodgkin's lymphoma especially in immunocompromised patients.

B. The staging of Hodgkin's is based on nodal involvement. It is rare to get NHL in patients under the age of 40. Most young patients with lymphoma tend to have Hodgkin's. See Table 6.1.

C. Reed–Sternberg cells are binucleate or multinucleate malignant B-lymphocytes in a background of multiple benign small lymphocytes and histiocytes. Their presence is pathognomonic of Hodgkin's lymphoma and helps differentiate histologically between NHL.

ᴸ

D. Correct answer: Approximately 70% cases of lymphoma are of B-cell in origin and 30% are T-cell in origin.

Table 6.1 Hodgkin's staging

Stage	Definition
I	Single lymph node or single extra-nodal organ or site.
II	≥2 node regions/extra-nodal sites on the same side of the diaphragm.
III	Lymph nodes involved on either side of the diaphragm ± splenic/localized extra-nodal involvement.
IV	Diffuse or disseminated involvement of ≥ extra-nodal tissue ± lymph node involvement.

Ballinger A (2012). Malignant disease. In: Kumar P, Clark M (Eds.), *Essentials of Kumar and Clark's Clinical Medicine*, 5th edition. Philadelphia, PA: Saunders Elsevier.

Haile-Mariam T, Polis MA (2010). Viral illnesses. In: Marx J, Hockberger RS, Walls RM (Eds.), *Rosen's Emergency Medicine*, 8th edition (pp. 75–80). Philadelphia, PA: Saunders Elsevier.

20. C. Callus formation is reduced in bones where periosteum is deficient.

A. Callus is formed from deposition of calcium phosphate which aids in identification of bone healing on plain radiographs.

B. Remodelling first starts at the periosteal and endosteal surfaces acting as a biological splint. The outer periosteal layer contains fibroblasts and the inner (cambium) layer consists of progenitor cells for osteoblasts and chondroblasts, responsible for increasing the width of bone.

C. Correct answer: Bones such as the skull or neck of femur are not prone to callus formation due to lack of periosteum as this is where callus formation first begins.

D. Procallus is a result of reabsorption of the initial haematoma that forms with the rupturing of blood vessels at the fracture site. It is a result of inflammation and granulation tissue on the fracture surfaces. As such, it provides little structural rigidity and support to the fractured bone.

E. Exercise increases the rate of healing as it increases blood supply (and consequently oxygen supply) to the musculoskeletal system. It also puts stress onto the bone, aiding it to remodel the callous along weight bearing lines. Chronic hypoxia slows repair.

Geiderman JM, Katz D (2010). General principles of orthopaedic injuries. In: Marx J, Hockberger RS, Walls RM (Eds.), *Rosen's Emergency Medicine*, 8th edition (pp. 75–80). Philadelphia, PA: Saunders Elsevier.

21. D. Schwann cells help macrophages clear debris from degeneration.

A. Axonal injury results in calcium-dependent acute axonal degeneration distal to the injury. The proximal and distal parts of the injured nerve separate within 30 minutes of the insult. The axolemma is the first to swell, followed by complete granular degradation of the axonal skeleton and its organelles.

B. Myelin is a phospholipid membrane produced by Schwann cells in the PNS and oligodendrocytes in the CNS. Myelin needs to be cleared quickly post injury to allow efficient degeneration and subsequent regeneration.

C. Repair in the CNS takes far longer for one main reason: Oligodendrocytes produce myelin sheaths in the CNS, not Schwann cells, and require axonal signals to survive. They undergo apoptosis or enter dormancy when there are no signals, and, unlike Schwann cells, are unable to clear myelin. Consequently, there is a failure to recruit macrophages to aid myelin clearance.

D. Correct answer: Schwann cells are crucial in the first few hours in degrading their own myelin and phagocytosing the remaining extracellular myelin. They release inflammatory cytokines and chemokines in response to sensing injury to attract macrophages, but this can take a few days, and so Schwann cells have a key role in myelin clearance until then.

E. The neuron's neurolemma distal to the injury does not degenerate and remains as a hollow tube. Approximately four days post injury, the proximal neuron to the lesion sprouts towards the remaining tube attracted by growth factors released by Schwann cells. When it makes contact, the sprout can reinnervate the target tissue. This can be hindered by the size of the injury or by the presence of scar tissue.

Kerschensteiner, Schwab ME, Lichtman JW, Misgeld T (2005). *In vivo* imaging of axonal degeneration and regeneration in the injured spinal cord. *Nat Med*, **11**(5), 572–7.

Vargas ME, Barres BA (2007). Why is the Wallerian degeneration of the CNS so slow? *Ann Rev Neurosci*, **30**(1), 153–79.

1. **A 25-year-old man has attended the emergency department (ED) with an injury to his left little finger. He has a dislocation of the proximal interphalangeal joint. A reduction is planned under ulnar nerve block. Which is the single most appropriate site to inject the local anaesthetic agent?**
   A. 1–2 cm proximal to the crease of the wrist between palmaris longus and flexor carpi ulnaris
   B. 1–2 cm proximal to ulnar styloid process
   C. 1–2 cm distal to the crease of the wrist between the tendons of palmaris longus
   D. 3–5 cm distal to the lateral epicondyle on the flexor surface of the forearm
   E. 3–5 cm proximal to the crease of the wrist between palmaris longus and flexor carpi radialis

2. **A 53-year-old man is brought to the ED in cardiac arrest. He has a history of cocaine use but had no other medical history. Pulseless electrical activity is confirmed, and you proceed along the non-shockable side of the cardiac arrest algorithm by delivering IV adrenaline. Spontaneous return of circulation is achieved, and you note sinus rhythm on the monitor. Considering cardiac myocyte action potentials, when does an electrical equilibrium between the movement of potassium and calcium ions occur?**
   A. Phase 0
   B. Phase 1
   C. Phase 2
   D. Phase 3
   E. Phase 4

3. **A 65-year-old man has a dislocation of the right ankle joint after a fall by missing a couple of steps. It needs manipulation and reduction under sedation. Which single statement about propofol is correct?**
   A. Has analgesic properties
   B. Highly lipophilic
   C. Imidazole derivative
   D. Onset of action is usually in two minutes
   E. Patients >55 years of age require 20% higher dose

4. **A 42-year-old male from South East Asia has had weight loss, night sweats, and haemoptysis. Which test is mostly likely to confirm the diagnosis of tuberculosis (TB)?**
   A. Cavitations on chest X-ray (CXR)
   B. Consolidation on CXR
   C. Egg-based culture of bacteria
   D. Thick and thin blood films
   E. Ziehl–Neelsen negative cells on sputum culture

5. **An 82-year-old male has had a fall at home. He could not get up from the floor for about 48 hours because of lack of strength and pain in his right hip joint. In the ED, he is clinically dehydrated. The serum creatinine phosphokinase (CPK) is 7,500 IU/L and he is suspected to have rhabdomyolysis. Which is the single most correct statement with regards to this clinical situation?**
   A. Absence of blood on urine dipstick rules out rhabdomyolysis
   B. Creatine kinase (CK) peaks during the first 12 hours
   C. Decrease in cytoplasmic calcium concentration
   D. Failure of adenosine triphosphate (ATP) dependent cellular transport
   E. Reduction in permeability of sodium ions

6. **A new test is introduced to the department, and trailed. Analysis shows a specificity of 99% and a sensitivity of 22%. In a population of 100 patients who require this test, which of the following statements is true?**
   A. False negatives 1 patient, false positives 78 patients
   B. False negatives 99 patients, false positives 22 patients
   C. True negatives 1 patient, true positives 78 patients
   D. True negatives 99 patients, true positives 22 patients
   E. True positive 99 patients, false positives 22 patients

7. **A 30-year-old tree surgeon has had a laceration to his left forearm. There is a suspicion of median nerve injury. Which single movement is most likely to be affected?**
   A. Adduction of the little finger
   B. Adduction of the wrist joint
   C. Extension of the metatarsophalangeal (MTP) joints
   D. Making a ring with the thumb to the index finger
   E. Supination of the forearm

8. **A 58-year-old homeless man is brought to the ED after being found unconscious in the street. He is a known alcoholic. On arrival, he is maintaining his own airway with normal breath sounds, but his peripheries are cool. He is given fluids and blood glucose measurement is 1.1 mmol/L, therefore intramuscular (IM) glucagon is administered. A repeat blood glucose shows very little improvement. Which of the following is MOST LIKELY to explain the cause of the hypoglycaemia?**

   A. Excessive gluconeogenesis
   B. Exhaustion of hepatic glycogen stores
   C. Hyperinsulinism
   D. Increased glycogen synthase activity
   E. Peripheral tissue resistance to glucagon

9. **A 27-year-old man has sustained a laceration on his left forearm requiring cleaning and suturing. This procedure has been planned to perform under local anaesthesia using lidocaine. Which single statement about lidocaine is correct?**

   A. Allows initiation and propagation of action potential
   B. Conduction is blocked at afferent nerve endings
   C. Larger nerve fibres are affected first followed by the smaller nerves
   D. Stimulates passage of sodium through voltage-gated sodium ion channels
   E. The effect on central nervous system (CNS) is depression

10. **A 30-year-old man has had progressive ascending myopathy. He had diarrhoea with abdominal pain about a week ago. Which is the single most likely organism responsible for the symptoms?**

    A. *Campylobacter jejuni*
    B. *Entamoeba hystolytica*
    C. *Escherichia coli*
    D. *Salmonella typhi*
    E. *Shigella spp*

11. **A 29-year-old male has been brought to the ED following stab injury to his abdomen. His BP is 70/55 mmHg, HR 126 bpm, and RR 28 breaths/min. The massive haemorrhage protocol has been initiated and group O-negative blood requested. Which statement is true?**

    A. Cross-match blood takes a minimum of 45 minutes to be ready
    B. O-negative blood does not have antibodies against A and B
    C. O-negative blood takes 15 minutes to be ready
    D. Type AB blood has antibodies for both
    E. Type specific blood takes a minimum of 30 mins to be ready

12. **A 40-year-old builder has had fall sustaining a supracondylar fracture of the left elbow joint. There is a suspicion of ulnar nerve injury. Which single movement is most likely to be affected?**

A. Reduced adduction of the little finger against resistance

B. Reduced resistance of the forearm when flexing the elbow joint

C. Reduced resistance of the wrist on abduction

D. Weak adduction of the index finger against resistance

E. Weaker supination of the forearm

13. **A five-year-old boy is brought to the ED with cough and coryza. Further questioning reveals several months of fatigue and recurrent ear and throat infections. On examination, he is pale with enlarged cervical and axillary lymph nodes. You note several petechiae across the trunk and hepatosplenomegaly. Blood tests taken on a previous attendance demonstrate the following: WCC 40 x 10^9/L, Hb 76 g/L, Plt 34 x 10^9/L. What is the most likely diagnosis?**

A. Acute lymphoblastic leukaemia

B. Fanconi's anaemia

C. Henoch-Schönlein purpura

D. Idiopathic thrombocytopaenic purpura

E. Non-accidental injury

14. **A 35-year-old man is feeling suicidal. He is bought to the ED where he is found to have lip-smacking and facial twitching. He is on risperidone for schizophrenia. Which single neurotransmitter is associated with his extra-pyramidal features?**

A. Acetylcholine

B. Dopamine

C. Histamine

D. Noradrenaline

E. Serotonin

15. **An 18-month-old male has had a fever, maculopapular rash, and cough. He received some vaccinations until the age of six months, but thereafter, has not received any. At the nursery, he has a friend who recently had same symptoms. What is the single most likely causative organism?**

A. Bordetella pertussis

B. Corynebacterium diphtheriae

C. Haemophilus influenzae

D. Measles

E. Respiratory syncytial virus

16. **A 72-year-old male has had cough and fever. There is right lower lobe consolidation on CXR. Which is the INCORRECT mechanism as a predisposing factor in development of pneumonia?**
    A. Cigarette smoking decreases pulmonary secretions
    B. Diabetes mellitus decreases the white blood cell (WBC) function
    C. Excess alcohol intake affects migration of WBCs
    D. Malnutrition weakens the immune system
    E. Renal disease decreases the antibody formation

17. **A 45-year-old builder has had a fall, sustaining a Monteggia fracture of the left forearm. There is a suspicion of radial nerve injury. Which single movement is most likely to be affected?**
    A. Extension of the elbow
    B. Flexion of the fingers
    C. Flexion of the wrist
    D. Pronation of the forearm
    E. Supination of the forearm

18. **An 18-year-old man is brought to the ED with shortness of breath. He has a history of viral-induced wheeze as a child but is otherwise well. On auscultation, widespread expiratory wheeze is heard. He responds well to nebulized salbutamol and is discharged home with inhalers. Which one of the following results shows his expected pulmonary function tests at the time of the attack?**
    A. FEV_1 is decreased; forced vital capacity (FVC) is decreased; FEV_1:FVC <0.7
    B. FEV_1 is decreased; FVC is unchanged; FEV_1:FVC >0.7
    C. FEV_1 is increased; FVC is decreased; FEV_1:FVC >0.7
    D. FEV_1 is increased; FVC is increased; FEV_1:FVC <0.7
    E. FEV_1 is unchanged; FVC is increased; FEV_1:FVC <0.7

19. **A 35-year-old man has been brought to the ED with alcohol intoxication. He has alcohol dependency. Which is the least likely effect of acute alcohol ingestion?**
    A. Blocks glucose uptake in initial stages
    B. Degradation of adenine nucleotides may cause acute gout
    C. Diuresis is because of inhibition of pituitary antidiuretic hormone (ADH) secretion
    D. Hyperactivity occurs because of removal of inhibitory effects
    E. Vomiting is solely because of local gastric effect

20. **A 22-year-old builder has been bitten on his right arm by a bat while doing construction work in a derelict building. He has a puncture wound on the right arm. What should be the next immediate step?**

    A. Administer antirabies antibodies

    B. Administer tetanus booster only

    C. Administer tetanus booster and immunoglobulin

    D. Commence rabies vaccination

    E. Thorough wound cleaning in soapy water

21. **An 82-year-old male has been brought to the ED by his daughter, who informs you that he has had fever and cough. His BP is 162/94 mmHg, HR 116 bpm, RR 22 breaths/min, T 38°C. His Abbreviated Mental Test Score (AMTS) is 4 out of 10, which according to his daughter, is new. In the above patient, which is the high-risk criteria for sepsis?**

    A. AMTS

    B. Blood pressure

    C. Heart rate

    D. Respiratory rate

    E. Temperature

22. **A 45-year-old housekeeper has had had injury to the tip of her right middle finger while tucking in a bed sheet. Her tip of the finger is in flexed position and she is unable to extend her distal phalanx. Damage to which structure is most likely to cause the finger deformity?**

    A. Digital nerve

    B. Extensor digitorum longus

    C. Flexor digitorum profundus tendon

    D. Flexor digitorum superficialis tendon

    E. Fracture through the shaft of the distal phalanx

23. **A 25-year-old man attends the ED with dizziness, fatigue, and shortness of breath. He has a past medical history of Crohn's disease. On examination, he appears pale. His blood results are as follows: Hb 68 g/L, MCV 102 fL/cell, vitamin B12 120 ng/L. At which of the following sites does the majority of vitamin B12 absorption occur?**

    A. Descending duodenum

    B. Distal jejunum

    C. Proximal ileum

    D. Stomach

    E. Terminal ileum

24. **A 50-year-old man has had ventricular tachycardia. He is alert and has stable observations. Intravenous lidocaine has been prescribed. What is the most likely mechanism of action of this drug?**
    A. Calcium channel blockade
    B. Lengthening of refractoriness due to potassium channel blockade
    C. Sodium channel blockade with lengthened refractoriness
    D. Sodium channel blockade with minimal effect on refractoriness
    E. Sodium channel blockade with shortened refractoriness

25. **A 72-year-old woman in a care home has had diarrhoea and vomiting. She has been suspected to have contracted *Clostridium difficile* infection. Which is the most effective method to prevent transmission to the other residents?**
    A. Clean your hands with alcohol gel
    B. Isolation of the patient
    C. Prescribe oral metronidazole
    D. Use protective apron and gloves when in contact with the discussed patient
    E. Wash hands with soap and water

26. **A two-year-old boy has had fever and coughs but able to drink and communicate. His HR 160 bpm, RR 45 breaths/min, T 38°C, capillary refill of two seconds, and SaO$_2$ is 95% on air. In the above patient, which is the high-risk criteria for sepsis?**
    A. Capillary refill
    B. Heart rate
    C. Respiratory rate
    D. SaO$_2$
    E. Temperature

27. **A 41-year-old man has had chronic back pain. He attends the ED experiencing altered sensation to the lateral aspect of the mid-thigh. Damage to which structure is most likely to cause the sensory symptoms?**
    A. Femoral nerve
    B. Ilioinguinal nerve
    C. Lateral femoral cutaneous nerve
    D. Obturator nerve
    E. Saphenous nerve

28. **A 16-year-old girl has concealed her pregnancy and delivers her baby in the ED with an estimated gestation of 38 weeks. At delivery, the baby is flexed and screaming but remains cyanosed. Fortunately, after 30 seconds of stimulation, the baby's colour changes from blue to pink. Which physiological mechanism underlies the rapid colour change in this baby?**
    A. Basal metabolic rate is lowest in the neonatal period
    B. Foetal circulation prevents right-to-left shunts
    C. Interaction of foetal haemoglobin with 2,3-DPG is greater than in adults
    D. Lung compliance is greatest in the neonatal period
    E. P50 value of foetal haemoglobin is lower than in adults

29. **A 20-year-old man has had massive haemothorax and bedside focused assessment sonography test (FAST) positive abdominal scan following a fall from a tall tree of about 10 metres height. His BP is 80/50 mmHg and HR 124 bpm. He has been given tranexamic acid, massive blood transfusion protocol has been activated and operating theatre been arranged. Which single most likely mechanism of action of tranexamic acid in this situation?**
    A. Activation of coagulation protein
    B. Delays fibrinolysis
    C. Enhances vitamin K-dependent coagulation factors
    D. Promotes ADP-dependent platelet aggregation
    E. Stimulates anticoagulant regulatory proteins (C and S)

30. **A 24-year-old man has had a cough. He had recurrent chest infections in the near past. He suffers from HIV and in non-compliant with his medication. His CD4 count is very low. Which of the pathogens is the most likely responsible for his infection?**
    A. *Candida albicans*
    B. Cytomegalovirus
    C. *Klebsiella pneumoniae*
    D. *Mycobacterium tuberculosis*
    E. *Pneumocystis jirovecii*

31. **A 28-year-old male has had a fall of his bicycle and sustained an irregular and dirty laceration in the front of his right knee. Which is the least likely risk factor for developing wound infection?**
    A. Closure of the wound with sutures
    B. Contamination with foreign matter
    C. Injury more than 12 hours old
    D. Laceration produced with a knife
    E. Local anaesthesia with adrenaline

32. **A 32-year-old man has had a fall from a ladder onto concrete floor. He has back pain. He is unable to dorsiflex the big toe and has reduced fine touch and pinprick on the anterolateral surface of the left leg. Which is the single most likely nerve root involved?**

    A. L3
    B. L4
    C. L5
    D. S1
    E. S2

33. **A 68-year-old gentleman is brought to ED with chest pain and difficulty breathing. He suffered an ST-elevation myocardial infarction (STEMI) last month and had been getting on well with medication and physiotherapy when the symptoms started suddenly. On examination, he has a pan-systolic murmur heard throughout the praecordium but loudest at the left sternal edge in the fifth intercostal space. His chest radiograph demonstrates prominent lung vasculature and evidence of pulmonary oedema. Which one of the following answers regarding cardiac cycle is true?**

    A. Aortic pressure is always greater than left ventricular pressure
    B. Aortic valve opening coincides with mitral valve closure
    C. Left atrial pressure is greater than or equal to left ventricular pressure while the mitral valve is open
    D. Mitral valve closure causes the second heart sound
    E. Venous C wave is caused by atrial contraction

34. **A 30-year-old man has had injury to the left knee in a high-speed car collision. His knee had a forceful impact from lateral side because of the intrusion of the dashboard of the car. Which is the single most likely injury sustained?**

    A. Foot drop
    B. Fracture of the patella
    C. Patellar dislocation
    D. Rupture of the anterior cruciate ligament
    E. Rupture of the posterior cruciate ligament

35. **A 21-year-old man is brought to the ED as a trauma call following a high-speed road traffic accident (RTA). On examination, he is maintaining his airway, with normal breath and heart sounds. His Glasgow Coma Scale (GCS) is 15 and he is pale and cool peripherally. Initial observations in the ED are as follows: BP 142/87 mmHg, HR 131 bpm, RR 32 breaths/min, SaO$_2$ 100% (in room air). His capillary blood glucose is elevated, and his urine output is reduced. Secretion of which of the following co-ordinates this response?**

   A. Adrenaline
   B. Aldosterone
   C. Cortisol
   D. Corticotropin-releasing hormone
   E. Glucagon

36. **A 50-year-old man has had shortness of breath and pleuritic chest pain. He was previously treated for deep vein thrombosis. He is diagnosed to have pulmonary embolism. He has been started on warfarin. Which single most likely statement on warfarin is correct?**

   A. International normalized ratio (INR) reliably reflects anticoagulation effect in the initial three to four days
   B. It competitively stimulates vitamin K epoxide reductase
   C. It has the equal rate of action on all the vitamin K-dependent factors
   D. The therapeutic effect develops after four to five days
   E. Warfarin does not cross the placenta

37. **A 25-year-old man has in a high-speed car collision. Following a forceful impact of the intrusion of the dashboard of the car he is suspected to have injury to the left hip joint and sciatic nerve. He has difficulty in moving his left leg. Which is the least likely clinical feature associated with sciatic nerve injury?**

   A. Foot drop
   B. Loss of flexion of the knee joint
   C. Loss of planter flexion of the foot
   D. Sensory impairment on the medial side of the leg
   E. Sensory impairment on the sole of the foot

38. **A 70-year-old male has had a fever, and a cough with sputum similar to red-current jelly. What is the most likely infective organism?**

   A. *Escherichia Coli*
   B. *Klebsiella pneumoniae*
   C. *Legionella pneumophila*
   D. *Mycobacterium tuberculosis*
   E. *Streptococcus pneumoniae*

39. **A 65-year-old woman has had a fever, headache, and irritability in the left eye. On examination, her left eye is abducted and facing downward. The pupil is dilated in comparison to the right. The cavernous sinus thrombosis is suspected. Which is cranial nerve lesion is most likely to cause the signs?**
    A. Abducens
    B. Occulomotor
    C. Optic
    D. Trigeminal
    E. Trochlear

40. **A 17-year-old student attends the ED with fatigue, abdominal pain, and confusion. She gives a history of polyuria and polydipsia. Venous blood gas results are as follows: pH 6.89, K+ 6.9 mmol/L, glucose 31.2 mmol/L, ketones 5.4. Which of the following pancreatic cells is likely to be affected?**
    A. α cells
    B. δ cells
    C. β cells
    D. γ cells
    E. Acinar cells

41. **A 62-year-old woman has had bleeding from her varicose veins. She is on rivaroxaban. Which single most likely statement on rivaroxaban is correct?**
    A. It is direct competitive inhibitor of factor Xa
    B. It is direct thrombin inhibitor
    C. Inhibits vitamin K epoxide reductase
    D. Potent antidote is available to reverse the bleeding
    E. The drug may accumulate in the system if the glomerular filtration rate (GFR) is below 15 mL/min

42. **A 45-year-old man has had long-term neck pain. On a recent MRI scan he is found to have slipped intervertebral disc between C5 and C6 vertebrae compressing on the left nerve root. Which is the single most likely movement affected?**
    A. Abduction of the shoulder
    B. Adduction of the shoulder
    C. Extension of the elbow
    D. Extension of the wrist
    E. Flexion of the wrist

43. **An 82-year-old woman is brought to the ED with severe abdominal pain. She has a history of peptic ulcer disease and transient ischaemic attack. She previously took rabeprazole, but this was recently discontinued when she was prescribed clopidogrel by the stroke physician. On examination, she is exquisitely tender in the epigastric region with guarding. Several cells are involved in peptic ulcer formation. Which of the following secretes histamine?**
    A. Chief cells
    B. Enterochromaffin-like cells
    C. G cells
    D. Goblet cells
    E. Parietal cells

44. **A 72-year-old man presents with congestive cardiac failure with significant fluid overload. Intravenous furosemide has been planned to offload him. Which is the most likely site of action of this drug?**
    A. Ascending loop of Henle
    B. Descending loop of Henle
    C. Distal convoluted tubule
    D. Glormerulus
    E. Proximal convoluted tubule

45. **A 75-year-old male has had sudden onset of visual difficulty. On examination he has a right homonymous macular defect. Which is the most likely cause of the abnormality?**
    A. Left optic tract
    B. Left visual cortex
    C. Right optic tract
    D. Right visual cortex
    E. Tip of the left occipital lobe

46. **A 56-year-old man attends the ED with chest pain. On examination, the pain is reproducible on palpation and you suspect costochondritis. His electrocardiogram (ECG) from triage demonstrates a prolonged PR interval. Which part of the conductive pathway of the heart does the duration of the PR interval reflect?**
    A. Atrioventricular node
    B. Bundle of His
    C. Bundle of Kent
    D. Purkinje fibres
    E. Sinoatrial node

47. A 65-year-old male has had visual disturbances of sudden onset. On examination, he has homonymous hemianopia. The computed tomography (CT) scan of his brain confirms an occlusive cerebrovascular accident (CVA). Which artery is most likely occluded?

A. Anterior cerebral

B. Basilar

C. Middle cerebral artery

D. Pontine

E. Posterior cerebral

48. A 42-year-old woman has had watery diarrhoea 20 times and vomiting 15 times within the last eight hours. She has recently been treated with an antibiotic for a urinary tract infection. A diagnosis of infection by *C. difficile* is suspected. Which single most antibiotic is the least likely to predispose her present clinical symptoms?

A. Amoxycillin

B. Cefalexin

C. Ciprofloxacin

D. Clindamycin

E. Trimethoprim

49. A 27-year-old woman attends the ED feeling short of breath. She has a past medical history of eczema. On examination, she has increased work of breathing and bilateral expiratory wheeze. After supplemental oxygen is given her SaO_2 increases from 89% to 97%. What was the cause of the hypoxaemia?

A. Hypoventilation

B. Low inspired FiO_2

C. Right-to-left shunt

D. Thickened diffusion membrane

E. Ventilation:perfusion mismatch

50. A 17-year-old boy has a pre-auricular laceration to the right cheek after an alleged assault. Which function is least likely to be preserved following this injury?

A. Corneal reflex

B. Mastication

C. Raising eyebrows

D. Saliva production

E. Taste sensation in the anterior tongue

51. **A 25-year-old man has attended the ED in acute shock following diabetic ketoacedosis (DKA). He needs urgent resuscitation. Failing to obtain peripheral intravenous line, you have decided to access the femoral vein in the groin. Which statement is correct regarding femoral vein?**
    A. Is lateral to the artery
    B. It is within the femoral canal
    C. Shares the femoral sheath with the femoral artery
    D. Lies just medial to the femoral nerve
    E. Located at the mid-point between the anterior superior iliac spine (ASIS) and pubic symphysis

52. **A 4-year-old boy attends the ED with fever, cough and maculo-papular rash. The most probable diagnosis is measles. The mother is reassured that the boy has life-long immunity against measles. Which of the following is involved in both adaptive and innate immunity?**
    A. B-cells
    B. Macrophages
    C. Natural killer T-cells
    D. Neutrophils
    E. Plasma cells

53. **An 80-year-old woman has had shortness of breath, pedal oedema and bilateral pleural effusions. Intravenous furosemide has been prescribed. Which is the single most site of the following the drugs acts upon?**
    A. Epithelial sodium channel
    B. Potassium/ATPase channel
    C. Sodium/chloride transporter
    D. Sodium/potassium transport
    E. Sodium/potassium/chloride co-transporter

54. **A 35-year-old woman attends the ED after swallowing her boyfriend's house key. She is complaining of pain at the level of her manubriosternal joint. Compression at the level of which of the following structures is likely to be causing her dysphagia?**
    A. Aortic arch
    B. Cricoid cartilage
    C. Gastro-oesophageal junction
    D. Oesophageal hiatus of the diaphragm
    E. Right main bronchus

55. A 57-year-old man is brought to the ED with central, crushing chest pain. He has a history of type 2 diabetes mellitus, hypertension, and 60-a-day for 40 years of smoking. On examination, he is diaphoretic with enlarged body habitus. You request an ECG. Where are you most likely to see ischaemic changes on the ECG?

A. Anterior leads

B. Inferior leads

C. Lateral leads

D. Posterior leads

E. Septal leads

56. A 70-year-old woman has had generalized pain in the abdomen. She has been smoking for about 55 years and is T2DM. A computed tomography (CT) scan with contrast shows superior mesenteric occlusion. What single structure is most likely to be affected?

A. Ascending colon

B. Descending colon

C. Duodenum

D. Sigmoid colon

E. Stomach

57. A 25-year-old man has had a laceration on the occipital protuberance area, which requires cleaning and suturing. Which is the single nerve needs to be anaesthetized?

A. Accessory nerve

B. Auriculotemporal nerve

C. Great auricular nerve

D. Greater occipital nerve

E. Posterior auricular nerve

58. A two-year-old boy is brought to the ED with a respiratory infection. He has a diagnosis of Leigh syndrome that was diagnosed at one year of age after a period of developmental regression and is on a treatment protocol. The ED consultant on-call is quizzing the juniors on mitochondrial diseases following the admission. What is the function of mitochondria?

A. Degradation of phagocytosed foreign material

B. Packaging and secreting vesicles

C. Production of ATP via oxidative phosphorylation

D. Protein synthesis

E. Replication of DNA

59. An 81-year-old male has had sudden onset of right sided facial droop, arm, and leg weakness. He is alert and has no dysphasia. Which is the most likely site of abnormality?

A. Frontal lobe

B. Internal capsule

C. Parietal lobe

D. Temporal lobe

E. Thalamic lesion

60. A 21-year-old man walks in to Minors ED complaining of palpitations. He has a history of psychosis and is taking olanzapine. On examination, his heart sounds are normal with a regularly regular rhythm. His ECG demonstrates an irregular, polymorphic ventricular tachycardia and a QT interval of 520 mS. What is the single best explanation for how prolonged QT interval can lead to life-threatening arrhythmias?

A. Blockade of calcium channels in myocytes

B. Decreased refractory period of the myocytes due to adrenergic stimulation

C. Early depolarizations in the myocardium generating different refractory periods in the myocytes

D. Increased activity of the atrioventricular (AV) node

E. Myocardial stunning

61. A 30-year-old woman has had fever, headaches, photophobia, and neck stiffness. She is suspected to have encephalitis. Which is the single most sensitive and specific diagnostic test?

A. Blood culture

B. CT brain

C. Cerebrospinal fluid (CSF) analysis

D. CSF culture

E. CSF PCR

62. A 22-year-old male has had a high-speed car collision. He has been diagnosed to have a fracture of T4 vertebral body. At which level is the patient mostly likely to have sensory deficit to?

A. The apex beat

B. The manubriosternal joint

C. The nipple line

D. The shoulder

E. The umbilicus

63. **A 32-year-old diabetic man attends the ED with fever, headache, and visual disturbances. On examination he has right upper quadrantic homonymous hemianopia. A CT scan of the brain shows an abscess in the left temporal lobe. Which is the most likely anatomical explanation of the eye symptom and sign?**
    A. Lower fibres of left optic radiation
    B. Lower fibres of right optic radiation
    C. Optic chiasm
    D. Upper fibres of left optic radiation .
    E. Upper fibres of right optic radiation

64. **A 52-year-old local politician attends the ED with visual loss. He has a diagnosis of relapsing-remitting multiple sclerosis and is on a treatment protocol. The medical student shadowing your on-call shift enquires about demyelinating neurological conditions after the admission. What is the primary physiological effect of demyelination on the neuron?**
    A. Diffuse axonal injury
    B. Hyperpolarisation of the resting membrane potential
    C. Loss of saltatory conduction
    D. Reduced levels of neurotransmitter release from the pre-synaptic neuron
    E. Wallerian degeneration

65. **A 24-year-old male smoker has been having a cough with whitish sputum for the last one week. He has attended the ED after noticing streak of fresh blood in the phlegm. What is the most likely source of bleeding?**
    A. Bronchial artery
    B. Inflammation of the lung parenchyma
    C. Necrotizing infection of bronchiols
    D. Pulmonary artery
    E. Tracheobronchial capillaries

66. **A 72-year-old man has had generalized pain in the abdomen. He has a long-term history of smoking, atrial fibrillation, and T2DM. A CT with contrast shows inferior mesenteric artery occlusion. What single structure is most likely to be affected?**
    A. Ascending colon
    B. Descending colon
    C. Jejunum
    D. Terminal ileum
    E. Transverse colon

67. **A 35-year-old man has had a laceration on the front of the ear, which has been repaired by local anaesthetic injection in front of the auricle. Which single nerve has been blocked by the local anaesthetic agent?**
    A. Accessory nerve
    B. Auriculotemporal nerve
    C. Greater occipital nerve
    D. Lesser occipital nerve
    E. Posterior auricular nerve

68. **A 92-year-old man is brought to the ED from his sheltered accommodation following a fall. In the last year he has required more assistance with tasks such as getting dressed and making tea. Staff has noticed that he has become more aggressive and often has difficulty recognizing people, even family members. On examination, he is uncooperative but otherwise well. He scores 2/10 on the AMTS for his date of birth and the naming the current monarch. Given the most likely diagnosis, activity of which neurotransmitter is reduced?**
    A. Acetylcholine
    B. Dopamine
    C. GABA
    D. Noradrenaline
    E. Serotonin

69. **A 38-year-old female has had a fall while trying to run to board a bus. She could not get up on her own because of severe pain and deformity to her right ankle. She was given morphine intravenously by the ambulance crew following which she started vomiting. Ondansetron has been prescribed. Which single factor is the most accurate about the antiemetic drug?**
    A. A member of antihistamine group
    B. Absorption through oral route is unreliable
    C. Acts by blocking the dopaminergic receptors
    D. Antagonist to 5-HT3 receptor
    E. Mechanism of action of the antiemetic effect is unclear

70. **A two-year-old boy has been hit by a car while crossing the road. He is in pain and suspected to have injury to chest and abdomen. What is the most likely statement true regarding chest injury in this patient?**
    A. Compliance of the chest wall much greater than adults
    B. Increased chest wall pliability protects intrathoracic organs better
    C. Intrathoracic injuries are uncommon without external chest injuries
    D. Rib fractures are common in this patient
    E. Smaller body mass allows smaller force per unit body surface area

71. A 38-year-old man has been in a rear to front low-speed car collision. The next day, he developed a spasm of the left-sided sternocleidomastoid muscle. Which single movement is the most likely to be restricted?

A. Backward tilting of head
B. Forwards flexion of the head
C. Tilting the head towards the right shoulder
D. Turning the head towards the left shoulder
E. Turning the head to the right shoulder

72. A 41-year-old woman attends the ED with an abrasion to her knee sustained while rock climbing. On examination, the wound is no longer bleeding but has visible debris in the base of the wound. Which of the following immune cells is the first to arrive at the injured site?

A. B-cells
B. Macrophages
C. Natural killer T-cells
D. Neutrophils
E. Plasma cells

73. A 27-year-old woman has had sudden onset of spasmodic pain in the abdomen. She has been prescribed a hyoscine butylbromide (Buscopan) injection. Which statement about the drug is correct?

A. Able to reduce morphine-induced smooth muscle spasm
B. Can be used to dilate pupils
C. Effective relaxant of skeletal muscles
D. Has no function on autonomic ganglia
E. Unable to relax cardia in achalasia

74. A 71-year-old female has had sudden onset of right sided facial droop, and arm and leg weakness. Her right eye is in abducted position with inferior gaze. Which is the most likely site of abnormality?

A. Internal capsule
B. Mid-brain
C. Parietal lobe
D. Temporal lobe
E. Thalamic lesion

75. **A 62-year-old woman is brought to the ED following a collapse at home. She has a history of syncopal episodes. On examination, her pulse is irregular with periods of tachycardia followed by a pause and then a normal heart rate. What is the physiological cause of the pause following the period of tachycardia?**

    A. AV nodal block
    B. Beta blockade
    C. Overdrive suppression
    D. Parasympathetic stimulation
    E. Potassium channel blockade

76. **A 20-year-old female has had sudden onset of repeated jerking of the left arm. She is suspected to have focal seizure. Which is the most likely site of abnormality?**

    A. Motor cortex
    B. Occipital lobe
    C. Parietal lobe
    D. Temporal lobe
    E. Thalamus

77. **A 60-year-old man attends the ED with severe haematemesis. He has a long-term history of alcohol abuse, atrial fibrillation, and T2DM. What is single most likely source of bleeding?**

    A. Azygos vein
    B. Azygo-portal anastomosis
    C. Gastric vein
    D. Oesophageal artery
    E. Portal vein

78. **A 32-year-old man has been stabbed in his left chest. By the time he arrived in the ED, he was in cardiac arrest. A resuscitative thoracotomy has been performed. What structure is likely to be cut in while performing this procedure?**

    A. Diaphragm
    B. Inferior vena cava
    C. Intercostal neurovascular bundle
    D. Internal mammary artery
    E. Left vagus nerve

79. **A 17-year-old boy is brought to the ED with a 2-hour history of severe dyspnoea. He has asthma and in the previous days he has been using his salbutamol inhaler up to ten times a day. On examination, he is pale and clammy, he has increased work of breathing and very quiet breath sounds. Initial observations in the ED are as follows: HR 143 bpm, BP 102/63 mmHg, RR 42 breaths/min, T 36.8°C, SaO$_2$ 96% (on 15 L O$_2$). You request an arterial blood gas scan (ABG), which demonstrates the following: pH 7.47, PaO$_2$ 14.1 kPa, PaCO$_2$ 4.2 kPa. Which one of the following answers best explains the PaCO$_2$ value?**

A. PaCO$_2$ is high, due to air trapping
B. PaCO$_2$ is low, due to impaired gas exchange
C. PaCO$_2$ is normal, due to the patient tiring
D. PaCO$_2$ is low, due to hypoventilation
E. PaCO$_2$ is normal, due to hypoxic drive

80. **A 30-year-old man has had a fall from the roof of his house onto his back. He has fractured his L1 vertebral body. Which structure is the least likely to be injured?**

A. Body of pancreas
B. Duodenojejunal flexure
C. Hila of the kidneys
D. Pylorus ⌐
E. Tip of the spinal cord

81. **A 26-year-old woman attends ED with shortness of breath and productive cough. On examination, she is cyanotic with reduced air entry at the right lung base. You take an arterial sample for blood gas analysis that reveals her PaO$_2$ is reduced. The partial pressure of a gas is equal to which one of the following calculations?**

A. Alveolar partial pressure—arterial partial pressure
B. Fraction of gas in the gas mixture/total pressure
C. Fraction of gas in the gas mixture x total pressure ✓
D. Number of gases in the gas mixture/total pressure
E. Temperature of the gas × viscosity of the gas

82. **An 18-year-old female has neck stiffness, vomiting, and photophobia following a flu-like illness. The human papilloma virus (HSV) infection has been suspected. Treatment with which drug is the most appropriate?**

A. Aciclovir
B. Amphotericin
C. Capsofungin
D. Clotrimazole
E. Fluconazole

83. **A 40-year-old man has had long-term back pain. On a recent MRI scan he is found to have slipped intervertebral disc between L4 and L5 vertebrae compressing on the left nerve root. Which is the most likely clinical finding?**
    A. Loss of ankle jerk
    B. Loss of knee jerk
    C. Weak ankle planter flexion
    D. Weak dorsiflexion of the big toe
    E. Weak knee flexion

84. **A 49-year-old woman attends the ED with a history of abdominal discomfort and steatorrhoea. She reports unintentional weight loss of 5 kg in the last year and a 20-year history of alcohol excess with recurrent pancreatitis. Which of the following is LEAST likely to be affected in pancreatic exocrine insufficiency?**
    A. Bile acid secretion
    B. Carbohydrate metabolism → can 80% of amylase production is not dependent on pancreas.
    C. CCK activity
    D. Duodenal pH
    E. Pancreatic lipase function

85. **A 72-year-old man is referred to the ED when his GP detected significant anaemia and low vitamin B12 levels on his blood tests. He had been suffering from fatigue, shortness of breath, and chest pain. Autoimmune damage of which cells occurs in pernicious anaemia?**
    A. Chief cells
    B. Enterochromaffin-like cells
    C. G-cells
    D. Parietal cells
    E. Terminal ileal enterocytes

86. **A 20-year-old woman has been brought by the ambulance crew from a GP surgery with suspected meningitis. She has already been given benzylpenicillin by her GP. Which is the most likely action the drug has on bacteria?**
    A. Disrupts cell membrane integrity
    B. Inhibits cell wall synthesis
    C. Inhibits DNA replication
    D. Inhibits protein synthesis
    E. Interferes binding to the peptide chain

87. **A 54-year-old woman is brought to the ED after being found in the stairwell of her block of flats. She was last seen well five days before and the neighbour who found her describes a history of chronic alcohol abuse and depression. On examination, there is tender bruising along the left side of her body and she is neurologically intact. Initial blood tests demonstrate an acute kidney injury. Her urine appears dark and the dip is strongly positive for blood. What is the most likely diagnosis?**

    A. Blast transformation of chronic myelogenous leukaemia (CML)
    B. Compartment syndrome
    C. Disseminated intravascular coagulation
    D. Hepato-renal syndrome
    E. Rhabdomyolysis

88. **A 72-year-old diabetic man has had difficulty in swallowing. On examination his uvula is high lifted to the right side on asking the patient to say a prolonged 'Ah'. Which is the most likely nerve damage would cause the abnormality?**

    A. Facial
    B. Glossopharyngeal
    C. Hypoglossal
    D. Trigeminal
    E. Vagus

89. **A 36-year-old woman attends the ED with intermittent abdominal pain. On examination, she is obese and has a palpable suprapubic mass extending to above the umbilicus. Unexpectedly, she delivers a baby in the ED with an estimated gestation of 28 weeks. What is the function of surfactant in the lung?**

    A. Airway resistance is decreased
    B. Alveolar surface area is increased
    C. Lung compliance is reduced
    D. Pressure required to expand the alveoli is reduced
    E. Ventilation:perfusion ratio is improved

90. **A 72-year-old woman has sudden loss of vision in the left eye. Which is the most likely site may be affected?**
    A. Left optic nerve
    B. Left optic radiation
    C. Optic chiasm
    D. Right optic nerve
    E. Right optic radiation

91. **A 33-year-old man attends the ED with intermittent dizzy spells. The episodes are unpredictable and normally last a couple of minutes, but today have persisted for several hours. On examination, his pulse is rapid but regular and he is otherwise well. His ECG is shown in Figure 7.1.**

    In atrioventricular nodal re-entry tachycardia (AVNRT), vagal manoeuvres are the primary intervention. Which of the following is likely to occur with increased vagal tone?
    A. Fast response to intervention
    B. Increased AV nodal conduction
    C. Increased myocardial contractility
    D. Increased noradrenaline release
    E. Marked respiratory sinus arrhythmia

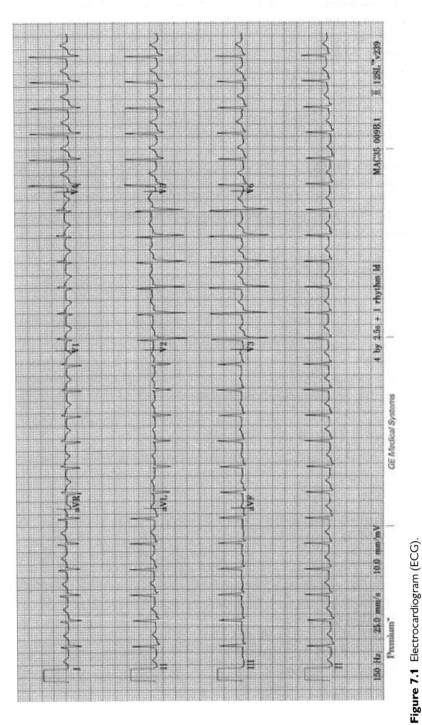

Figure 7.1 Electrocardiogram (ECG).
Courtesy of lifeinthefastlane.com. Copyright © 2007–2017.

92. **An 80-year-old female has had pain in the abdomen and dyspepsia. Her husband is worried as it might be due to her recently increased use of aspirin for rheumatic pain. Which single most likely mechanism for her symptoms?**
    A. Cytokine-induced prostaglandin synthesis
    B. Inhibition of COX-1 mediated prostaglandin synthesis
    C. Inhibition of COX-2 mediated prostaglandin synthesis
    D. Inhibition of thromboxane A2
    E. Stimulation of lipo-oxygenase pathway

93. **A 50-year-old male has had dizziness on standing position. He has also developed hiccoughs and urinary urgency, frequency, and incomplete bladder emptying. He is known to have T2DM and chronic alcoholism. It is suspected he is developing autonomic dysfunction. Which is the most likely site of abnormality?**
    A. Brainstem
    B. Cervical cord
    C. Frontal lobe
    D. Hypothalamus
    E. Thoracic cord

94. **A 76-year-old woman is brought to the ED after collapsing spontaneously while shopping. She had been complaining of increasing fatigue over the previous month. On examination, she has normal heart sounds. Initial observations in the ED are as follows: BP 92/48 mmHg, HR 41 bpm, RR 20 breaths/min, T 37.1°C, SaO$_2$ 97% (in room air). Her ECG demonstrates trifascicular block. Which one of the following sets of ECG findings demonstrates trifascicular block?**
    A. PR interval of 140 mS, left bundle branch block, and left axis deviation
    B. PR interval of 60 mS, left bundle branch block, and right axis deviation
    C. PR interval of 140 mS, right bundle branch block, and right axis deviation
    D. QRS interval of 160 mS, left bundle branch block, and right axis deviation
    E. QRS interval of 240 mS, right bundle branch block, and left axis deviation

95. **A 21-year-old student is being treated for an acute asthma attack. He has had two salbutamol nebulizers. It is decided that he may benefit from nebulized ipratropium. Which is the single most important site of action of this drug?**
    A. Alpha-adrenergic
    B. Antimuscarinic
    C. Beta-2 adrenergic
    D. Leukotriene receptor antagonist
    E. Nicotinic

96. **A 16-year-old boy has had itchy red scaliness between his toes in the web spaces. His toenails appear pitted. A diagnosis of Athletes foot is suspected. Which is the single best diagnostic test?**

A. Blood test

B. Gram stain and culture

C. Skin scrapings

D. Skin swab

E. Toenail clipping

97. **A 62-year-old man attends the ED with recurrent epistaxis. In the last year he has noticed easy bruising and bleeding gums when he brushes his teeth. On examination, he is haemodynamically stable. His blood tests show the following: partial thromboplastin time (APTT) 52 seconds (normal: 21–34 seconds), fibrinogen normal, PT normal. Which of the following diagnoses is most likely?**

A. Factor V Leiden

B. Factor XII deficiency

C. Haemophilia B

D. Protein S deficiency

E. Von Willebrand's disease

98. **A 28-year-old female has had constant tremor, difficulty in swallowing, swelling in the front of her neck, tachycardia, and a rash on her shins. Which single best anatomical option could contribute to the dysphagia?**

A. Direct involvement of oesophagus

B. Infiltration of inferior belly of omohyoid muscle

C. Infiltration of recurrent laryngeal nerve

D. Infiltration of superior belly of omohyoid muscle

E. Involvement of cricothyroid membrane

99. **A 56-year-old gentleman is brought to the ED complaining of central, crushing chest pain. He is a lifelong smoker with known hypertension and hypercholesterolaemia. On examination, he is diaphoretic and tachycardic. You request an ECG, by which time the gentleman is pain free. The ECG shows only deeply inverted, biphasic T waves in leads V2 and V3. What is the single most likely finding at coronary angiography?**

A. Complete occlusion of the left anterior descending artery

B. Complete occlusion of the proximal left circumflex artery

C. Normal coronary arteries

D. Severe proximal stenosis of the left anterior descending artery

E. Widespread moderate coronary artery disease

100. **A 45-year-old woman attends ED complaining of difficulty in eating and drinking for two days. She has swelling of the anterior pillar of the tonsil on the left side. She is suspected to have peritonsillar abscess, and referred to the Ears, Nose, and Throat department (ENT) for urgent aspiration. Which lymph nodes are most likely to be typically involved in this patient?**

A. Jugulodigastric
B. Mastoid
C. Preauricular
D. Submental
E. Superficial cervical

1. B. 1–2 cm proximal to ulnar styloid process.

The ulnar nerve lies just medial to the ulnar artery and immediately lateral to the flexor carpi ulnaris (FCU) tendon. By injecting 5 mL of local anaesthetic 1–2 cm proximal to the ulnar styloid process between the ulnar artery pulsation and the FCU tendon would cause the ulnar nerve block. The dorsal branch of the ulnar nerve may be blocked by subcutaneous (SC) infiltration of around the ulnar border of the wrist.

Wyatt J, Illingworth RN, Graham CA, et al. (2012). *Oxford Handbook of Emergency Medicine*, 4th edition (p. 296). Oxford, UK: Oxford University Press.

2. C. Phase 2.

An electrical equilibrium occurs as potassium ion efflux via various types of potassium channels matches calcium ion influx. This is visualized as the plateau phase of the action potential.

Koeppen BM (2015). *Berne & Levy Physiology*, 6th edition. Maryland Heights, MO: Elsevier Mosby.

3. B. Highly lipophilic.

   A. Propofol does not have any analgesic property and can cause pain during injection.
   B. Correct answer: It is highly lipophilic, hence readily crosses the blood–brain barrier.
   C. Propofol is a phenol derivative.
   D. The onset of action is about 40 seconds and duration of action is usually six minutes.
   E. Patients over the age of 55 years are particularly sensitive to propofol. The dose in older patients should be reduced by 20%.

UpToDate (2017). Procedural sedation in adults outside the operating room. Available at: https://www.uptodate.com/contents/procedural-sedation-in-adults-outside-the-operating-room

4. C. Egg-based culture of bacteria.

Culture helps in identification of mycobacterium and drug susceptibility. It takes about six to eight weeks, as the growth is slower in the egg-medium. Growth in liquid media (Middlebrook 7H12) tends to be rapid.

UpToDate (2017). Diagnosis of pulmonary tuberculosis in HIV uninfected. Available at: https://www.uptodate.com/contents/diagnosis-of-pulmonary-tuberculosis-in-hiv-uninfected-patients

5. D. Failure of ATP-dependent cellular transport.

   A. Although myoglobin is pathognomic of rhabdomylysis, the absence of plasma or urine myoglobin (tested as urine dipstick positive for blood) does not rule out rhabdomyolysis as the serum half-life is only one to three hours and is completely absent after 24 hours.

B. CK starts rising within the first 12 hours, reaches peak at 24 hours and remains at this level for about three days. Elevated level of CK is the hallmark of rhabdomyolysis (five times of the upper limit of the normal).

C. The final common pathway in the pathogenesis of rhabdomyolysis is same though the causes may be diverse. There is an increase in the cytoplasmic Ca+ concentration leading to myocyte destruction and release of muscle contents in to the circulation. The direct cell wall damage and ATP depletion are two primary mechanisms that result into accumulation of Ca+ in the cytoplasm.

D. Correct answer: ATP depletion results in the malfunctioning of ATP-dependent cell membrane ion pumps causing the increased Ca+ in the cytoplasm.

E. As a result of the failure of energy-dependent ion pumps, there increased permeability of Na+ ions.

Parekh R (2014). Rhabdomyolysis. In: Marx J, Hockberger RS, Walls RM (Eds.), *Rosen's Emergency Medicine*, 8th edition (pp. 1667–75). Philadelphia, PA: Elsevier.

6. D.   True negatives 99 patients, true positives 22 patients.

Sensitivity = proportion of true positives who are test positive

Specificity = proportion of true negatives who are test negative

Harris M, Taylor G (2008). *Medical Statistics Made Easy*, 3rd edition. Bloxham, UK: Scion Publishing.

7. D.   Making a ring by the thumb to the index finger.

Paralysis or paresis of the flexor pollicis longus (FPL) and lateral half of flexor digitorum profundus (FDP) as a result on injury to the anterior osseous branch of median nerve in the forearm may result into hyperextension of the terminal phalanges of the thumb and index finger.

McRae R (2012). *Clinical Orthopaedic Examination*, 5th edition (p. 25). Edinburgh, UK Churchill Livingstone.

8. B.   Exhaustion of hepatic glycogen stores.

Chronic alcohol excess in the fasting state has multiple effects on the liver and pancreas, the two organs responsible for maintaining blood glucose concentration. These include inhibition of gluconeogenesis due to alcohol metabolism depleting enzyme stores, impaired counter-regulatory response to hypoglycaemia and depletion of hepatic stores of glycogen over one to two days.

Koeppen BM, Stanton, BA (2015). *Berne & Levy Physiology*, 6th edition. Maryland Heights, MO: Elsevier Mosby.

9. B.   Conduction is blocked at afferent nerve endings.

Lidocaine impedes the initiation and propagation of the action potential (nerve impulses). The threshold of excitability is increased by reducing the transit of sodium through voltage-gated sodium ion channels. As a result, the conduction is blocked at the afferent nerve endings. The smallest fibres (autonomic, sensory) are affected first followed by the larger nerves (motor). The effect on the CNS is stimulation.

Nolan J (2012). Anaesthesia and neuromuscular block. In: Brown MJ, Bennett PN (Eds.), *Clinical Pharmacology*, 11th edition (pp. 303–4). Edinburgh, UK: Churchill Livingstone Elsevier.

10. A. *Campylobacter jejuni.*

The infections with *Campylobacter jejuni* are common. The symptoms last for about one to two weeks. The patients usually have abdominal pain, diarrhoea with occasional rectal bleeding. Complications are rare which may include reactive arthritis, Guillain-Barré syndrome, and so on.

Ramrakha PS, Moore KP, Sam A (2010). Gastroenterological emergencies. In: *Oxford Handbook of Acute Medicine*, 3rd edition. Oxford, UK: Oxford University Press.

11. A. Cross-match blood takes a minimum of 45 minutes to be ready.

A. Correct answer.
B. Type O blood has antibodies for both A and B groups, negative is for absence of Rhesus typing.
C. O-negative blood has no preparation time; it is available immediately in emergency.
D. Blood group AB does not have any antibodies against A or B.
E. Type specific blood takes a minimum of 15 minutes to get ready.

Emery M (2014). Blood and blood components. In: Marx J, Hockberger RS, Walls RM (Eds.), *Rosen's Emergency Medicine*, 8th edition (pp. 75–80). Philadelphia, PA: Saunders Elsevier.

12. A. Reduced adduction of the little finger against resistance.

In cases of the injury of the ulnar nerve at the elbow joint, the FCU and the medial half of the FDP are affected. When the FCU is tested by applying the resistance to the flexion of the wrist joint, it may deviate towards the ulnar side or a weaker contraction of the tendon is felt just above the wrist.

McRae R (2012). *Clinical Orthopaedic Examination*, 5th edition (p. 24). Edinburgh, UK: Churchill Livingstone.

13. A. Acute lymphoblastic leukaemia (ALL).

ALL is characterized by bone marrow failure with overproduction of lymphoblasts. Peak age of incidence is two to five years and the survival rate is approximately 80% in children. Signs include organ infiltration and non-specific signs of pancytopaenia, while diagnosis is histological.

Koeppen BM (2015). *Berne & Levy Physiology*, 6th edition. Maryland Heights, MO: Elsevier Mosby.

14. B. Dopamine.

Blockade of dopamine D2 receptors in the nigrostriatal pathway producing extrapyramidal symptoms by the antipsychotics is more common with the classical agents than the atypical agents like risperidone, which may result into such symptoms in high dosage.

Nutt D et al. (2008). Respiratory system. In: Brown MJ, Bennett PN (Eds.), *Clinical Pharmacology*, 11th edition (p. 327). Edinburgh, UK: Churchill Livingstone Elsevier.

15. D. Measles.

The Department of Health (DoH) recommends for routine vaccination, injection of measles, mumps, and rubella (MMR) at the age of one year and the second dose at about three years of age. Despite receiving his initial vaccines at the age of 8, 12, and 16 weeks, he has missed this.

Measles is caused by a morbillivirus of the paramyxovirus family. The symptoms at the early stages are fever, malaise, coryza, conjunctivitis, and cough. It is a notifiable disease. It is highly communicable infectious disease and the spread may occur following coughing, sneezing, close personal contact, or direct contact with infected nasal or throat secretions.

NHS, Vaccination Schedule. Available at: http://www.nhs.uk/Conditions/vaccinations/Pages/vaccination-schedule-age-checklist.aspx

Measles: symptoms, diagnosis, complications and treatment (factsheet). Available at: https://www.gov.uk/government/publications/measles-symptoms-diagnosis-complications-treatment/measles-symptoms-diagnosis-complications-and-treatment-factsheet

16. A. Cigarette smoking decreases pulmonary secretions.

Cigarette smoking increases the pulmonary secretions and damages the ciliary action. All other statements are true and act as predisposing factors for pneumonia.

Lee G, Andrew IS (2016). Goldman-Celil Medicine, 25th edition. Philadelphia, PA: Elsevier Saunders.

17. E. Supination of forearm.

If the radial nerve injured in Monteggia fractures (fracture of the proximal third of the ulna and dislocation of the radial head) in the supinator tunnel, the nerve supply to the supinator may be affected resulting in weaker or loss of supination in extended elbow (which eliminates the supinating action of the biceps).

McRae R (2012). *Clinical Orthopaedic Examination*, 5th edition (p. 20). Edinburgh, UK: Churchill Livingstone.

18. A. FEV_1 is decreased; FVC is decreased; FEV_1:FVC <0.7.

Asthma is an obstructive respiratory disease, which will cause a reduced FEV_1:FVC ratio. Similar to reduced peak flow, the reduced FEV_1 reflects increased airway resistance on expiration, while the reduced FVC is the result of widespread bronchoconstriction.

Koeppen BM (2015). *Berne & Levy Physiology*, 6th edition. Maryland Heights, MO: Elsevier Mosby.

19. E. Vomiting is solely because of local gastric effect.

Vomiting, in addition to the local gastric effect, it may be caused by a central effect. It has general depressant effect mediated through particular membrane ion channels and receptors. The ethanol influences neurotransmitter release and activity.

Haydock S (2012). Drug dependence. In: Brown MJ, Bennett PN (Eds.), *Clinical Pharmacology*, 11th edition (pp. 142–5). Edinburgh, UK: Churchill Livingstone Elsevier.

20. E. Thorough wound toileting in soapy water.

Following a bat bite, the wound should be washed thoroughly with soap and running tap water for at least 15 minutes. Apply antiseptic and leave the wound open. It is a notifiable disease.

NHS Guidance, Rabies in bats: how to spot it and report it. Available at: http://www.nhs.uk/Conditions/Rabies/Pages/Introduction.aspx

21. A. AMTS.

According to the National Institute for Health and Care Excellence (NICE) guidelines (NG 51) published in 2016, objective evidence of the altered mental state is high-risk criteria in risk stratification tool for suspected sepsis. The other clinical observations are also included from low to moderate to high risk. For more detail, please refer to the reference.

NICE guidance, NG51, Sepsis: recognition, diagnosis and early management. Available at: https://www.nice.org.uk/guidance/NG51/chapter/Recommendations#risk-factors-for-sepsis

22. B. Extensor digitorum longus.

The patient has mallet finger deformity. The extensor digitorum tendon in each finger is attached to the base of the distal phalanx. In the above situation, the tendon ruptured with or without an avulsion fracture of the base of the distal phalanx resulting in the deformity.

Wyatt J, Illingworth RN, Graham CA, et al. (2012). *Oxford Handbook of Emergency Medicine*, 4th edition (pp. 432–6). Oxford, UK: Oxford University Press.

23. E. Terminal ileum.

Vitamin B12, or cobalamin, is a water-soluble vitamin found only in animal products. In the acidic stomach environment, B12 binds to chaperone R proteins released in saliva until the complex is cleaved by pancreatic lipase. Intrinsic factor is released by parietal cells and binds the free B12. Only bound B12 triggers cubilin receptors in the distal ileal brush border and is absorbed.

Koeppen BM (2015). *Berne & Levy Physiology*, 6th edition. Maryland Heights, MO: Elsevier Mosby.

24. E. Sodium channel blockade with shortened refractoriness.

Lidocaine is a class 1B drug, which acts by blocking the sodium channel and shortens the refractoriness. It shortens the action potential duration. It is particularly useful in ventricular arrhythmias.

Grace A (2008). Cardiac arrhythmia. In: Brown MJ, Bennett PN (Eds.), *Clinical Pharmacology*, 11th edition (pp. 430–3). Edinburgh, UK: Churchill Livingstone Elsevier.

25. E. Wash hands with soap and water.

Isolation of patients, using protective apron and gloves and washing hands with soap and water are all of paramount importance in prevention of such infection. However, the hand washing with soap and water is the most effective way to prevent the spread.

Department of Health (2006). *Clostridium difficile* infection: How to deal with the problem. Available at: https://www.gov.uk/government/uploads/system/uploads/attachment_data/file/340851/Clostridium_difficile_infection_how_to_deal_with_the_problem.pdf

Gerding DN, Muto CA, Owens Jr. RC (2008). Measures to control and prevent *Clostridium difficile* infection. *Clinical Infectious Diseases*, **46**, S43–9.

26. B. Heart rate.

According to the NICE guidelines (NG 51) published in 2016, heart rate of >150 bpm in children aged one to two years is a high-risk criterion in the risk stratification tool for suspected sepsis. The other clinical observations are also included from low to moderate to high risk. For more detail, please refer to the reference.

NICE guidance, NG51, Algorithm for managing sepsis in children under 5 years in an acute hospital setting. Available at: https://www.nice.org.uk/guidance/ng51/resources/algorithm-for-managing-suspected-sepsis-in-children-aged-under-5-years-in-an-acute-hospital-setting-91853485527

27. C. Lateral cutaneous nerve of the thigh.

The lateral cutaneous nerve of the thigh, a direct branch from the lumbar plexus supplies the lateral aspect of the thigh. Femoral nerve, through medial and intermediate cutaneous branches, supplies the anterior and medial surface of the thigh and through the saphenous branch, supplies to the medial side of the leg, ankle, and foot to the great toe.

Ellis H, Mahadevan V (2013). *Clinical Anatomy: Applied Anatomy for Students and Junior Doctors*, 13th edition (pp. 272–3). Oxford, UK: John Wiley & Sons Ltd.

28. E. P50 value of foetal haemoglobin is lower than in adults.

P50 is the partial pressure of oxygen required to saturate 50% of available haemoglobin. Foetal haemoglobin has greater affinity for oxygen than adult haemoglobin, which is necessary in *utero* for foetal blood to displace and bind oxygen from maternal blood. The oxygen dissociation curve is shifted to the left by foetal haemoglobin, but to the right by increased 2,3-DPG levels.

Koeppen BM (2015). *Berne & Levy Physiology*, 6th edition. Maryland Heights, MO: Elsevier Mosby.

29. B. Delays fibrinolysis.

Tranexamic acid, an antifibrinolytic agent, competitively inhibits the binding of plasminogen and tPA to fibrin and effectively blocks conversion of plasminogen to plasmin thus delaying fibrinolysis.

Baglin T (2008). Drugs and haemostasis. In: Brown MJ, Bennett PN (Eds.), *Clinical Pharmacology*, 11th edition (pp. 492). Edinburgh, UK: Churchill Livingstone Elsevier.

30. E. *Pneumocystis jirovecii.*

Pneumocystis jirovecii (previously called *Pneumocystis carinii*) is yeast-like fungus causing opportunistic infection in the lung (pneumocystis pneumonia—PCP) in the immune-depressive patients (HIV infected or organ transplant patients).

Miller RF, Huang L (2015). Pneumocystis jirovecii. In: Warrell DA, Cox TM, Firth JD (Eds.), *Oxford Textbook of Medicine*, 5th edition. Oxford, UK: Oxford University Press.

31. D. Laceration produced with a knife.

  A. Closure of the wound with sutures has the higher risk of infection than staples or tape.
  B. Contamination with devitalized tissue, foreign matter, saliva, or stool has high risk of developing infection in the wound.
  C. Injury more than 8 to 12 hours may be high risk of developing infection, but also depends on the other various factors.
  D. Correct answer: Clean laceration made with a sharp object can be safely closed in some patients even 24 hours or later.
  E. Ischaemia produced by adrenaline in local anaesthesia may promote settling of infections in the wound.

Simon BC, Hern HG (2014). Wound management principles. In: Marx J, Hockberger RS, Walls RM (Eds.), *Rosen's Emergency Medicine*, 8th edition (pp. 751–66). Philadelphia, PA: Elsevier.

32. C. L5.

The paralysis or paresis of the extensor hallucis longus (EHL), supplied by the deep peritoneal (fibular) branch (L5) of the common peroneal nerve (L4, L5, S1, S2). Weakness of dorsiflexion of the big toe when resistance is applied is a useful index of injury to the L5 anterior ramus and spinal nerve. The sensory supply of L5 is to the anterolateral side of the leg and medial side of the foot.

Ellis H, Mahadevan V (2013). *Clinical Anatomy: Applied Anatomy for Students and Junior Doctors*, 13th edition (pp. 278–9). Oxford, UK: John Wiley & Sons Ltd.

Sinnatamby CS (2011). *Last's Anatomy: Regional and Applied*, 12th edition. London, UK: Churchill Livingstone.

33. C. Left atrial pressure is greater than or equal to left ventricular pressure while the mitral valve is open.

Consider that blood will only move from an area of higher pressure to one of lower pressure. As such, valves from one chamber to the next will only be open while the pressure difference keeps them open. This gentleman is likely to be suffering a late complication of STEMI, either a ventricular septal defect or a ruptured papillary muscle as the result of his infarct. These complications are rare in the era of primary coronary intervention.

Koeppen BM (2015). *Berne & Levy Physiology*, 6th edition. Maryland Heights, MO: Elsevier Mosby.

34. D. Rupture of the anterior cruciate ligament.

The anterior cruciate ligament (ACL) is commonly injured in sports, but other mechanisms as previously described (a direct blow to the flexed knee during car collisions) may also cause ACL tears. The ACL injuries are usually associated with meniscal tears, mostly lateral in acute injuries.

Pallin DJ (2014). Knee and lower leg. In: Marx J, Hockberger RS, Walls RM (Eds.), *Rosen's Emergency Medicine*, 8th edition (Chapter 57, pp. 698–722). Philadelphia, PA: Elsevier.

35. D. Corticotropin-releasing hormone.

The body's response to stress is triggered by recognition of a stressful stimulus in the amygdala. The hypothalamus then secretes corticotropin-releasing hormone (CRH) which activates the sympathetic nervous system and stimulates secretion of the adrenal hormones via adrenocorticotropic hormone (ACTH). They combine to increase heart rate and blood pressure, blood flow to muscles, blood glucose, and conservation of fluid and salts.

Koeppen BM (2015). *Berne & Levy Physiology*, 6th edition. Maryland Heights, MO: Elsevier Mosby.

36. D. The therapeutic effect develops after four to five days.

Warfarin, the name derived from Wisconsin Alumni Research Foundation with the suffix from 'coumarin'. The therapeutic anticoagulant effect takes four to five days to develop. The INR is not reliable in the initial stages as the vitamin K-dependent factors diminish at different rates. The INR is particularly sensitive to the level of factor VII. It competitively inhibits vitamin K epoxide reductase.

Baglin T (2008). Drugs and haemostasis. In: Brown MJ, Bennett PN (Eds.), *Clinical Pharmacology*, 11th edition (pp. 485–6). Edinburgh, UK: Churchill Livingstone Elsevier.

37. D. Sensory impairment on the medial side of the leg.

The sciatic nerve may be injured in posterior dislocation of the hip joint or fracture of the posterior part of the acetabulum. Damage to the sciatic nerve is associated with the paralysis of the hamstrings and all the muscles of the leg and foot. There is also loss of all movements below the knee joint including the foot drop. The sensory loss is also extensive sparing the area on medial side of the leg, over the medial malleolus and big toe, which are supplied by the saphenous branch of the femoral nerve.

Ellis H, Mahadevan V (2013). *Clinical Anatomy: Applied Anatomy for Students and Junior Doctors*, 13th edition (p. 277). Oxford, UK: John Wiley & Sons Ltd.

38. B. *Klebsiella pneumoniae.*

Klebsiella pneumoniae in an important cause of both community acquired pneumonia and nosocomial pneumonia. It is often associated with chronic alcoholism, diabetes mellitus, and chronic obstructive pulmonary disease. The characteristic sign is red coloured sputum (the colour of red-current jelly). Lung abscess and empyema are more frequent with K pneumonia that other organisms.

Tosh PK, Berbari EF (2016). Pulmonary and mycobacterial infection. In: Ficalora RD (Ed.), *Mayo Clinic Internal Medicine Board Review*, 11th edition (Chapter 45). Oxford, UK: Oxford University Press.

39. B. Occulomotor.

In the cranial nerve III lesions, there is ptosis of the upper eyelid due to the paralysis of the levator. The eye looks down and out when the eyelid is lifted up due to the unopposed actions of the lateral rectus and superior oblique. Because of the paralysis of superior, medial, and inferior recti, the eye could not be turned upwards. There is also interruption of parasympathetic nerve supply resulting in pupillary dilatation and unreactive to light or accommodation though the consensual light reflex to the other eye is preserved.

Sinnatamby CS (2011). Head and neck and spine. In: *Last's Anatomy: Regional and Applied*, 12th edition (p. 397). London, UK: Churchill Livingstone.

40. A. α-cells.

This patient has attended in diabetic ketoacidosis, the consequence of lack of insulin in untreated diabetes mellitus. Acinar cells are pancreatic exocrine cells, while 4 cell types have been detected in the islets of Langerhans: α cells produce glucagon, α cells produce insulin, β cells produce somatostatin and γ cells produce pancreatic polypeptides.

Koeppen BM (2015). *Berne & Levy Physiology*, 6th edition. Maryland Heights, MO: Elsevier Mosby.

41. A. It is direct competitive inhibitor of factor Xa.

Rivaroxaban, one of the oral direct anticoagulants, is a direct competitive inhibitor of factor Xa and limits generation of thrombin in dose dependent manner. It has no antidote. It is metabolized in the liver and renal excretion is minimal. There is no accumulation of the drug even if the GFR is below 15 mL/min.

Baglin T (2008). Drugs and haemostasis. In: Brown MJ, Bennett PN (Eds.), *Clinical Pharmacology*, 11th edition (pp. 488). Edinburgh, UK: Churchill Livingstone Elsevier.

42. A. Abduction of the shoulder.

Abduction and lateral rotation is weaker against resistance if the C5 nerve root is impinged. There may be associated sensory loss on the lateral aspect of the upper arm.

Sinnatamby CS (2011). *Last's Anatomy: Regional and Applied*, 12th edition (pp. 14–17). London, UK: Churchill Livingstone.

43. B. Enterochromaffin-like cells.

Chief cells contain zymogen granules and secretes chymosin and pepsinogen, which is activated to pepsin by gastric acid. G cells secrete gastrin and enterochromaffin-like cells (ECL) cells secrete histamine, both of which act on parietal cells to stimulate gastric acid release. Goblet cells secrete mucus, which contributes to the gastric mucosal barrier to prevent ulcer formation.

Koeppen BM (2015). *Berne & Levy Physiology*, 6th edition. Maryland Heights, MO: Elsevier Mosby.

44. A. Ascending loop of Henle.

Furosemide, one of the 'loop' diuretics, impairs the urine-concentrating mechanism of the loop of Henle and has a high efficacy. It acts on the thick portion of the ascending limb of the loop of Henle to produce the discussed effect. It may cause up to 25% of the filtered sodium to be excreted. The drug may result in to low potassium, magnesium, calcium, and sodium. It acts within an hour if taken orally and 30 minutes if given intravenously. It relieves acute pulmonary oedema by its venodilator action, which precedes the diuresis.

Aliyu S (2008). Viral, fungal, protozoal and helminthic infections. In: Brown MJ, Bennett PN (Eds.), *Clinical Pharmacology*, 11th edition (pp. 213–14). Edinburgh, UK: Churchill Livingstone Elsevier.

45. E. Tip of the left occipital lobe.

Traumatic lesion to the tip of the left occipital lobe (i.e. to the macular area) results in a right homonymous macular defect.

Sinnatamby CS (2011). Head and neck and spine. In: *Last's Anatomy: Regional and Applied*, 12th edition (pp. 496–7). London, UK: Churchill Livingstone.

46. A. Atrioventricular node.

The P wave represents atrial depolarization, while the QRS complex reflects ventricular depolarization. As such, the PR interval reflects the transmission of the atrial impulse to the ventricles via the AV node, which is normally 120–200 milliseconds. Causes of prolonged PR interval include hypertrophy of cardiac muscle, myocarditis, and ischaemic heart disease.

Koeppen BM (2015). *Berne & Levy Physiology*, 6th edition. Maryland Heights, MO: Elsevier Mosby.

47. C. Middle cerebral artery.

The middle cerebral artery (MCA) supplies most of the sensory and motor cortex, internal capsule, and optic radiation. Complete occlusion of MCA may result in dense flaccid hemiparesis, homonymous hemianopia, aphasia (if dominant hemisphere is involved), and marked inattention or neglect (if non-dominant side is affected).

Fuller G, Manford M (2000). *Neurology* (p. 66). Edinburgh, UK: Churchill Livingstone.

48. E. Trimethoprim.

The following antibiotics, which may result in *Clostridium difficile* diarrhoea and colitis, are listed in Table 7.1:

Table 7.1 Drugs that may cause *Clostridium difficile* diarrhoea and colitis

Frequently associated	Occasionally associated	Rarely associated
Fluoroquinolones	Macrolides	Aminoglycosides
Clindamycin	Trimethoprim-sulfamethoxazole	Tetracyclines
Broad spectrum cephalosporins		Metronidazole
Penicillins		Vancomycin

UpToDate (2017). *Clostridium difficile* infection in adults: Clinical manifestations and diagnosis. Available at: https://www.uptodate.com/contents/clostridium-difficile-infection-in-adults-clinical-manifestations-and-diagnosis

49. E. Ventilation:perfusion mismatch.

This is the most common cause of hypoxaemia and comprises conditions such as asthma, COPD, pneumonia, PE, and pulmonary oedema. The Aa gradient will be high but the patient should respond to oxygen supplementation.

Koeppen BM (2015). *Berne & Levy Physiology*, 6th edition. Maryland Heights, MO: Elsevier Mosby.

50. C. Raising eyebrows.

Injury to facial nerve at this level may result in asymmetry of the corner of the mouth, flattening of skin folds, and inability to close the eye or wrinkle the forehead. On the face, sometimes depending on the particular branch, which is severed, one of these functions may only be affected.

Sinnatamby CS (2011). Head and neck and spine. In: *Last's Anatomy Regional and Applied*, 12th edition (pp. 496–7). London, UK: Elsevier Ltd.

51. E. Located at the mid-point between the ASIS and pubic symphysis.

The femoral artery, when the hip is slightly flexed and laterally rotated, lies at the mid-point between ASIS and symphysis pubis. The femoral sheath is the prolongation of transversalis fascia in the front and psoas fascia at the back. It contains the femoral vessels. The femoral nerve is outside and lateral to the femoral sheath. Within the sheath, a space medial to the femoral vein is called femoral canal, which contains a lymph node (of Cloquet) draining the lymph from clitoris in female and glans in male.

Sinnatamby CS (2011). *Last's Anatomy: Regional and Applied*, 12th edition (pp. 111–78). London, UK: Churchill Livingstone.

52. C. Natural killer T-cells.

Natural killer T-cells display characteristics of both T-cells, which participate in adaptive immunity, and natural killer cells that are involved in innate immunity. Possessing the ability to recognize antigen-presenting molecules, these cells allow a rapid response to virally infected cells but also play a role in antibody formation and memory cell development.

Koeppen BM (2015). *Berne & Levy Physiology*, 6th edition. Maryland Heights, MO: Elsevier Mosby.

53. E. Sodium/Potassium/Chloride co-transporter.

In the thick segment of the ascending limb, sodium and chloride ions are transported from the tubular fluid to the interstitial fluid by the three-ion co-transporter system ($Na^+/K^+/2Cl^-$) driven by the sodium pump. The loop diuretics work at this level by inhibiting the three-ion transporter preventing sodium ion reabsorption and lowering the osmotic gradient between cortex and medulla. This causes production of large volume of dilute urine.

O'Shaughnessy KM (2008). Kidney and genitourinary tract. In: Brown MJ, Bennett PN (Eds.), *Clinical Pharmacology*, 11th edition (pp. 452–5). Edinburgh, UK: Churchill Livingstone Elsevier.

54. C. Aortic arch.

There are four constrictions in oesophagus where the foreign bodies may get stuck. These may be the cricopharyngeal sphincter, sites crossed by aortic arch, the left principal main bronchus, and when it passes through the diaphragm.

Sinnatamby CS (2011). *Last's Anatomy: Regional and Applied*, 12th edition. London, UK: Churchill Livingstone.

55. A. Anterior leads.

The most common site of coronary artery occlusion is the left anterior descending artery, referred to as the 'widowmaker' due to the high incidence of morbidity and mortality resulting from anterior myocardial infarction. The anterior leads are V3–4, though any of the chest leads may be affected.

Koeppen BM (2015). *Berne & Levy Physiology*, 6th edition. Maryland Heights, MO: Elsevier Mosby.

56. A. Ascending colon.

The superior mesenteric artery is a branch from aorta arising at the level of L1. It supplies the distal duodenum, jejunum, ileum, caecum, ascending colon, and transverse colon.

Ellis H, Mahadevan V (2013). *Clinical Anatomy: Applied Anatomy for Students and Junior Doctors*, 13th edition (p. 94). Oxford, UK: John Wiley & Sons Ltd.

57. D. Greater occipital nerve.

The skin of the back of the head (occipital area) is supplied by the greater occipital nerve, which is primarily formed from the root of C2 (posterior rami). This nerve with the lesser occipital nerve could be blocked by local anaesthesia for posterior scalp surgery or wound repairs.

Yin W (1996). General surgery and trauma. In: Brown DL (Ed.), *Regional Anaesthesia and Analgesia* (p. 505). Philadelphia, PA: W. B. Saunders Company.

58. C. Production of ATP via oxidative phosphorylation.

These are the cellular functions of lysosomes, the Golgi apparatus, mitochondria, endoplasmic reticulum, and the nucleus, respectively. Mitochondria are the engines of the cell, producing a supply of ATP to support the other cellular functions. Mitochondria carry maternal DNA only in the form of plasmids.

Koeppen BM (2015). *Berne & Levy Physiology*, 6th edition. Maryland Heights, MO: Elsevier Mosby.

59. B. Internal capsule.

Occlusion of the small branches of the anterior and posterior circulation may result various types of lacunar infarcts. Pure motor hemiparesis affecting the face, arm, and leg with no other deficit is usually an internal capsule lesion.

Fuller G, Manford M (2000). *Neurology: An Illustrated Colour Text* (p. 67). Edinburgh, UK: Churchill Livingstone.

60. C. Early depolarizations in the myocardium generating different refractory periods in the myocytes.

This can lead to Torsades de pointes and increases the risk of re-entrant ventricular arrhythmias and ventricular fibrillation. Early repolarizations occur more frequently in the presence of adrenergic stimulation, which is why many patients with long QT syndrome suffer arrhythmias while exercising or under stress. Above 500 milliseconds, the risk of fatal arrhythmias such as Torsades de pointes increases significantly.

Koeppen BM (2015). *Berne & Levy Physiology*, 6th edition. Maryland Heights, MO: Elsevier Mosby.

61. E. CSF PCR.

The most common cause of encephalitis is HSV—1 virus. The initial test is neuroimaging (CT or MRI) in suspected cases for potential cerebral oedema or to exclude space occupying lesion. This is followed by lumbar puncture (LP) if safe to do so. In addition to standard CSF analysis and culture, a sample is also sent for HSV PCR, which is much more sensitive and specific for HSV—1, HSV—2 and enteroviruses.

Martinez T (2016). Encephalitis. In: Chanmugam AS, Rothman R, Desai S, Putman S (Eds.), *Infectious Diseases Emergencies* (Chapter 7). Oxford, UK: Oxford University Press.

62. C. The nipple line.

There is considerable overlap of dermatome on the trunk and the limbs. The dermatomes are organized in orderly numerical sequence. The clinically useful guidelines are available to examine the specific dermatome. The sensation across the nipple line is supplied by the T4 in most of the situations. Please see the reference for further detail.

Sinnatamby CS (2011). Introduction to regional anatomy. In: *Last's Anatomy: Regional and Applied*, 12th edition. London, UK: Churchill Livingstone.

63. A. Lower fibres of left optic radiation.

An abscess in the temporal lobe may produce lesions in the lower fibres in the left optic radiation resulting in the right upper quadrantic homonymous hemianopia as the upper part of the visual field is represented through the lower fibres in the optic radiation (from the lower part of the retina).

Sinnatamby CS (2011). Head and neck and spine. In: *Last's Anatomy: Regional and Applied*, 12th edition (pp. 496–7). London, UK: Churchill Livingstone.

64. C. Loss of saltatory conduction.

Myelin-containing Schwann cells line single neurons of the peripheral nervous system, while oligodendrocytes perform this function for multiple neurons in the central nervous system. Myelination allows significantly increased rate of impulse transmission as action potentials 'leap' between the nodes of Ranvier.

Koeppen BM (2015). *Berne & Levy Physiology*, 6th edition. Maryland Heights, MO: Elsevier Mosby.

65. E. Tracheobronchial capillaries.

A. Disruption of bronchial artery may occur in arteritis, trauma, or malignant erosions resulting in massive and sudden haemoptysis.
B. Inflammation of bronchial wall and dilation with necrotizing infection in bronchiectasis may result in massive haemoptysis.
C. See answer B.
D. Bleeding from pulmonary artery if affected centrally may result in massive haemoptysis.
E. Correct answer: Tracheobronchial capillaries are the source of bleeding in vigorous coughing or minor bronchial infections.

Brown CA, Raja AS (2014). Haemoptysis. In: Marx J, Hockberger RS, Walls RM (Eds.), *Rosen's Emergency Medicine*, 8th edition (Chapter 24). Philadelphia, PA: Elsevier.

66. B. Descending colon.

The inferior mesenteric artery is a branch from aorta arising at the level of L3. It supplies the hindgut derivatives namely descending colon, sigmoid, and rectum.

Ellis H, Mahadevan V (2013). *Clinical Anatomy: Applied Anatomy for Students and Junior Doctors*, 13th edition (p. 94). Oxford, UK: John Wiley & Sons Ltd.

67. B. Auriculotemporal nerve.

The auriculotemporal nerve, a branch from trigeminal nerve supplies sensation to the superior two-thirds of the anterior surface of the ear. It may be blocked by injecting local anaesthetic agent at the anterior aspect of the auricle, forwards of the external auditory meatus.

Yin W (1996). General surgery and trauma. In: Brown DL (Ed.), *Regional Anaesthesia and Analgesia* (p. 505). Philadelphia, PA: W. B. Saunders Company.

68. A. Acetylcholine.

Impairment of acetylcholine pathways is implicated in Alzheimer's disease, which is the most common form of dementia in the United Kingdom. Acetylcholine is synthesized in the basal nucleus of Meynert and is involved in all motor neurons, all pre-ganglionic autonomic neurons, and multiple central pathways related to emotion and memory.

Koeppen BM (2015). *Berne & Levy Physiology*, 6th edition. Maryland Heights, MO: Elsevier Mosby.

69. D. Antagonist to 5-HT$_3$ receptor.

- Ondansetron, currently the anti-emetic of choice, is a serotonin 5-HT$_3$ receptor antagonist, which blocks the serotonin stimulation centrally in the chemoreceptor trigger zone and peripherally in the vagal nerve terminals, both of which stimulate vomiting.
- The mechanism of action that produces the antiemetic effect of antihistamines is unclear.
- Phenothiazines produce their antiemetic effects by blocking the dopaminergic receptors in the chemoreceptor trigger zone in the brain. It may also directly depress the vomiting centre.
- All types of antiemetics are absorbed well through gastrointestinal tract.

Eckman M, Labus D (Eds.) (2009). *Clinical Pharmacology Made Incredibly Easy* (eBook from OVID), 3rd edition. Philadelphia, PA: Lippincott Williams & Wilkins.

UpToDate (2017). Ondansentron drug information. Available at: https://www.uptodate.com/contents/ondansetron-drug-information

70. A. Compliance of the chest wall much greater than adults.

There are differences between the features of thoracic trauma in children and adult. Smaller the body mass of a child causes application of greater force per unit body surface area. Pliability of chest wall/ ribs may result in significant intrathoracic organ injuries without much external sign of trauma. Compliance of the child's chest is much greater than that of the adult.

Medscape, Pediatric Thoracic Trauma. Available at: http://emedicine.medscape.com/article/905863-overview

71. E. Turning the head to the right shoulder.

Contraction of the left sternocleidomastoid muscle would tilt the head towards the ipsilateral shoulder, and rotate the head to the opposite side. If both muscles act together, the head is flexed forwards.

Sinnatamby CS (2011). Head and neck and spine. In: *Last's Anatomy: Regional and Applied*, 12th edition (pp. 329–454). London, UK: Churchill Livingstone.

72. D. Neutrophils.

Neutrophils are the most plentiful immune cells in the bloodstream and respond to signalling molecules, such as histamine, and adhesion molecules presented by damaged endothelial cells. Increased capillary permeability allows the neutrophils to enter the injured tissue, where they engulf pathogens and foreign material by phagocytosis for intracellular degradation by lysomes.

Koeppen BM (2015). *Berne & Levy Physiology*, 6th edition. Maryland Heights, MO: Elsevier Mosby.

73. A. Able to reduce morphine-induced smooth muscle spasm.

Hyoscine butylbromide blocks autonomic ganglia. It is an effective smooth muscle relaxant including cardia in achalasia and the pyloric antrum. It is also used for spasm of smooth muscle and reduces morphine-induced smooth muscle spasm.

O'Shaughnessy KM (2012). Cholinergic and antimuscarinic (anticholinergic) mechanisms and drugs. In: Brown MJ, Bennett PN (Eds.), *Clinical Pharmacology*, 11th edition (pp. 380–1). Edinburgh, UK: Churchill Livingstone Elsevier.

74. B. Mid-brain.

Lesion on the left mid-brain area would cause hemiparesis on the contralateral side (here on the right side) and features of III nerve involvement also on the contralateral side.

Fuller G, Manford M (2000). *Neurology: An Illustrated Colour Text* (p. 67). Edinburgh, UK: Churchill Livingstone.

Ramrakha PS, Moore K, Sam, A (2010). *Oxford Handbook of Acute Medicine*, 3rd edition (pp. 342–3). Oxford, UK: Oxford University Press.

75. C. Overdrive suppression.

Overdrive suppression describes the phenomenon by which cardiac pacemaker cells that depolarize at a lower frequency do not trigger their own cardiac impulses when a faster pacemaker cell is doing so. When the faster pacemaker cells stop pacing, the slower pacemaker cells undergo a refractory period, or pause, before they begin to depolarize and trigger their own cardiac impulse.

Koeppen BM (2015). *Berne & Levy Physiology*, 6th edition. Maryland Heights, MO: Elsevier Mosby.

76. A. Motor cortex.

In focal seizures, which may occur at any age, the abnormal stimulation starts in one part of the brain. The focal symptoms indicate the abnormal area of the cortex. This pattern of jerking of one limb may be from abnormal discharges in the motor cortex. Occipital lobe involvement would cause visual hallucination. Discharges in the temporal lobe may cause swallowing or chewing movement, or olfactory or gustatory hallucinations.

Fuller G, Manford M (2000). *Neurology: An Illustrated Colour Text* (p. 67). Edinburgh, UK; Churchill Livingstone.

77. B. Azygo-portal anastomosis.

The distal part of oesophagus has connections between the portal and systemic venous system, which opens up because of rise in the pressure in the portal veins (portal hypertension) in cirrhosis. Haematemesis in the discussed situation occurs because of the rupture of these veins.

Ellis H, Mahadevan V (2013). *Clinical Anatomy: Applied Anatomy for Students and Junior Doctors*, 13th edition (p. 96). Oxford, UK: John Wiley & Sons Ltd.

78. D. Internal mammary artery.

While performing the 'clam-shell' thoracotomy in the ED, the chest is opened by an incision, which runs across the front of the chest at the level of nipple line from one infra-axillary area to other. The incision is made in the intercostal muscles just above the ribs avoiding the neurovascular bundle. While dividing the sternum, the internal mammary arteries (IMAs) are identified and ligated to avoid bleeding later on. The left vagus nerve runs on the anterior surface of the pericardium, which should be identified and avoided while incising the pericardium.

Chikwe J, Cooke DT, Weiss A (2013). Chest trauma. In: *Cardiothoracic Surgery*, 2nd edition (Chapter 17). Oxford University Press.

79. C. $PaCO_2$ is normal, due to the patient tiring.

This is a medical emergency and it is important to recognize that a normal $PaCO_2$ during an asthma attack can indicate exhaustion in the patient and necessitates urgent escalation to HDU/ITU.

Koeppen BM (2015). *Berne & Levy Physiology*, 6th edition. Maryland Heights, MO: Elsevier Mosby.

80. A. Body of pancreas.

The transpyloric plane passes through the lower border of L1 vertebral body, pylorus, pancreatic neck, duodenojejunal flexure, fundus of the gall bladder, tip of the ninth costal cartilages and hila of the kidneys.

Ellis H, Mahadevan V (2013). *Clinical Anatomy: Applied Anatomy for Students and Junior Doctors*, 13th edition (p. 61). Oxford, UK: John Wiley & Sons Ltd.

81. C. Fraction of gas in the gas mixture x total pressure.

Dalton's gas law states that the sum of the partial pressures (or fractions) of the individual gases in a mixture must equal the total pressure (or 1.0).

Koeppen BM (2015). *Berne & Levy Physiology*, 6th edition. Maryland Heights, MO: Elsevier Mosby.

82. A. Aciclovir.

Aciclovir is a nucleoside analogue, which inhibits viral replication by acting as a substrate for viral DNA polymerase. It is against herpes viruses. The drug is indicated in herpes simplex and Varicella zoster virus infections.

Aliyu S (2008). Viral, fungal, protozoal and helminthic infections. In: Brown MJ, Bennett PN (Eds.), *Clinical Pharmacology*, 11th edition (pp. 213–14). Edinburgh, UK: Churchill Livingstone Elsevier.

83. B. Loss of knee jerk.

The nerve root affected is that of L4, which results in weak quadriceps power and knee jerk. The sensory loss is on the lower medial leg area. Great toe extension is affected by L5 lesions. Loss of ankle jerk and weak planter flexion of the foot are found when S1 nerve root is affected.

Drake R (2004). *Gray's Anatomy for Students* (p. 71). London, UK: Churchill Livingstone.

Wyatt J, Illingworth RN, Graham CA, et al. (2012). Oxford Handbook of Emergency Medicine, 4th edition (p. 492). Oxford, UK: Oxford University Press.

84. B. Carbohydrate metabolism.

Pancreatic exocrine insufficiency is the loss of digestive enzymes and bicarbonate secretion from tissue damaged by chronic inflammation, leading to malabsorption. Lipid digestion is first affected due to decreased duodenal pH. Bile production and release are inhibited. Gastric lipase is the only means of lipid digestion. Approximately 80% of carbohydrate digestion occurs in the absence of pancreatic amylase.

Koeppen BM (2015). *Berne & Levy Physiology*, 6th edition. Maryland Heights, MO: Elsevier Mosby.

85. D. Parietal cells.

Pernicious anaemia specifically refers to the macrocytic anaemia that occurs due to insufficient intrinsic factor release as the result of autoimmune destruction of the parietal cells. However, many people use the term more generally to refer to all cases of anaemia due to low vitamin B12. Pernicious means 'deadly' and describes the prognosis of the condition before B12 injections were available. Incidence in over-60s is 1 in 1,000.

Koeppen BM (2015). *Berne & Levy Physiology*, 6th edition. Maryland Heights, MO: Elsevier Mosby.

86. B. Inhibit cell wall synthesis.

Penicillin containing beta-lactam ring acts by inhibiting cell wall synthesis resulting in osmotic rupture. It is bactericidal. The bacteria, which are resting organisms not making new walls, are not affected by penicillins. The resistant bacteria produce beta-lactamases, which hydrolyses the beta-lactam ring.

Farrington M (2008). Antibacterial drugs. In: Brown MJ, Bennett PN (Eds.), *Clinical Pharmacology*, 11th edition (pp. 173–5). Edinburgh, UK: Churchill Livingstone Elsevier.

87. E. Rhabdomyolysis.

Muscle breakdown secondary to a crush injury or long lie causes release of myoglobin and other muscle products (e.g. creatine kinase) into the bloodstream, which are nephrotoxic in high concentrations. Compartment syndrome and disseminated intravascular coagulation (DIC) are associated with rhabdomyolysis.

Koeppen BM (2015). *Berne & Levy Physiology*, 6th edition. Maryland Heights, MO: Elsevier Mosby.

88. E. Vagus.

The motor innervation of soft palate may be affected in high lesions of vagus nerve. It may also affect difficulty in swallowing and vocal cord defects. The unaffected side of the soft palate moves upward pulling the uvula towards the normal side.

Sinnatamby CS (2011). Head and neck and spine. In: *Last's Anatomy: Regional and Applied*, 12th edition (pp. 496–7). London, UK: Churchill Livingstone.

89. D. Pressure required to expand the alveoli is reduced.

Surfactant develops from week 24–28 of gestation, reaching normal terms levels by approximately week 35. Surfactant reduces the surface tension of the air:alveolus interface preventing collapse during expiration. According to the Law of Laplace, pressure required to expand the alveolus is proportional to surface tension and inversely proportional to alveolar radius.

Koeppen BM (2015). *Berne & Levy Physiology*, 6th edition. Maryland Heights, MO: Elsevier Mosby.

90. A. Left optic nerve.

A complete blindness to one eye is because of total lesion in the optic nerve. Specific areas of visual field defect occur because of pathology at different sites. The right optic nerve lesion would result in total visual loss in the right eye.

Sinnatamby CS (2011). Head and neck and spine. In: *Last's Anatomy: Regional and Applied*, 12th edition (pp. 496–7). London, UK: Churchill Livingstone.

91. A. Fast response to intervention.

Vagal stimulation releases acetylcholine to act on muscarinic receptors that are prevalent at the sinoatrial and atrioventricular nodes. These receptors directly interact with K^+ channels, without any intervening second messenger. As such vagal responses occur quickly.

Koeppen BM (2015). *Berne & Levy Physiology*, 6th edition. Maryland Heights, MO: Elsevier Mosby.

92. B. Inhibition of COX-1 mediated prostaglandin synthesis.

PGI_2 and PGE_2 are cytoprotective mucosal prostaglandins, which inhibit acid secretion in the stomach, promote mucus production, and enhance mucosal perfusion. The non-steroidal anti-inflammatory drugs (NSAIDs) inhibits the COX-1 mediated production of these prostaglandins.

Thornton C, Mason JC (2008). Drugs for inflammation and joint disease. In: Brown MJ, Bennett PN (Eds.), *Clinical Pharmacology*, 11th edition (pp. 243–5). Edinburgh, UK: Churchill Livingstone Elsevier.

93. A. Brainstem.

The diabetes and alcohol are responsible for most of the autonomic dysfunction. Some may be caused by drugs (e.g. antihypertensive agents). The site of lesion often dictates the symptoms and signs. In the organs, which are innervated by both the sympathetic nervous system (SNS) and parasympathetic nervous system (PSNS), the net effects depend on the balance of abnormality affecting the two systems. The hypothalamus and brainstem lesions where the autonomic signals are integrated, may lead to abnormality in the spontaneous activities such as respiration (Cheyne-Stokes respiration or hiccoughs in brainstem lesions). Please see the reference for detail symptoms and signs affected as a result of pathology in different anatomical locations.

Fuller G, Manford M (2000). *Neurology: An Illustrated Colour Text* (pp. 114–15). Edinburgh, UK: Churchill Livingstone.

94. C. PR interval of 140 mS, right bundle branch block and right axis deviation.

Trifascicular block is an ECG diagnosis characterized by prolonged PR interval (>120 mS), right bundle branch block, and left anterior or posterior fascicular block. Left anterior fascicular block manifests as left axis deviation on the ECG while left posterior fascicular block manifests as right axis deviation.

Koeppen BM (2015). *Berne & Levy Physiology*, 6th edition. Maryland Heights, MO: Elsevier Mosby.

95. B. Antimuscarinic.

Bronchoconstriction is caused by release of acetylcholine from the vagal nerve endings in the airways activating the muscarinic receptors on the bronchial smooth muscles. Blockage of these receptors by inhaled ipratropium causes bronchodilatation. They are also useful if used in conjunction with beta2 agonists in acute severe asthma.

O'Shaughnessy KM (2008). Respiratory system. In: Brown MJ, Bennett PN (Eds.), *Clinical Pharmacology*, 11th edition (pp. 474–5). Edinburgh, UK: Churchill Livingstone Elsevier.

96. C. Skin scrapings.

Athlete's foot is caused by dermatophytes, filamentous fungi. The most common clinical subtype is Tinea pedis as in this case. The diagnosis can be confirmed by detecting segmented hyphae in the skin scrapings from the affected skin with a potassium hydroxide preparation. Gram stain and culture is required when a secondary bacterial infection is suspected.

UpToDate (2017)., Dermatophyte (tinea) infections. Available at: https://www.uptodate.com/contents/dermatophyte-tinea-infections

97. E. Von Willebrand's disease.

This is the most common bleeding disorder in humans and can be hereditary or acquired. It is associated with aortic stenosis, hypothyroidism, and Wilm's tumour. Factor V Leiden and protein S deficiency increase risk of clots. Haemophilia A & B present early with significant bleeds. Patients with Factor XII deficiency have prolonged APTT but are asymptomatic.

Koeppen BM (2015). *Berne & Levy Physiology*, 6th edition. Maryland Heights, MO: Elsevier Mosby.

98. D. Infiltration of superior belly of omohyoid muscle.

A. The direct involvement of oesophagus from extension of thyroid gland tumours are extremely rare.

B. Inferior belly of omohyoid muscle is situated in the posterior triangle of the neck, hence, possibility of its infiltration is remote.

C. Recurrent laryngeal nerve involvement results in aphonia or hoarseness of voice.

D. Correct answer: Infiltration of superior belly of omohyoid muscle, is the only plausible option in this situation.

E. Involvement of cricothyroid membrane may cause hoarseness or stridor.

Sinnatamby CS (2011). Head and neck and spine. In: *Last's Anatomy: Regional and Applied*, 12th edition (pp. 496–7). London, UK: Churchill Livingstone.

99. D. Severe proximal stenosis in the left anterior descending artery.

Wellen's syndrome is suggested by the finding of deeply inverted or biphasic T waves in the anterior chest leads, typically V2 and V3, in a patient with chest pain. The diagnosis portends a significant, but incomplete, stenosis in the proximal left anterior descending (LAD) coronary artery. In the original study group, 75% of patients with Wellen's syndrome went on to have anterior myocardial infarctions within one week.

Koeppen BM (2015). *Berne & Levy Physiology*, 6th edition. Maryland Heights, MO: Elsevier Mosby.

100. A. Jugulodigastric.

The jugulodigastric group of lymph nodes, a variety of superior deep cervical nodes, are typically involved in tonsillitis.

Standring S (2016). Neck. In: *Gray's Anatomy*, 41st edition (Chapter 29; p. 442–74). London, UK: Elsevier Ltd.

INDEX

Note: Page numbers followed by *q* refer to questions and *a* to answers. Tables are indicated by (*t*), and figures by (*f*).

2,3-diphosphoglycerate 87*q*, 128*a*
5-HT3 receptor antagonists 196*q*, 215*a*

A

Aa gradient 84*q*, 124*a*
A band 82*q*, 122*a*
Abbreviated Mental Test Score (AMTS) 266*q*, 292*a*
abdominal aorta 19*q*, 56*a*
abdominal X-ray 19*q*(*f*)
abducent nerve 33*q*, 75*a*
abductor pollicis brevis 2*q*, 36*a*
abductor pollicis longus 38*a*
ablation therapy 90*q*, 132–3*a*
absolute risk reduction (ARR) 230*q*, 234*a*, 235*a*
acanthosis nigricans 155*a*
accessory pathway 93*q*, 136*a*
ACE (angiotensin converting enzyme) 150*a*
ACE (angiotensin converting enzyme) inhibitors 103*q*, 149*a*
acetaldehyde 200*q*, 222*a*
acetazolamide 196*q*, 216*a*
acetylcholine 81*q*, 83*q*, 101*q*, 120*a*, 122–3*a*, 101*q*, 146*a*
    Alzheimer's disease 278*q*, 301*a*
    gastric acid secretion 80*q*, 118*a*
    vomiting 102*q*, 148*a*
aciclovir 167*q*, 173*q*, 177*a*, 183*a*, 281*q*, 303*a*
acidosis 127–8*a*
    lactic 220*a*
    metabolic 103*q*, 148*a*
    respiratory 103*q*, 125*a*, 148*a*
acinar cells 296*a*
ACL (anterior cruciate ligament) 9*q*, 43*a*, 269*q*, 295*a*
acoustic neuroma 72*a*, 77*a*
acquired immune deficiency syndrome (AIDS) 171*q*, 184*a*
acromegaly 111*q*, 159*a*
ACTH see adrenocorticotrophic hormone
actin filaments 81*q*, 119*a*, 122*a*
action potentials 79*q*, 81*q*, 83*q*, 116*a*, 119–20*a*, 122*a*
    cardiac myocyte 261*q*, 289*a*
activated partial thromboplastin time (APTT) 79*q*, 117*a*
actrapid insulin 193*q*, 211*a*
acute lymphoblastic leukaemia (ALL) 264*q*, 291*a*
acute myeloid leukaemia (AML) 257*a*

AD (Alzheimer's disease) 27*q*, 67*a*, 120*a*, 278*q*, 301*a*
Addisonian crisis 156*a*
Addison's disease 102*q*, 148*a*, 156*a*, 157*a*
adductor pollicis 2*q*, 36*a*
adenosine 94*q*, 137*a*, 204*q*, 227*a*
adenosine triphosphate (ATP) 84*q*, 123*a*, 275*q*, 299*a*
    cellular transport, failure of 262*q*, 289*a*, 290*a*
ADH see antidiuretic hormone
adipose tissue 80*q*, 114*q*, 117*a*, 162*a*
adrenal crisis 114*q*, 163*a*
adrenal gland, layers of 109*q*, 156*a*
adrenal haemorrhage, bilateral 114*q*, 163*a*
adrenaline 94*q*, 137*a*, 195*q*, 213*a*(*t*), 214*a*
    anaphylaxis 192*q*, 209*a*
    cardiopulmonary resuscitation 204*q*, 227*a*
    production/secretion 114*q*, 156*a*, 162*a*, 163*a*
    side effects 195*q*, 213*a*
adrenal medulla 114*q*, 162–3*a*
adrenocorticotrophic hormone (ACTH)
    ACTH-secreting pituitary adenoma 158*a*
    hypothalamic–pituitary–adrenal axis 112*q*, 159–60*a*
    removal of negative feedback to secretion of 109*q*, 155*a*, 156*a*
    secretion 163*a*
    stress response 295*a*
adventitia (serosa) 97*q*, 141*a*, 142*a*
Aedes mosquito 165*q*, 174*a*
AF (atrial fibrillation) 90*q*, 132–3*a*
afferent nerve from appendix 16*q*, 52*a*
African Burkitt's lymphoma 257*a*
afterload 135*a*
ageing
    pneumonia risk 245*q*, 255*a*
    reduced arterial compliance secondary to 95*q*, 138*a*
agonal breathing 86*q*, 127*a*
AICA (anterior inferior cerebellar artery) 26*q*, 65*a*, 66*a*
AIDS (acquired immune deficiency syndrome) 171*q*, 184*a*
airway resistance 84*q*, 124*a*
albumin, serum 103*q*, 149*a*
alcohol/alcoholism
    anaemia 246*q*, 256*a*
    autonomic dysfunction 286*q*, 305*a*

alcohol/alcoholism (cont.)
  cephalosporin 202q, 224a
  effects 265q, 292a
  gabapentin 202q, 224a
  hypoglycaemia 198q, 218a, 263q, 290a
  intoxication 102q, 148a, 200q, 222a
  metformin 199q, 220a
  nitrous oxide 200q, 221a
  warfarin 201q, 223a
  wound healing 243q, 252a
aldehyde dehydrogenase 200q, 222a
aldosterone 103q, 104q, 149a, 150a, 156a
alfentanil 193q, 211a(t)
alkalosis
  metabolic 95q, 103q, 138a, 149a
  respiratory 103q, 138a, 149a
ALL (acute lymphoblastic leukaemia) 264q, 291a
α1-adrenergic receptors 83q, 122a
α2-adrenergic receptors 122a
α cells (pancreas) 271q, 296a
alpha thalassaemia 246q, 256a
alteplase 257a
altitude, living at 87q, 128a
alveolar air equation 124a
Alzheimer's disease (AD) 27q, 67a, 120a, 278q, 301a
aminoglycosides 191q, 199q, 206a, 221a
amiodarone 204q, 227a
AML (acute myeloid leukaemia) 257a
amlodipine 212a
amoebic dysentery 187a
amoxicillin 173q, 188a, 191q, 199q, 207a, 220a
  neonatal sepsis 165q, 174a
  resistance 191q, 207a
ANA (antinuclear antibodies) 243q, 251–2a
anaemia
  Down's syndrome 87q, 127a
  folate deficiency 246q, 256a
  iron deficiency 246q, 256a
  macrocytic 100q, 144–5a, 256a, 304a
  microcytic 256a
  normocytic 256a
  pernicious 100q, 144–5a, 282q, 304a
  sickle cell 87q, 128a
anal canal 17q, 54a
anal fissure 17q, 54a
analgesia 194q, 212a
  evidence-based medicine 231q, 236–7a
  nitrous oxide 200q, 221a
  NSAIDs 198q, 200q, 219a, 221a, 305a
  opiate 193q, 211a
  procedural sedation and 202q, 224–5a
anal sphincters
  external 17q, 54a
  internal 98q, 142a
  nerve supply 20q, 58a
anal verge 17q, 54a
anaphylaxis 192q, 209a
anatomical shunts 84q, 88q, 124a, 129a

anatomical snuffbox 3q, 38a
anatomy 1–34q, 35–77a
androgen production 156a
androstenedione production 156a
angina 134a
angiotensin 107q, 154a
angiotensin converting enzyme (ACE) 150a
angiotensin converting enzyme (ACE) inhibitors 103q, 149a
angiotensin I 103q, 149a
angiotensin II 104q, 149a, 150a
angle of Louis 10q, 45a
anion gap 102q, 148a
ankle
    jerk 20q, 58a, 281q, 303a
    plantar flexion 281q, 303a
    sprain 9q, 44a
ANP (atrial natriuretic peptide) 150a, 152a
antecubital fossa 2q, 36a
anterior cerebral artery 27q, 68a
anterior communicating artery 27q, 68a
anterior cruciate ligament (ACL) 9q, 43a, 269q, 295a
anterior ethmoid artery 20q, 58a
anterior inferior cerebellar artery (AICA) 26q, 65a, 66a
anterior pituitary gland 26q, 66a
anterior talofibular ligament 9q, 44a
anterior tibiofibular ligament 9q, 44a
anterior triangle of neck 22q, 32q, 61a, 74a
anthrax 172q, 175a, 187–8a
antibiotics 199q, 220–1a
    classes 206a(t)
antidiuretic hormone (ADH) 103q, 104q, 149a, 150a
    functions 150a
    psychogenic polydipsia 108q, 154a
antiemetics 196q, 215a, 278q, 301a
antiepileptics 197q, 217a
antinuclear antibodies (ANA) 243q, 251–2a
aortic arch 14q, 49a
    foreign body 274q, 298a
aortic dissection 12q, 48a, 231q, 236a
aortic flow 91q, 134a
aortic valve 91q, 134a
apneustic breathing 86q, 127a
appendicitis, acute 16q, 52a
appendicular artery 16q, 52a
appendix 16q, 52a
APTT (activated partial thromboplastin time) 79q, 117a
aquaporin 1: 84q, 123a
aquaporin 2: 103q, 149a, 150a
aquaporin 3: 103q, 149a
aqueduct of Sylvius 28q, 68a
arachidonic acid pathway 242q, 250a
arachnoid 69a
arboviruses 177a
arm
    Monteggia fracture 265q, 292a
    nerve supply 4q, 38a
    paraesthesia 4q
ARR (absolute risk reduction) 230q, 234–5a

arterial compliance, reduced 95*q*, 138*a*
arthritis
    acute gouty 203*q*, 225*a*
    juvenile 169*q*, 180*a*
aryepiglottic fold 22*q*, 60*a*
Ascaris lumbricoides 168*q*, 180*a*
ascending cholangitis 123*a*
ascending reticular activating system (ARAS) 67*a*
ascorbic acid see vitamin C
aspirin 204*q*, 227*a*, 286*q*, 305*a*
asplenia 243*q*, 252*a*
asthma
    acute 13*q*, 48*a*, 281*q*, 303*a*
    adenosine contraindicated in 227*a*
    airway resistance 84*q*, 124*a*
    intravenous magnesium 199*q*, 220*a*
    ipratropium 286*q*, 305*a*
    lung function 87*q*, 128*a*, 265*q*, 292*a*
    severity classification 208*a*(t)
atelectasis 125*a*
atenolol 217*a*
athlete's foot 185*a*, 287*q*, 306*a*
ATP see adenosine triphosphate
atrial fibrillation (AF) 90*q*, 132–3*a*
atrial flutter 136*a*, 140*a*
atrial natriuretic peptide (ANP) 150*a*, 152*a*
atrial systole 91*q*, 134*a*
atrioventricular nodal re-entry tachycardia (AVNRT) 136*a*,
    284–5*q*, 305*a*
atrioventricular node (AV node) 96*q*, 139–40*a*
    ablation therapy 90*q*, 132*a*
    adenosine 204*q*, 227*a*
    post-repolarization refractoriness 96*q*, 139*a*, 140*a*
    PR interval 272*q*, 297*a*
    second degree heart block 96*q*, 139*a*
attrition bias 232*q*, 237*a*
auriculotemporal nerve 278*q*, 301*a*
autonomic dysfunction 286*q*, 305*a*
AV node see atrioventricular node
AVNRT (atrioventricular nodal re-entry tachycardia) 136*a*,
    284–5*q*, 305*a*
axilla 1*q*, 4*q*, 35*a*, 38*a*
axillary artery 1*q*, 35*a*
axillary nerve 4*q*, 38*a*, 39*a*
axonal skeleton 248*q*, 258*a*
azathioprine 243*q*, 252*a*
azygo-portal anastomosis 280*q*, 302*a*

B

Bacillus anthracis 165*q*, 172*q*, 175*a*, 187*a*
bacterial meningitis 28*q*, 68*a*, 177*a*
bariatric surgery 100*q*, 144–5*a*
basal ganglia 26*q*, 66*a*
basal metabolic rate 111*q*, 159*a*, 160*a*
basal skull fracture 34*q*, 77*a*
basilar artery occlusive disease 77*a*
bat bite 266*q*, 292*a*
Battle sign 77*a*

Beck's triad 123*a*
beef tapeworm 180*a*
Bell's palsy 30*q*, 71*a*
bendroflumethazide 198*q*
benzodiazepines 194*q*, 212*a*(t)
benzylpenicillin 165*q*, 169*q*, 174*a*,
    181*a*, 282*q*, 304*a*
beta-agonists 83*q*, 122*a*
beta-blockers 197*q*, 217*a*
β cells (pancreas) 296*a*
beta-lactamases 304*a*
bias in clinical trials 231–2*q*, 236*a*, 237–8*a*
bicarbonate 85*q*, 125*a*, 162*a*
biceps 4*q*, 38*a*, 83*q*
biceps femoris 7*q*, 41*a*, 42*a*
bile 97*q*, 140*a*
    content 16*q*, 51*a*, 97*q*, 140*a*
    pancreatic exocrine insufficiency 304*a*
    salts 97*q*, 101*q*, 140*a*, 146*a*, 147*a*
biliary system 16*q*, 51*a*
bilirubin 245*q*, 254*a*
binasal hemianopia 30*q*, 72*a*
bisoprolol 197*q*, 217*a*
bitemporal hemianopia 30*q*, 72*a*
bladder
    anatomy 18*q*, 55*a*
    'automatic' 58*a*
    distension 18*q*, 55*a*
    dysfunction 106*q*, 152*a*
    nerve supply 58*a*
blast crisis 247*q*, 257*a*
blood glucose 81*q*, 92*q*, 119*a*, 135*a*
blood pressure 135*a*
blood transfusion 263*q*, 291*a*
BNP (brain natriuretic peptide) 152*a*
BOAST (British Orthopaedic Association Standards for
    Trauma) 215*a*
body temperature regulation 242*q*, 250*a*
Bohr shift 127–8*a*
bone marrow
    failure 246*q*, 256*a*
    suppression 243*q*, 252*a*
bone turnover 109*q*, 156–7*a*
Bordetella pertussis 168*q*, 179*a*, 186*a*
botulism 179*a*
Bowman's capsule 106*q*, 152*a*
Bowman's glands 31*q*, 73*a*
brachial artery 2*q*, 36*a*
brachial plexus 5*q*, 39*a*
brachioradialis 2*q*, 4*q*, 36*a*, 38*a*
bradykinesia 27*q*, 68*a*
bradykinin 103*q*, 149*a*
brain CT scan 28*q*(f)
brain natriuretic peptide (BNP) 152*a*
brainstem
    autonomic dysfunction 286*q*, 305*a*
    lesion 26*q*, 67*a*
breast 14*q*, 50*a*

British Orthopaedic Association Standards for Trauma (BOAST) 215*a*
bronchial artery 277*q*, 300*a*
bronchiectasis 87*q*, 128*a*, 300*a*
bronchiolitis 168*q*, 179*a*
bronchitis, chronic
   differential diagnosis 89*q*, 131*a*
   lung compliance 126*a*
   lung function 89*q*, 131*a*
   ventilation and perfusion 85*q*, 125*a*
Brunner's glands 162*a*
bulbar urethra 18*q*, 54*a*
bundle of His 90*q*, 132*a*
bundle of Kent 90*q*, 133*a*
Buscopan (hyoscine butylbromide) 279*q*, 302*a*

C

C3a complement 242*q*, 251*a*
C3 complement 243*q*, 251*a*
C4 complement 243*q*, 251*a*
C5a complement 242*q*, 251*a*
C5 nerve root 271*q*, 296*a*
caecum 16*q*, 52*a*, 98*q*, 142*a*
calcaneofibular ligament 9*q*, 44*a*
calcitonin 112*q*, 160*a*
calcium
   absorption 203*q*, 226*a*
   metabolism 112*q*, 160*a*
calcium channel blockers 194*q*, 212*a*
calcium channels
   L-type 79*q*, 94*q*, 116*a*, 117*a*, 137*a*
   supraventricular tachycardia 95*q*, 138*a*
calcium chloride 211*a*
calcium gluconate 153*a*, 193*q*, 211*a*
callus formation 248*q*, 258*a*
Calot's triangle 16*q*, 51*a*
cAMP 83*q*, 122*a*
Campylobacter jejuni 172*q*, 186*a*, 263*q*, 291*a*
candida 171*q*, 185*a*
Candida albicans 167*q*, 172*a*, 178*a*
capsule (adrenal gland) 109*q*, 156*a*
carbamazepine 197*q*, 217*a*
carbapenems 206*a*
carbohydrate 100*q*, 145*a*, 282*q*, 304*a*
carbon dioxide
   diffusion capacity for (DLCO$_2$) 87*q*, 89*q*, 131*a*
   metabolic hyperaemia 94*q*, 137*a*
   partial pressure of (PaCO$_2$) 87*q*, 92*q*, 128*a*, 136*a*, 281*q*, 303*a*
   perfusion-limited gas 129*a*
   poisoning 88*q*, 129*a*
   transport 85*q*, 125–6*a*
carbonic anhydrase 85*q*, 125*a*
carbon monoxide
   affinity for haemoglobin 88*q*, 129*a*
   diffusion capacity for (DLCO) 128*a*
   diffusion-limited gas 129*a*

carboxylpolypeptidase 147*a*
cardiac action potential 79*q*, 116–17*a*
cardiac α adrenergic receptors 113*q*, 161*a*
cardiac axis 90*q*, 133*a*
cardiac cycle 91*q*, 134*a*, 269*q*, 295*a*
cardiac muscle 81*q*, 119*a*
cardiac myocyte action potentials 261*q*, 289*a*
cardiac output 91*q*, 134–5*a*
   hyperthyroidism 112*q*, 113*q*, 160*a*, 161*a*
   hypoxaemia 88*q*, 130*a*
cardiac pacemaker cells 302*a*
cardiac tamponade 123*a*
Cardiobacterium hominis 167*q*, 178–9*a*
cardiopulmonary resuscitation (CPR)
   adrenaline 204*q*, 227*a*
   amiodarone 204*q*, 227*a*
   pulseless electrical activity 204*q*
   ventricular fibrillation 204*q*
carotid cavernous fistula 34*q*, 77*a*
carpal bones 3*q*, 37*a*
case–control studies 229*q*, 232*q*, 233*a*, 238*a*, 239*a*
catastrophic haemorrhage 91*q*, 134*a*
catecholamines 114*q*, 156*a*, 162*a*, 163*a*
   comparison 213*a*(t)
cauda equina syndrome 20*q*, 58*a*
cavernous sinus thrombosis 271*q*, 296*a*
cavitating pneumonia 165*q*, 175*a*
CCK (cholecystokinin) 97*q*, 140*a*, 162*a*
CCS (central cord syndrome) 25*q*, 65*a*
cefalexin 166*q*, 176*a*, 191*q*
cefotaxime 165*q*, 174*a*
ceftriaxone 165*q*, 169*q*, 174*a*, 181*a*
cefuroxime 195*q*, 202*q*, 215*a*, 224*a*
cellulitis 166*q*, 176*a*, 199*q*, 220–1*a*
Centor Criteria 254*a*
central cord syndrome (CCS) 25*q*, 65*a*
central diabetes insipidus 104*q*, 150*a*
central sleep apnoea 86*q*, 127*a*
cephalic vein 3*q*, 38*a*
cephalosporins 202*q*, 206*a*, 224*a*
cerebellar stroke 25*q*, 65–6*a*
cerebellum 30*q*, 34*q*, 71*a*, 77*a*
cerebral blood flow 200*q*, 204*q*, 221*a*, 227*a*
cerebral cortex 27*q*, 67*a*
cerebral palsy 92*q*, 135–6*a*
cerebral perfusion pressure (CPP) 92*q*, 135–6*a*
cerebrospinal fluid (CSF)
   encephalitis 276*q*, 299–300*a*
   meningitis 28*q*, 68–9*a*, 167*q*, 177*a*(t)
cerebrovascular accident (CVA) 216*q*, 273*q*, 297*a*
cervicoaxillary opening 1*q*, 35*a*
cGMP 83*q*, 122*a*
Charcot's triad 123*a*
chemotherapy 253*a*
chest wall compliance in children 278*q*, 301*a*
chest X-rays 12*q*(f), 13*q*(f)
Cheyne–Stokes breathing 86*q*, 127*a*

chickenpox 170q, 183a
chief cells 296a
chlamydia
    diagnosis 244q, 253a
    microbiology 176a
    pelvic inflammatory disease 173q, 189a
    and perihepatitis 173q, 189a
    treatment 181a
Chlamydia trachomatis 166q, 176a, 244q, 253a
chloride administration 102q, 148a
chloride shift 85q, 125a
chloride transporter mutation 88q, 130a
cholecystitis, acute 16q, 202q, 224a
cholecystokinin (CCK) 97q, 140a, 162a
cholesterol 101q, 114q, 115q, 146a, 162a, 163a
choline 83q, 122a, 123a
chronic kidney disease (CKD) 198q, 219a
chronic liver disease (CLD) 242q, 250a
chronic myeloid leukaemia (CML) 247q, 257a
chronic obstructive pulmonary disease (COPD)
    carbon dioxide transport 85q, 125a
    lung compliance 86q, 126a
    lung function 88q, 89q, 129a, 131a
    premature airway closure in expiration 87q, 128a
    steroid medications 192q, 209a
chyme 98q, 142a, 147a
chymosin secretion 296a
CI (confidence intervals) 231q, 237a
cigarette smoking 222a, 265q, 292a
cilia, immotile 88q, 130a
ciliated columnar epithelial cells 89q, 131a
ciliated cuboidal epithelial cells 89q, 131a
ciprofloxacin 166q, 176a, 177a
circumflex artery 14q, 50a, 51a, 92q, 136a
cirrhosis 302a
cisterna magna 69a
cisterna pontis 69a
CK (creatine kinase) 262q, 290a
CKD (chronic kidney disease) 198q, 219a
clarithromycin 173q, 199q, 220a
    interaction with cyclosporine 199q, 221a
    Mycoplasma pneumoniae 166q, 177a
clavicle fracture 5q
clindamycin 165q, 174a, 195q, 215a
clonidine 230q(t), 235a(t)
clopidogrel 257a
Clostridium botulinum 168q, 179a
Clostridium difficile 167q, 253a, 267q, 273q, 293a, 297a(t)
Clostridium histolyticum 168q, 179a
Clostridium perfringens 166q, 168q, 172q, 176a, 179a, 186a
Clostridium septicum 168q, 179a
Clostridium tetani 168q, 179a
CMV (cytomegalovirus) 169q, 180a
coagulation 79q, 80q, 117a, 118a
co-amoxiclav 169q, 173q, 181a, 191q, 199q, 221a
    contraindications 166q, 177a
    open fracture 195q, 215a

pyelonephritis 166q, 176a
    tetanus 200q, 222a
cobalamin (vitamin B12) 100q, 144–5a, 266q, 293a, 304a
cocaine use 12q, 48a, 194q
codeine 193q, 194q, 211a(t), 212a
coeliac disease 251a
cohort studies 232q, 238a, 239a
    prospective 229q, 232q, 233a, 238a
    retrospective 229q, 233a, 238a
colchicine 203q, 225a
colitis 297a(t)
collagen deposition 243q, 252a
collecting duct 105q, 107q, 151a, 153a, 154a
colloid production 113q, 161a
colomycin 173q
colon 98q, 142a
    descending 19q, 56a, 277q, 300a
    sigmoid colon 19q, 57a
    superior mesenteric occlusion 275q, 299a
    transverse 17q, 53a
coma 26q, 67a
common peroneal nerve 8q, 9q, 42a, 44a, 294a
compartment syndrome 283q, 304a
complement deficiencies 243q, 252a
complete spinal cord injury 29q, 70a
compliance of chest wall in children 278q, 301a
confidence intervals (CIs) 231q, 237a
congestive heart failure 123a
conjunctiva 24q, 64a
Conn syndrome 110q, 157a
contact activation pathway 117a
Coomb's test 246q, 256a
COPD see chronic obstructive pulmonary disease
coronary artery 92–3q, 136a, 275q, 299a
    territories and ECG changes 51a(t)
corticosteroids see steroids
corticotropin-releasing hormone (CRH) 112q, 114q, 160a,
        163a, 270q, 295a
cortisol
    effects 110q, 157a
    hypothalamic–pituitary–adrenal axis 112q, 159a, 160a
    production 156a
    secretion 163a
    serum 111q, 159a
Corynebacterium diphtheriae 245q
costovertebral pleura 49a
COX-1 mediated prostaglandin synthesis 286q, 305a
Coxiella burnetii 167q, 179a
Coxsackievirus 167q, 177a
C-peptide, serum 111q, 113q, 158a, 159a, 162a
CPP (cerebral perfusion pressure) 92q, 135–6a
CPR see cardiopulmonary resuscitation
crack cocaine 12q, 48a
cranberry juice 201q, 223a
cranial diabetes insipidus 26q, 66a
C-reactive protein (CRP) 242q, 243q, 250a, 251a
creatine kinase (CK) 262q, 290a

CRH (corticotropin-releasing hormone) 112q, 114q, 160a, 163a, 270q, 295a
cricothyroid membrane 23q, 61a, 306a
cricothyroidotomy 23q, 61a
critical appraisals 232q, 238a
cross-matching of blood 263q, 291a
cross-sectional surveys 232q, 239a
CRP (C-reactive protein) 242q, 243q, 250a, 251a
cruciate anastomosis 6q, 41a
cruciate ligaments 9q, 43a
cryptococcus 171q, 185a
CSF see cerebrospinal fluid
cuboidal epithelium with glandular cells 89q, 131a
curriculum (Emergency Medicine 2015) xvii
Curtis–Fitz–Hugh syndrome (perihepatitis) 173q, 189a
Cushing's disease 110q, 158a
Cushing's syndrome 110q, 157–8a
Cushing's triad 123a, 135a
cutaneous nerve 11q, 46a
CVA (cerebrovascular accident) 216a, 273q, 297a
cyanide 84q, 102q, 148a
cyanosis 87q, 127a
cyclizine 196q, 198q, 215a, 219–20a
cyclophosphamide 252a
cyclosporine 199q, 221a
cystic fibrosis 89q, 130a
cytochrome P450 195q, 215a
cytomegalovirus (CMV) 169q, 180a
cytoplasmic calcium concentration, rhabdomyolysis 262q, 290a

D

D2 receptor antagonists 196q, 215a
Dalton's gas law 303a
DAT (direct antiglobulin test/Coomb's test) 246q, 256a
DC cardioversion 90q, 132a
DCT1 co-transporter 99q, 143a
dead space 84q, 88q, 125a, 130a
deafness 31q, 73a
deep circumflex iliac artery 17q, 52a
deep inferior epigastric artery 17q, 53a
deep peroneal nerve 8q, 42a
deep vein thrombosis (DVT) 12q, 47a
defaecation reflex 98q, 142a
dehydroepiandrosterone (DHEA) production 156a
delirium 27q, 67a
deltoid ligament complex 9q, 44a
dementia 26q, 67a
demyelination, physiological effect 277q, 300a
dengue fever 165q, 167q, 174a
dermatomes 10q, 45a
descending colon 19q, 56a, 277q, 300a
desmoglein-1: 84q, 123a
detection bias 232q, 237–8a
detrusor muscle 106q, 152a
dexamethasone 160a, 192q, 209a(t)
dexamethasone suppression test 110q, 158a

dextrose 193q, 211a
DHEA (dehydroepiandrosterone) production 156a
diabetes insipidus (DI) 26q, 66a, 104q, 150a
diabetes mellitus (DM)
    autonomic dysfunction 286q, 305a
    nephrotic syndrome 153a
    type 1: 111q, 158a, 162a
        113q, 161–2a
diabetic ketoacidosis (DKA) 111q, 158a, 197q, 218a, 271q, 296a
diabetic neuropathy 9q, 44a
diagnostic tests 229q, 230q, 231q, 233–6a, 262q, 290a
diaphragmatic pleura 13q, 49a
diarrhoea
    acute 244q, 253a
    anion gap metabolic acidosis 102q, 148a
    Campylobacter jejuni 263q, 291a
    Clostridium difficile 273q, 297a(t)
    inflammatory 253a
    osmotic 101q, 145–6a, 244q, 254a
    secretory 101q, 145a, 146a, 244q, 253a
diastole 91q, 134a
diazepam 194q, 212a(t)
diffusion capacity
    for carbon dioxide (DLCO$_2$) 87q, 89q, 131a
    for carbon monoxide (DLCO) 128a
digestive enzymes 162a
digoxin 90q, 132a, 196q, 216–17a
    side effects 216a
    toxicity 196q, 216a, 217a
dilated cardiomyopathy 91q, 134–55a
diltiazem 194q, 212a
diphtheria, pertussis, and tetanus vaccine 169q
diphtheria, tetanus, pertussis, and polio (DTaP/IPV) vaccine 203q, 226a
direct antiglobulin test (DAT, Coomb's test) 246q, 256a
disc prolapse 20q, 58a
disseminated intravascular coagulation (DIC) 283q, 304a
distal convoluted tubule 107q, 154a, 155a
distal radius 3q, 37a
distal tubule 107q, 153a
disulfiram 200q, 222a
diuretics 196q, 216a
DKA (diabetic ketoacidosis) 111q, 158a, 197q, 218a, 271q, 296a
DM see diabetes mellitus
dobutamine 195q, 213a(t), 214a
dopamine 81q, 111q, 120a, 159a
    extrapyramidal symptoms 264q, 291a
    vomiting 102q, 148a
dorsalis pedis pulse 6q, 41a
double-stranded DNA (dsDNA) antibodies 243q, 251a
Down's syndrome 87q, 127a
doxycycline 169q, 173q, 181a, 188a, 191q
dsDNA (double-stranded DNA) antibodies 243q, 251a
DTaP/IPV (diphtheria, tetanus, pertussis, and polio) vaccine 203q, 226a

Duchenne muscular dystrophy 81*q*
duodenum
    anatomy 19*q*, 56*a*
    lipid metabolism 102*q*, 147*a*
    pH 97*q*, 140*a*
    secretions 114*q*, 162*a*
dura 69*a*
DVT (deep vein thrombosis) 12*q*, 47*a*
dysentery 253*a*

E

eardrum, perforation 31*q*, 73*a*
EBV (Epstein–Barr virus) 169*q*, 180*a*, 247*q*, 257*a*
ECF (extracellular fluid) 80*q*, 117*a*
ECG see electrocardiogram
ECL (enterochromaffin-like) cells 272*q*, 296*a*
ectopic pacemaker function 136*a*
ectopic pregnancy 20*q*, 57*a*
EHL (extensor hallucis longus) paralysis/paresis 294*a*
Eisenmenger syndrome 87*q*, 127*a*
elastase 147*a*
elastin fibres 102*q*, 147*a*
elbow 3*q*, 38*a*, 264*q*, 291*a*
electrocardiogram (ECG)
    cardiac axis 90*q*, 133*a*(f)
    coronary artery occlusion 275*q*, 299*a*
    examples 15*q*(f), 93*q*(f), 96*q*(f), 205*q*(f), 285*q*(f)
    PR interval 272*q*, 286*q*, 297*a*, 305*a*
    P wave 91*q*, 134*a*, 297*a*
    QRS complex 297*a*
    QT interval 94*q*, 137*a*, 276*q*, 299*a*
    second degree heart block 96*q*, 139*a*
    STEMI 92–3*q*, 136*a*
    trifascicular block 286*q*, 305*a*
    Wellen's syndrome 287*q*, 306*a*
ELISA (enzyme-linked immunosorbent assay) 241*q*, 249*a*
Emergency Medicine 2015 Curriculum xvii
emphysema
    dead space 125*a*
    differential diagnosis 89*q*, 131*a*
    lung compliance 86*q*, 126*a*
    lung function 86*q*, 87*a*, 89*q*, 126*a*, 128*a*, 131*a*
    physiology 84*q*, 125*a*
encephalitis 177*a*, 276*q*, 299–300*a*
endocarditis 167*q*, 178–9*a*
endocrine pancreas 114*q*, 162*a*
endothelin 107*q*, 154*a*
endotracheal intubation 22*q*, 60*a*
Entamoeba histolytica 172*q*, 187*a*
Entamoeba spp. 253*a*
enteric plexus 98*q*
Enterobacter aerogenes 173*q*
Enterobius vernicularis 168*q*, 180*a*
enterochromaffin-like (ECL) cells 272*q*, 296*a*
enzyme-linked immunosorbent assay (ELISA) 241*q*, 249*a*
eosinophils 243*q*
ephedrine 213*a*(t)

epidemic parotitis see mumps
epigastrium 17*q*, 52–3*a*
epiglottis 22*q*, 60*a*
epistaxis 20*q*, 58*a*
epithelialization 243*q*, 252*a*
epithelium (gastrointestinal tract) 97*q*, 141*a*
eponychium 2*q*, 37*a*
Epstein–Barr virus (EBV) 169*q*, 180*a*, 247*q*, 257*a*
erythema infectiosum 170*q*, 183*a*
erythrocyte sedimentation rate (ESR) 242*q*, 243*q*, 250*a*, 251*a*
erythromycin 186*a*
Escherichia coli 166*q*, 176*a*
    O157:H7 172*q*, 186*a*
esmolol 197*q*, 217*a*
ESR (erythrocyte sedimentation rate) 242*q*, 243*q*, 250*a*, 251*a*
ethambutol 182*a*
event rate 230*q*, 235*a*
evidence-based medicine 229–32*q*, 233–9*a*
excitable tissues 79*q*, 116*a*
exocrine pancreas 114*q*, 162*a*
expectation bias 232*q*, 237*a*
extensor digitorum longus injury 266*q*, 293*a*
extensor hallucis longus (EHL) paralysis/paresis 294*a*
extensor pollicis brevis 3*q*, 38*a*
external anal sphincter 17*q*, 54*a*
external urinary sphincter 106*q*, 152*a*
extracellular fluid (ECF) 80*q*, 117*a*
extrinsic pathway see tissue factor pathway
eye
    anatomy 24*q*, 63–4*a*
    examination 33*q*(f)
    foreign body in 24*q*, 63–4*a*

F

facial nerve
    anatomy 23*q*, 31*q*, 33*q*, 34*q*, 62*a*, 74*a*, 75*a*, 76*a*
    injury 273*q*, 298*a*
    palsies 30*q*, 71*a*
factor V Leiden 287*q*, 306*a*
factor VII 295*a*
factor Xa 271*q*, 296*a*
factor XII deficiency 287*q*, 306*a*
Fallopian tubes 20*q*, 57*a*
false ribs 10*q*, 45–6*a*
fascia iliaca block 5*q*, 39*a*
FCU (flexor carpi ulnaris) 291*a*
FDP (flexor digitorum profundus) 2*q*, 36*a*, 290*a*, 291*a*
FDS (flexor digitorum superficialis) 2*q*, 36*a*
femoral canal 298*a*
femoral nerve 9*q*, 44*a*, 293–4*a*, 298*a*
    fascia iliaca block 5*q*, 39*a*
    saphenous branch 295*a*
femoral sheath 298*a*
femoral vein 274*q*, 298*a*

femur
  avascular necrosis of head 6q, 41a
  forwards prominence of lateral condyle 8q, 42a
  fractured neck of 5q, 6q, 108q, 231q, 236–7a
fentanyl 193q, 211a(t)
festinant gait 68a
FEV₁ see forced expiratory volume in one second
FEV₁/FVC ratio see forced expiratory volume in one second/
  forced vital capacity ratio
fever 242q, 250a
fibrin 80q, 118a
fibrinolysis 268q, 294a
fibroblast proliferation 243q, 252a
fibula 9q, 44a
fibular nerve see common peroneal nerve
Fick's law 129a
fifth disease (erythema infectiosum) 170q, 183a
fingers
  blood supply 2q, 37a
  dislocated interphalangeal joint 261q, 289a
  extensor digitorum longus injury 266q, 293a
  flexors 4q, 38a
  nailbeds 2q, 37a, 92q, 135a
  severed tendon 2q, 36a
fissure-in-ano 17q, 54a
fistulae, perianal 243q
flexor carpi ulnaris (FCU) 291a
flexor digitorum profundus (FDP) 2q, 36a, 290a, 291a
flexor digitorum superficialis (FDS) 2q, 36a
flexor pollicis brevis 36a
flexor pollicis longus (FPL) 290a
floating ribs 10q, 45a
flu see influenza
flucloxacillin 173q, 188a, 195q, 199q, 220a, 221a
focal seizure 280q, 302a
foetal haemoglobin 87q, 127a, 128a, 268q, 294a
folate deficiency 246q, 256a
food intolerance 242q, 251a
food poisoning 172q, 186a
forced expiratory volume in one second
  (FEV₁) 87q, 128a
  asthma 265q, 292a
  COPD 88q, 89q, 129a, 131a
forced expiratory volume in one second/forced vital capacity
  ratio (FEV₁/FVC) 87q, 128a
  asthma 265q, 292a
  COPD 88q, 89q, 129a, 131a
forced vital capacity (FVC) 87q, 128a
  asthma 265q, 292a
  COPD 88q, 89q, 129a, 131a
foreign body
  aortic arch 274q, 298a
  eye 24q, 63–4a
  inhaled 11q, 46a
fourth ventricle 69a
FPL (flexor pollicis longus) 290a
Francisella tularensis 172q, 187a

FRCEM Primary examination xvii–xviii
  mock exam paper 261–88q, 289–306a
frontal sinus 21q, 59a
frontotemporal dementias 26q, 67a
fructose 100q, 145a
functional residual capacity 86q, 126a
funny current 79q, 94q, 95q, 116a, 137a, 139a
furosemide 196q, 216a, 272q, 274q, 297a, 298a
FVC see forced vital capacity

G
G6PD (glucose-6-phosphate dehydrogenase) 246q, 256a
GABA see gamma-aminobutyric acid
gabapentin 202q, 224a
GABHS (group A β-haemolytic streptococcus) 245q, 254a
galactorrhoea 110q, 158a
gallbladder 16q, 51a, 97q, 140a
gallstones 101q, 146a, 254a
gamma-aminobutyric acid (GABA) 81q, 120a
  receptors 29q, 69a, 194q, 212a
γ cells (pancreas) 296a
gas gangrene 168q, 176a, 179a
gas transfer 88q, 129a
gastric bypass surgery 100q, 144a, 145a
gastric emptying 97q, 140–1a
gastric secretions 80q, 101q, 118a, 146a
gastrin 101q, 146a
  gastric emptying 97q, 140a
  secretion 80q, 118a, 140a, 296a
  Zollinger–Ellison syndrome 115q, 164a
gastrocnemius 41a
gastro-colic reflex 142a
gastrointestinal (GI) tract
  blood supply 17q, 53a
  layers 98q, 141a
  peristalsis 97q, 100q, 141a, 144a
Gaviscon 215a
GBS (group B streptococcal) infection 165q, 167q, 169q,
  174a, 177a, 180–1a
G cells 115q, 140a, 164a, 296a
gelofusine 4% 90q, 132a
gemelli 6q
genitofemoral nerve 5q, 39a
gentamicin 165q, 166q, 174a, 176a, 191q, 206a
German measles see rubella
GFR (glomerular filtration rate) 104q, 105q, 107q, 150–1a,
  152a, 154a
ghrelin 101q, 146a
GI tract see gastrointestinal (GI) tract
glandular fever 169q, 180–1a
glomerular filtration rate (GFR) 104q, 105q, 107q, 150–1a,
  152a, 154a
glossopharyngeal nerve 31q, 32q, 74a, 75a
glucagon 111q, 159a, 162a
glucokinase 111q, 158a
gluconeogenesis 113q, 161a
glucose-6-phosphate dehydrogenase (G6PD) 246q, 256a

GLUT1 transporter 80*q*, 118*a*
GLUT2 transporter 80*q*, 84*q*, 118*a*, 123*a*, 145*a*
GLUT3 transporter 80*q*, 118*a*
GLUT4 transporter 80*q*, 118*a*
GLUT5 transporter 80*q*, 118*a*, 145*a*
glutamate 81*q*, 120*a*
gluteus maximus 6*q*, 40*a*
gluteus medius 6*q*, 40*a*
gluteus minimus 6*q*, 40*a*
glycerol suppositories 201*q*, 223*a*
glycopeptides 206*a*
goblet cells 89*q*, 130*a*, 296*a*
goitre 25*q*, 64*a*, 112–13*q*, 160–1*a*
gonorrhoea
    diagnosis 244*q*, 253*a*
    microbiology 176*a*
    pelvic inflammatory disease 173*q*, 189*a*
    treatment 169*q*, 181*a*
gouty arthritis, acute 203*q*, 225*a*
G proteins 80*q*, 118*a*
Grave's disease 92*q*, 135*a*
greater occipital nerve 275*q*, 299*a*
greater sac 17*q*, 53*a*
great palatine artery 20*q*, 58*a*
great saphenous vein 6*q*, 9*q*, 41*a*, 45*a*
group A β-haemolytic streptococcus (GABHS) 245*q*, 254*a*
group A streptococcus 173*q*
group B streptococcal (GBS) infection 165*q*, 167*q*, 169*q*,
    174*a*, 177*a*, 180–1*a*
gut, surface area 98*q*, 142*a*

H
H₁ receptor antagonists 198*q*, 219*a*, 220*a*
H₂ receptor antagonists 195*q*, 215*a*
haematuria 106*q*, 153*a*
haemochromatosis, hereditary 156*a*
haemoglobin 85*q*, 125*a*, 246*q*, 256*a*
    carbon monoxide's affinity for 88*q*, 129*a*
    foetal 87*q*, 127*a*, 128*a*, 268*q*, 294*a*
haemolytic uraemic syndrome 167*q*, 178*a*
haemophilia 287*q*, 306*a*
    Type B 257*a*
Haemophilus influenzae 165*q*, 168*q*, 173*q*, 175*a*, 179*a*
Haemophilus influenzae type B (Hib) 167*q*, 177*a*
    vaccine 203*q*, 226*a*
haemorrhage, renal autoregulation of 104*q*, 151*a*
haemostasis 80*q*, 118*a*
haemotympanum 34*q*, 77*a*
Haldane effect 85*q*, 125–6*a*
hamstrings 6*q*, 7*q*, 41*a*, 42*a*
hand
    fall injury 2*q*, 3*q*
    lacerated palm 2*q*, 36*a*
    nerve supply 1*q*, 35*a*
    paraesthesia 1*q*
    tendons 2*q*, 36*a*
    see also fingers

hanging 23*q*, 62*a*
haptoglobin 246*q*, 256*a*
Hartmann's pouch 16*q*, 51*a*
Hartmann's solution 201*q*, 211*a*, 222*a*, 223*a*
haustrae 142*a*
headache 29*q*, 71*a*
head injury
    basal skull fracture 34*q*, 77*a*
    bleeding 21*q*, 59*a*
    cranial diabetes insipidus 26*q*, 66*a*
    haematoma 28*q*, 69*a*
    healing process 243*q*, 252*a*
    penetrating 21*q*, 59*a*
hearing disturbance 31*q*, 73*a*
heart block 96*q*, 139*a*
heart sounds 91*q*, 134*a*
Heinz bodies 246*q*, 256*a*
heme 245*q*, 254*a*
Henderson–Hasselbalch equation 105*q*, 151*a*
heparin 257*a*
    low molecular weight 202*q*, 223–4*a*
    unfractionated 202*q*, 223*a*
hepatitis B 171*q*, 185*a*, 203*q*, 225*a*
hepatitis C 171*q*, 185*a*
hepatocytes 245*q*, 254*a*
hepatorenal pouch 17*a*, 53*a*
hepatosplenomegaly 241*q*, 249*a*
hereditary haemochromatosis 156*a*
Hering–Breuer inspiratory–inhibitory reflex 131*a*
herpes simplex encephalitis 167*q*, 177*a*
herpes simplex virus (HSV) 20*q*, 57*a*, 169*q*, 181*a*
    HSV-1 167*q*, 177*a*, 181*a*, 299–300*a*
    HSV-2 177*a*, 181*a*, 300*a*
    treatment 281*q*, 303*a*
Hesselbach's triangle 53*a*
Hib see *Haemophilus influenzae* type B
hierarchy of evidences triangle 231*q*, 232*q*, 237*a*, 238*a*
hip
    fascia iliaca block 5*q*, 39*a*
    muscles 6*q*, 40*a*
    nerve supply 5*q*, 39–40*a*
    weak adduction 5*q*
His–Purkinje system 93*q*, 96*q*, 136*a*, 139*a*
histamine 101*q*, 146*a*
    secretion 80*q*, 118*a*, 272*q*, 296*a*
    vomiting 102*q*, 148*a*
historical (retrospective) cohort studies 229*q*, 233*a*, 238*a*
HIV see human immunodeficiency virus
Hodgkin's lymphoma 247*q*, 257–8*a*
    staging 258*a*(t)
homonymous hemianopia 30*q*, 72*a*, 273*q*,
    277*q*, 297*a*, 300*a*
homonymous macular defect, right 272*q*, 297*a*
hookworm 180*a*
HPV (human papillomavirus) vaccine 169*q*, 226*a*
HSV see herpes simplex virus
human herpes virus-4 180*a*

human immunodeficiency virus (HIV) 167q, 170–1q, 184a
  needle-stick injury 171q, 185a
  opportunistic infection 268q, 294a
  transmission 170q, 171q, 184a
human papillomavirus (HPV) vaccine 169q, 226a
human tetanus immunoglobulin 170q, 182a
humeroradial joint 3q, 38a
humeroulnar joint 3q, 38a
hydrocortisone 192q, 209a(t)
hydroxylysine 109q, 156a
hydroxyproline 109q, 156a
hyoscine butylbromide (Buscopan) 279q, 302a
hyperbilirubinaemia 254a
hypercalcaemia 155a, 198q, 218a
hyperkalaemia 153a, 193q, 211a, 219a
hyperleukocytosis 257a
hyperparathyroidism 108q, 155a
hyperpigmentation 109q, 155–6a
hypersensitivity 242q, 251a
hypertension
  cardiac output 91q, 135a
  nephritic syndrome 106q, 153a
  nephrotic syndrome 106q, 153a
  reduced arterial compliance secondary to 95q, 138a
  white coat 95q, 138a
hyperthyroidism 112–13q, 160–1a
hypocapnia 158a
hypogastric nerve 20q, 57a
hypoglossal nerve 31q, 32q, 74a, 75a
hypoglycaemia 198q, 218a, 263q, 290a
hypokalaemia 110q, 157a, 198q, 219a
hyponychium 2q, 37a
hypotension 29q, 70a, 114q, 163a
hypothalamic ischaemia in hypotension 114q, 163a
hypothalamic–pituitary–adrenal axis 112q, 159–60a
hypothalamus 28q, 68q, 114q, 162a, 286q, 305a
hypoventilation 84q, 88q, 124a, 129a
hypovolaemia 105q, 152a
hypoxaemia 12q, 47a, 84q, 124–5a, 129a
  pneumothorax 88q, 129–30a
  ventilation:perfusion mismatch 273q, 298a

I

I band 82q, 122a
ibuprofen 194q, 199q, 200q, 212a, 221a
IC (intercostal) drain 11q, 46a
IC (intercostal) muscles 11q, 46a
IC (intercostal) nerves 13q, 49a
ICBN (intercostobrachial nerve) 4q, 38a
ICF (intracellular fluid) 80q, 117a
ICP see intracranial pressure
IgE (immunoglobulin E) 242q, 251a
IgG (immunoglobulin G) 88q, 130a, 241q, 242q, 249a, 251a
IgM (immunoglobulin M) 241q, 242q, 249a, 251a
ileum 19q, 56–7q, 266q, 293a
ileus 141a
iliohypogastric nerve 5q, 39a

ilioinguinal nerve 5q, 20q, 40a, 57a
immune response 279q, 301–2a
immunity 273q, 298a
immunization schedule 203q, 226a(t)
immunoglobulin E (IgE) 242q, 251a
immunoglobulin G (IgG) 88q, 130a, 241q, 242q, 249a, 251a
immunoglobulin M (IgM) 241q, 242q, 249a, 251a
immunosuppression 243q, 252a
infectious mononucleosis 257a
inferior epigastric artery 17q, 53a
inferior mesenteric artery 17q, 53a, 277q, 300a
inferior mesenteric vein 17q, 53a
inferior oblique 30q, 72a
inferior radioulnar joint 3q, 37a
inferior rectus 30q, 72a
inflammatory bowel disease 253a
inflammatory markers 242q, 250a
influenza 171q, 185a
  vaccine 245q, 255a
infranodal block 96q, 139a
infraspinatous 4q, 38a
inguinal hernia 16q, 52a
inositol 1,4,5-triphosphate (InsP3) 83q, 122a
inotropes 213a(t)
INR (international normalized ratio) 79q, 117a, 201q, 223a, 270q, 295a
InsP3 (inositol 1,4,5-triphosphate) 83q, 122a
insulin 113q, 161–2a
  diabetic ketoacidosis 197q, 218a
  secretion 162a
  therapy 111q, 159a
insulin-dextrose 153a
insulin growth factor (IGF) 111q, 159a
intercostal (IC) drain 11q, 46a
intercostal (IC) muscles 11q, 46a
intercostal (IC) nerves 13q, 49a
intercostobrachial nerve (ICBN) 4q, 38a
internal anal sphincter 98q, 142a
internal capsule 25q, 26q, 65a, 66a, 276q, 299a
internal iliac arteries 20q, 57a
internal iliac veins 20q, 57a
internal jugular vein 23q, 62a
internal mammary artery 280q, 303a
international normalized ratio (INR) 79q, 117a, 201q, 223a, 270q, 295a
interstitial fibrosis 88q, 129a
intestine see gastrointestinal (GI) tract
intracellular fluid (ICF) 80q, 117a
intracranial pressure (ICP)
  cerebral perfusion pressure 92q, 135a
  nitrous oxide, effect on 200q, 221a
  raised 123a, 135a, 193q, 210a
intranasal influenza vaccine 169q, 180a
intravenous drug use 167q, 178–9a
intrinsic factor 100q, 118a, 144–5a
intrinsic pathway see contact activation pathway
ipratropium 192q, 208a, 286q, 305a

iron absorption 99*q*, 143*a*
irritant receptors 89*q*, 131*a*
islets of Langerhans 16*q*, 51*a*, 296*a*
isoniazid 182*a*

J

jaundice 245*q*, 254*a*
jejunum 19*q*, 56*a*
jugular venous pressure (JVP) 92*q*, 135*a*
jugulodigastric lymph nodes 288*q*, 306*a*
juvenile arthritis 169*q*, 180*a*
juxtaglomerular apparatus 105*q*, 106*q*, 151*a*, 152*a*
JVP (jugular venous pressure) 92*q*, 135*a*

K

Kartagener syndrome 88*q*, 130*a*
ketamine 192*q*, 210*a*
    contraindications 210*a*
    procedural sedation and analgesia 202*q*, 224–5*a*
    side effects 192*q*, 202*q*, 210*a*, 224*a*
ketogenic diet 111*q*, 159*a*
kidney disease, chronic (CKD) 198*q*, 219*a*
Klebsiella pneumoniae 165*q*, 172*q*, 175*a*, 186*a*, 270*q*, 296*a*
knee
    anatomy 6–7*q*, 41*a*
    anterior cruciate ligament 9*q*, 43*a*, 269*q*, 295*a*
    jerk, loss of 281*q*, 303*a*
    lateral patellar dislocation 8*q*, 42*a*
    medial collateral ligament 8*q*, 43*a*
    popliteal cyst 8*q*
    popliteal fossa 8*q*, 42–3*a*
    X-ray 7*q*(*f*)
Kussmaul breathing 86*q*, 111*q*, 127*a*, 158*a*

L

L1 fracture 281*q*, 303*a*
L4 lesions 303*a*
L5 lesions 303*a*
L5 nerve root 269*q*, 294*a*
labia majora 5*q*, 39*a*
labium majus 20*q*, 57*a*
labour, nitrous oxide in 221*a*
labyrinth 30*q*, 34*q*, 71*a*, 77*a*
lacrimal glands 24*q*, 64*a*
lactate dehydrogenase (LDH) 246*q*, 255*q*, 256*a*
lactic acid 94*q*, 137*a*
lactic acidosis 220*a*
lactose 100*q*, 145*a*
    intolerance 145*a*
lactulose 201*q*, 223*a*
lacular stroke 66*a*
LAD artery see left anterior descending (LAD) artery
lamina propria 98*q*, 141*a*, 142*a*
Lange–Nielsen syndrome 136*a*
lansoprazole 195*q*, 215*a*
Laplace's Law 134*a*, 304*a*
large intestine 98*q*, 142*a*

laryngoscopy 60*a*
lateral cutaneous nerve of thigh 5*q*, 40*a*
lateral femoral cutaneous nerve (LCFN) 5*q*, 9*q*, 39*a*, 44*a*,
    267*q*, 293*a*
lateral rectus 30*q*, 72*a*
lateral superior cerebellar artery 26*q*, 65*a*, 66*a*
lateral ventricle 28*q*, 68*a*, 69*a*
Law of Laplace 134*a*, 304*a*
laxatives 198*q*, 201*q*, 219*a*, 223*a*
LCFN (lateral femoral cutaneous nerve) 5*q*, 9*q*, 39*a*, 44*a*,
    267*q*, 293*a*
LDH (lactate dehydrogenase) 246*q*, 255*q*, 256*a*
lecithin 147*a*
left anterior descending (LAD) artery
    anatomy 10*q*, 14*q*, 45*a*, 50*a*
    ECG 92*q*, 136*a*
    myocardial infarction 10*q*, 14*q*, 45*a*, 50*a*, 51*a*, 92*q*, 136*a*
    normal variant 92*q*, 136*a*
    occlusion 299*a*
    severe proximal stenosis 287*q*, 306*a*
    type III variant 92*q*, 136*a*
left circumflex artery 10*q*, 45*a*
left coronary artery 14*q*, 50*a*
left main bronchus 11*q*, 46–7*a*
left main stem 92*q*, 136*a*
left optic radiation, lower fibres of 277*q*, 300*a*
left vagus nerve 303*a*
leg
    meralgia paraesthetica 5*q*, 40*a*
    midshaft fibular fracture 9*q*, 44*a*
    muscles 7*q*, 41–2*a*
    nerve supply 5*q*, 39–40*a*
    road traffic accident 6–7*q*, 41*a*
    veins 9*q*, 45*a*
legionella 173*q*, 188*a*
Legionella pneumophila 188*a*
Leigh syndrome 275*q*
length constant 81*q*, 120*a*
leptin secretion 114*q*, 162*a*
leptospirosis 173*q*, 188*a*
lesser sac (Omental busa) 17*q*, 53*a*
lethal triad (trauma triad of death) 84*q*, 123*a*
leukaemia
    acute lymphoblastic (ALL) 264*q*, 291*a*
    acute myeloid (AML) 257*a*
    chronic myeloid (CML) 247*q*, 257*a*
levator palpebrae superioris muscle 24*q*, 63*a*
levothyroxine 198*q*, 218–19*a*
Lewy bodies 68*a*
lidocaine 263*q*, 267*q*, 290*a*, 293*a*
light band (I band) 82*q*, 122*a*
likelihood ratios of a diagnostic test 230*q*, 234–5*a*
lincosamides 206*a*
lingual nerve 31*q*, 32*q*, 74*a*, 75*a*
lipase 102*q*, 147*a*
lipids 102*q*, 147*a*, 304*a*
lipopolysaccharide (LPS) 242*q*, 250*a*

lipoprotein lipase 111q, 158a
liquid paraffin 201q, 223a
lithium 194q, 213a
lithium heparin bottles 79q, 117a
Little's area 58a
live attenuated vaccines 169q, 180a
liver disease, chronic (CLD) 242q, 250a
LMWH (low molecular weight heparin) 202q, 223–4a
local anaesthesia
    auriculotemporal nerve 278q, 301a
    occipital laceration 275q, 299a
    ulnar nerve 261q, 289a
long QT syndrome 136a, 299a
loop diuretics 196q, 216a
loop of Henle
    ascending 105q, 107q, 108q, 151a, 154a, 155a,
        272q, 297a
    descending 105q, 106q, 107q, 108q, 151a, 152a, 154a
lorazepam 194q, 212a(t)
Lowenstein–Jensen agar 169q, 181a
lower fibres of left optic radiation 277q, 300a
low molecular weight heparin (LMWH) 202q, 223–4a
LP see lumbar puncture
LPS (lipopolysaccharide) 242q, 250a
L-type calcium channels 79q, 94q, 116a, 117a, 137a
lumbar plexus 39a
lumbar puncture (LP)
    encephalitis 300a
    meningitis 167q, 177a
    tissue layers 25q, 64a
lumbricals 2q, 36a
lunate 3q, 37a
lung
    anatomy 13q, 48–9a
    compliance 86q, 87q, 126a, 128a
    epithelium 89q, 130a
    fibrosis 126a
    function 86q, 87q, 88q, 89q, 126a, 128a, 129a, 131a,
        265q, 292a
    parenchyma, inflammation of 277q, 300a
    pneumonia, consolidation site 11–12q, 47a
    surfactant 283q, 304a
    volume 84q, 124a
Lyme disease 241q, 249a
lymphoedema 220a
lymphoma 243q, 247q, 252a, 257–8a
lymphopenia 243q, 252a
lyssaviruses 170q, 183a

M
macrocytic anaemia 100q, 144–5a, 256a, 304a
macrogols 201q, 223a
macrolides 199q, 206a, 221a
macrophages 252a
macular defect, right homonymous 272q, 297a
magnesium, intravenous 199q, 220a
malaria 168q, 179a, 241q, 249a

Mallampati scoring 22q, 60a
mallet finger deformity 266q, 293a
maltose 100q, 145a
mandible 24q, 63a
mandibular nerve 32q, 75a
mannitol 193q, 210a
manubrium 45a
maple syrup urine disease (MSUD) 107q
marginal artery of Drummond 53a
mast cells 242q, 251a
MCA (middle cerebral artery) 27q, 66a, 68a, 273q, 297a
McBurney's point 52a
MCL (medial collateral ligament) 8q, 43a
MCV (mean corpuscular volume) 246q, 256a
mean arterial pressure 92q, 136a
mean corpuscular volume (MCV) 246q, 256a
measles 170q, 177a, 183a, 264q, 291–2a
measles, mumps, and rubella (MMR) vaccine 203q,
    226a, 291a
medial collateral ligament (MCL) 8q, 43a
medial patellofemoral ligament 8q, 42a
medial rectus 30q, 72a
medial retinaculum 8q, 42a
median nerve 2q, 4q, 36a, 38a, 262q, 290a
mediastinal pleura 13q, 48–9a
medulla 109q, 156a
meiosis 243q, 252a
membrane potential, resting 79q, 116a, 120a
membranous urethra 18q, 54a
Men C (meningococcal C conjugate) vaccine 169q,
    203q, 226a
meninges 69a
meningitis
    bacterial 28q, 68a, 177a
    microbiology 167q, 177a
    viral 177a
meningococcal C conjugate (MenC) vaccine 169q,
    203q, 226a
meralgia paraesthetica 5q, 40a, 44a
meropenem 166q, 177a
MERS-CoA (Middle East respiratory syndrome
    coronavirus) 167q
meta-analyses 229q, 231q, 233a, 236a
metabolic acidosis 103q, 148a
metabolic alkalosis 95q, 103q, 138a, 149a
metabolic hyperaemia 94q, 137a
metaraminol 213a(t)
metformin 198q, 199q, 218a, 220a
methaemoglobin 88q, 129a
methicillin-resistant Staphylococcus aureus (MRSA) 255a
methotrexate 252a
metoclopramide 196q, 199q, 215a, 221a
metoprolol 191q, 197q, 207a, 217a
metronidazole 169q, 181a, 222a
microbiology 165–73q, 174–90a
microcytic anaemia 256a
micturition 106q, 152a

midazolam 194*q*, 212*a*(*t*)
mid-brain lesion 279*q*, 302*a*
middle cerebral artery (MCA) 27*q*, 66*a*, 68*a*, 273*q*, 297*a*
middle ear 30*q*, 34*q*, 71*a*, 77*a*
Middle East respiratory syndrome coronavirus
    (MERS-CoA) 167*q*
mid-inguinal point 5*q*, 16*q*, 39*a*, 52*a*
migraine 71*a*
minimal change disease 153*a*
minute ventilation 112*q*, 160*a*
mitochondria 275*q*, 299*a*
mitosis 252*a*
mitral valve 91*q*, 134*a*
MMR (measles, mumps, and rubella) vaccine 203*q*,
    226*a*, 291*a*
mock exam paper 261–88*q*, 289–306*a*
monoglycerides 102*a*, 147*a*
Monteggia fracture 265*q*, 292*a*
morphine 193*q*, 211*a*(*t*)
motor cortex 280*q*, 302*a*
movicol 201*q*, 223*a*
MRCP exam questions xvii
MRCS exam questions xvii
MRSA (methicillin-resistant *Staphylococcus aureus*) 255*a*
MS (multiple sclerosis) 29*q*, 70–1*a*, 81*q*, 277*q*, 300*a*
MSUD (maple syrup urine disease) 107*q*
mucociliary transport system 89*q*, 130*a*
mucosa (gastrointestinal tract) 98*q*, 141*a*
mucus 84*q*, 89*q*, 125*a*, 130*a*, 162*a*, 296*a*
multiple sclerosis (MS) 29*q*, 70–1*a*, 81*q*, 277*q*, 300*a*
mumps 170*a*, 177*a*, 183*a*
    MMR vaccine 203*q*, 226*a*, 291*a*
Murphy's sign 101*q*
muscularis externa 97*q*, 141*a*
muscularis mucosae 97*q*, 141*a*, 142*a*
myasthenia gravis 123*a*
Mycoplasma pneumoniae 166*q*, 177*a*
mycoplasma tuberculosis 169*q*, 181*a*
myelination 81*q*, 120*a*, 300*a*
myelin sheath 248*q*, 259*a*
myenteric plexus 98*q*, 142*a*
myocardial infarction 10*q*, 45*a*
    coronary arteries 14–15*q*, 50–1*a*
    evidence-based medicine 231*q*, 235–6*a*
    NSTEMI 82*q*
    STEMI 92–3*q*, 136*a*, 269*q*, 295*a*
myosin filaments 81*q*, 82*q*, 119*a*, 122*a*
myosin phosphorylation 83*q*, 122*a*

N
NAAT (nucleic acid amplification testing) 244*q*, 253*a*
nailbeds 2*q*, 37*a*, 92*q*, 135*a*
nasopharyngeal carcinoma 257*a*
National Institute for Health and Care Excellence (NICE)
    guidelines 182*a*, 216*a*, 292*a*, 293*a*
natural killer T-cells 273*q*, 298*a*
Necator americanus 168*q*, 180*a*

neck
    anterior triangle of 22*q*, 32*q*, 61*a*, 74*a*
    posterior triangle of 32*q*, 74*a*, 75*a*
neck of femur fracture 5*q*, 6*q*, 108*q*, 231*q*, 236–7*a*
necrotizing fasciitis 176*a*
needle-stick injury 171*q*, 185*a*, 203*a*
negative likelihood ratio of a diagnostic test 230*q*, 234–5*a*
negative predictive value of a diagnostic test 229*q*, 234*a*
Neisseria gonorrhoeae 166*q*, 176*a*, 244*q*, 253*a*
Neisseria meningitidis 167*q*, 177*a*
neonatal sepsis 165*q*, 174–5*a*
neovascularization 243*q*, 252*a*
nephritic syndrome 106*q*, 153*a*
nephrolithiasis 18*q*, 55–6*a*
nephron 105*q*, 106*q*, 107*q*, 151*a*, 152*a*, 154*a*
nephrotic syndrome 106*q*, 153*a*
nerve conduction 81*q*, 119–20*a*
neurohypophysis 26*q*, 66*a*
neurolemma 248*q*, 259*a*
neurovascular bundle 11*q*, 46*a*
neutropenia 190*a*
neutropenic sepsis 173*q*, 190*a*
neutrophils 279*q*, 301–2*a*
NHL (non-Hodgkin's lymphoma) 247*q*, 257*a*
NICE (National Institute for Health and Care Excellence)
    guidelines 182*a*, 216*a*, 292*a*, 293*a*
nicotinic acetylcholine receptor 84*q*, 123*a*
nifedipine 198*q*, 218*a*
nimodipine 194*q*, 212*a*
nitric acid 94*q*, 137*a*
nitric oxide 82*q*, 104*q*, 120–1*a*, 151*a*
nitrofurantoin 176*a*
nitrous oxide 200*q*, 221*a*
NNH (number needed to harm) 230*q*, 234*a*
NNT (number needed to treat) 230*q*, 234*a*, 235*a*
nodes of Ranvier 81*q*, 120*a*, 300*a*
non-group A β-haemolytic streptococcus 245*q*, 254*a*
non-Hodgkin's lymphoma (NHL) 247*q*, 257*a*
non-ST-elevation myocardial infarction (NSTEMI) 82*q*
non-steroidal anti-inflammatory drugs (NSAIDs) 198*q*, 200*q*,
    219*a*, 221*a*, 305*a*
noradrenaline 102*q*, 107*q*, 148*a*, 154*a*, 195*q*,
    213*a*(*t*), 214*a*
    production 156*a*
    release 114*q*, 163*a*
    supraventricular tachycardia 95*q*, 138*a*
    synthesis 162*a*
    vasovagal syncope 95*q*, 139*a*
normocytic anaemia 256*a*
nose 31*q*, 72*a*
nosebleed 20*q*, 58*a*
notifiable diseases 167*q*, 178*a*
NSAIDs (non-steroidal anti-inflammatory drugs) 198*q*, 200*q*,
    219*a*, 221*a*, 305*a*
NSTEMI (non-ST-elevation myocardial infarction) 82*q*
nuclear lesion 32*q*, 74*a*
nucleic acid amplification testing (NAAT) 244*q*, 253*a*

number needed to harm (NNH) 230q, 234a
number needed to treat (NNT) 230q, 234a, 235a

O

observational studies 238a
obturator artery 6q, 41a
obturator nerve 5q, 40a
occipital artery 21q, 59a
occipital lobe 272q, 280q, 297a, 302a
occipital protuberance, laceration 275q, 299a
oculomotor nerve (cranial nerve III) 33q, 75–6a, 271q, 296a
oesophageal phase, swallowing 100q, 144a
oesophagus
    anatomy 14q, 49a
    cricothyroidotomy 23q, 61a
    endotracheal intubation 22q, 60a
    muscle 100q, 144a
    rupture 14q, 49a
    thyroid gland tumours 306a
olfactory disturbance 31q, 72–3a
olfactory receptors 31q, 72a
oligodendrocytes 259a, 300a
oliguria 106q, 153a
omeprazole 195q, 215a
omohyoid muscle, infiltration of superior belly
        of 287q, 306a
ondansetron 196q, 215a, 278q, 301a
opiate analgesia 193q, 211a(t)
opponens pollicis 36a
optic chiasm 30q, 72a
optic nerve lesion 284q, 305a
optic radiation, lower fibres of left 277q, 300a
oral phase, swallowing 144a
orbicularis muscle 30q, 71a
organic matrix of bone 109q, 156a
oropharynx 24q, 63a
osmolality
    Hartmann's solution 201q, 222a
    plasma 104q, 150a, 155a
    saline 201q, 222a, 223a
osmoles 80q, 117a
osmosis 82q, 121a
osmotic diarrhoea 101q, 145–6a, 244q, 254a
osteoblasts 109q, 156–7a
osteoclasts 109q, 156a, 157a
osteocytes 156a
osteoid see organic matrix of bone
osteomalacia 160a
osteomyelitis 173q, 189a
    common organisms 189a(t)
osteoporosis 112q, 160a
otorrhea 34q, 77a
ovarian arteries 20q, 57a
ovarian veins 57a
overdose 26q, 67a, 103q
overdrive suppression 94q, 137–8a, 280q, 302a
oxygen 129a

oxyhaemoglobin dissociation curve 87q, 127–8a
oxytocin 66a

P

pacemaker channels see funny current
PaCO$_2$ (partial pressure of carbon dioxide) 87q, 92q, 128a,
        136a, 281q, 303a
palmaris longus 2q, 36a
palmer interosseous 2q, 36a
pancreas
    acinar cells 296a
    α cells 271q, 296a
    β cells 296a
    diabetic ketoacidosis 271q, 296a
    exocrine insufficiency 282q, 304a
    exocrine juice 99q, 142–3a
    γ cells 296a
    L1 fracture 281q, 303a
    lipases 102q, 147a
    secretions 114q, 162a
    venous drainage 16q, 51a
pancytopaenia 252a
PaO$_2$ (partial pressure of oxygen) 84q, 124a
P$_A$O$_2$ (alveolar partial pressure of oxygen) 84q, 124a
papillary muscle rupture 295a
paracetamol 194q, 212a
paraffin, liquid 201q, 223a
parainfluenza virus 168q, 179a
parasitic spread 241q, 249a
parathyroid glands 22q, 61a, 155a
parathyroid hormone (PTH) 112q, 155a, 160a, 203q, 226a
parathyroid hormone-secreting adenoma 155a
paratonsillar vein 24q, 64a
parietal cells 80q, 118a, 282q, 304a
Parkinson's disease (PD) 27q, 68a, 100q, 120a
parotid duct 23q, 62a
parotitis, acute 23q, 62a
partial pressure of a gas 281q, 303a
    alveolar partial pressure of oxygen (P$_A$O$_2$) 84q, 124a
    carbon dioxide (PaCO$_2$) 87q, 92q, 128a, 136a, 281q, 303a
    oxygen (PaO$_2$) 84q, 124a
parvovirus B19 183a
Pasteurella multocida 166q, 176a
patellar ligament 42a
pathology 241–8q, 249–59a
PCL (posterior cruciate ligament) 9q, 43a
PCO$_2$ 89q, 131a
PCR (polymerase chain reaction) 276q, 299–300a
PCV (pneumococcal conjugate) vaccine 169q, 203q, 226a
PD (Parkinson's disease) 27q, 68a, 100q, 120a
PE see pulmonary embolism
PEA (pulseless electrical activity) 204q, 227a
peak expiratory flow rate 84q, 124a
pelvic inflammatory disease (PID) 173q, 181a, 189a,
        244q, 253a
pelvic splanchnic nerve 20q, 57a
penicillin allergy 166q, 177a, 195q, 202q, 215a, 220a, 224a

penicillin G 222*a*

penicillins 206*a*

pepsin 147*a*

pepsinogen 144*a*, 296*a*

peptic ulcer 17*q*, 53–4*a*, 272*q*, 296*a*

performance bias 232*q*, 237*a*

perfusion 84*q*, 125*a*

perianal fistulae 243*q*

pericardial effusion 14*q*, 49*a*

pericardium, blood supply 14*q*, 49*a*

periciliary fluid 89*q*, 130*a*

perihepatitis 173*q*, 189*a*

peripheral chemoreceptors 89*q*, 131*a*

peripheral neuronal injury 248*q*, 258–9*a*

peristalsis 97*q*, 141*a*

   primary 100*q*, 144*a*

   secondary 100*q*, 144*a*

peritonsillar abscess 288*q*, 306*a*

pernicious anaemia 100*q*, 144–5*a*, 282*q*, 304*a*

pertussis see whooping cough

Peutz–Jeghers syndrome 156*a*

PGE₂ (prostaglandin E₂) 242*q*, 250*a*

pH

   duodenal 97*q*, 140*a*

   chemoreceptor response to changes in 89*q*, 131*a*

phaeochromocytoma 114*q*, 163*a*

pharmacology 191–205*q*, 206–27*a*

pharyngeal phase, swallowing 100*q*, 144*a*

pharyngitis, acute 24*q*

phenothiazines 301*a*

phenytoin 197*q*, 217*a*

Philadelphia chromosome 257*a*

phosphate enemas 201*q*, 223*a*

phrenic nerve 11*q*, 13*q*, 46*a*, 48*a*, 49*a*

physiological shunts 84*q*, 125*a*

physiology 79–115*q*, 116–64*a*

pia 69*a*

pica 101*q*

PICA (posterior inferior cerebellar artery) 34*q*, 65–6*a*, 68*a*, 71*a*, 77*a*

PID (pelvic inflammatory disease) 173*q*, 181*a*, 189*a*, 244*q*, 253*a*

pigeon fancier's lung (cryptococcus) 171*q*, 185*a*

piperacillin with tazobactam (tazocin) 173*q*, 166*q*, 177*a*, 190*a*

pituitary ischaemic crisis 114*q*, 163*a*

pituitary stalk 26*q*, 66*a*

plantar flexion of foot 281*q*, 303*a*

plasma

   calcium 203*q*, 226*a*

   osmolality 104*q*, 150*a*, 155*a*

Plasmodium falciparum 168*q*, 179*a*, 241*q*, 249*a*

Plasmodium knowlesi 168*q*, 179*a*

Plasmodium malariae 168*q*, 179*a*, 241*q*, 249*a*

Plasmodium ovale 168*q*, 179*a*, 249*a*

Plasmodium vivax 168*q*, 179*a*, 241*q*, 249*a*

platelet count 79*q*, 117*a*

pneumococcal conjugate (PCV) vaccine 169*q*, 203*q*, 226*a*

Pneumocystis jirovecii (formerly *Pneumocystis jirovecii*) 255*a*, 268*q*, 294*a*

pneumocystis pneumonia 246*q*, 255*a*, 294*a*

pneumonia

   cavitating 165*q*, 175*a*

   community-acquired 296*a*

   consolidation site 11–12*q*, 47*a*

   lung compliance 86*q*, 126*a*

   lung function 87*q*, 128*a*

   microbiology 175*a*

   nosocomial 296*a*

   pneumocystis 246*q*, 255*a*, 294*a*

   risk factors 245*q*, 255*a*, 265*q*, 292*a*

   treatment 166*q*, 177*a*

pneumothorax 13*q*, 48–9*a*, 88*q*, 129–30*a*

PO₂ 89*q*, 131*a*

podocytes 106*q*, 152*a*

Poiseuille's Law 82*q*, 121*a*, 124*a*, 126*a*

polio vaccine 203*q*, 226*a*

polycythaemia 87*q*, 127*a*

polydipsia, psychogenic 108*q*, 154*a*

polymerase chain reaction (PCR) 276*q*, 299–300*a*

pons 30*q*, 34*q*, 72*a*, 77*a*

popliteal fossa 8*q*, 42–3*a*

popliteal pseudoaneurysm 8*q*

pork tapeworm 180*a*

portal vein 16*q*, 17*q*, 51*a*, 53*a*

positive likelihood ratio of a diagnostic test 230*q*, 234–5*a*

positive predictive value of a diagnostic test 229*q*, 234*a*

posterior auricular artery 21*q*, 59*a*

posterior communicating artery 27*q*, 68*a*

posterior cranial fossa 30*q*, 34*q*, 71*a*, 72*a*, 77*a*

posterior cruciate ligament (PCL) 9*q*, 43*a*

posterior cutaneous nerve of the thigh 8*q*, 20*q*, 42*a*, 57*a*

posterior descending artery 14*q*, 50*a*

posterior inferior cerebellar artery (PICA) 34*q*, 65–6*a*, 68*a*, 71*a*, 77*a*

posterior pituitary gland 26*q*, 66*a*

posterior tibial nerve 9*q*, 44*a*

posterior triangle of neck 32*q*, 74*a*, 75*a*

post-exposure prophylaxis 171*q*, 185*a*

post-herpetic pain 202*q*

post-partum hypopituitarism (Sheehan syndrome) 163*a*

postural reflex, loss of 27*q*, 68*a*

potassium channels 93*q*, 116*a*, 136*a*

   voltage-gated 79*q*, 94*q*, 117*a*, 137*a*

potassium excretion 107*q*, 153*a*

PPIs (proton pump inhibitors) 195*q*, 215*a*

precentral gyrus 26*q*, 66*a*

prednisolone 160*a*, 192*q*, 209*a*(t)

pregnancy

   ectopic 20*q*, 57*a*

   nitrous oxide contraindicated in 200*q*, 221*a*

Prehn sign 18*q*, 55*a*

preload 91*q*, 134–5*a*

primary ciliary dyskinesia (Kartagener syndrome) 88*q*, 130*a*

PR interval 272*q*, 286*q*, 297*a*, 305*a*

procedural sedation and analgesia (PSA) 202q, 224–5a
prolactin 159a
pronator teres muscle 36a
propofol 193q, 202q, 210a, 225a, 261q, 289a
   contraindications 193q, 210a
   infusion syndrome 210a
   side effects 193q, 210a
prospective cohort studies 229q, 232q, 233a, 238a
prostacyclin 118a
prostaglandin E$_2$ (PGE$_2$) 242q, 250a
prostaglandins 107q, 154a
protein digestion 102q, 147a
protein S deficiency 287q, 306a
proteinuria 106q, 153a
proton pump inhibitors (PPIs) 195q, 215a
proximal convoluted tubule 105q, 107q, 151a, 154a, 155a
PSA (procedural sedation and analgesia) 202q, 224–5a
Pseudomonas aeruginosa 166q, 176a, 255a
psorophora mosquitoes 241q, 249a
psychogenic polydipsia 108q, 154a
PTH (parathyroid hormone) 112q, 155a, 160a, 203q, 226a
PTH-secreting adenoma 155a
pudendal nerve 5q, 20q, 40a, 54a, 57a, 106q, 152a
pufferfish 79q
pulmonary artery 90q, 132a, 277q, 300a
pulmonary embolism (PE) 12q, 47a
   Aa gradient 124a
   hypoxaemia 125a
   LMWH 202q
   thrombolysis 230q, 234a
   warfarin 201q
pulmonary fibrosis 87q, 128a
pulmonary mechanoreceptors 89q, 131a
pulmonary oedema 91q, 135a
pulmonary veins 90q, 132a
pulseless electrical activity (PEA) 204q, 227a
purple urine bag syndrome 172q, 186a
p values 231q, 237a
P wave 91q, 134a, 297a
pyelonephritis 176a
pylorus 97q, 141a
pyrazinamide 182a
pyrogens 242q, 250a

Q

QRS complex 297a
QT interval 94q, 137a, 276q, 299a
quadratus femoris 6q
quadriceps femoris 42a
quadriceps tendon 8q, 42a
quinolones 206a

R

rabeprazole 90q, 132a
rabies 170q, 183a
'raccoon eyes' 34q, 77a
radial artery 2q, 3q, 36a, 37a, 38a

radial nerve 4q, 38a, 265q, 292a
radial styloid process 3q, 37a
radius 3q, 37a
ramipril 90q, 132a
Ramsay Hunt syndrome 30q, 71a
randomized controlled trials (RCTs) 229q, 232q, 233a, 239a
   appraisal 231q, 236–7a
   bias, sources of 232q, 237–8a
   and cohort studies, comparison between 232q, 238a
   meta-analyses 231q, 236a
ranitidine 195q, 198q, 215a, 218a
RASS (Richmond Agitation-Sedation Scale) 230q, 235a
R-binder protein 100q, 144a
RCTs see randomized controlled trials
rectosigmoid junction 53a
rectum 53a
recurrent laryngeal nerve 306a
Reed–Sternberg cells 247q, 257a, 258a
re-entrant ventricular arrhythmias 299a
'regiment batch' area 4q, 39a
renal artery 19q, 56a
renal autoregulation 104q, 150–1a
renal tubular acidosis 102q, 148a
renin 103q, 106q, 149a, 152a
renin–angiotensin–aldosterone system 105q, 152a
reporting bias 232q, 237a
residual volume (RV) 87q, 128a
respiratory acidosis 103q, 125a, 148a
respiratory alkalosis 103q, 138a, 149a
respiratory syncytial virus (RSV) 83q, 122a, 168q, 179a
respiratory tract 89q, 131a
resting membrane potential 79q, 116a, 120a
resuscitation see cardiopulmonary resuscitation
retrospective cohort studies 229q, 233a, 238a
reverse triiodothyronine (rT$_3$) 112q, 161a
revision tips xvii
rhabdomyolysis 80q, 262q, 283q, 289–90a, 304a
ribavarin 171q, 185a
ribs 10q, 45–6a
Richmond Agitation-Sedation Scale (RASS) 230q, 235a
Rickettsia rickettsii 172q, 187a
rifampicin 169q, 182a
right bundle branch block 286q, 305a
right coronary artery 10q, 14q, 45a, 50a, 51a
right homonymous macular defect 272q, 297a
right main bronchus 11q, 46a
right marginal branch 10q
right subhepatic space 17q, 54a
right subphrenic space 17q, 54a
Ringer's solution 223a
ringworm 185a
Rinne's test 31q, 73a
risperidone 291a
rivaroxaban 271q, 296a
Rocky Mountain spotted fever 187a
Romano–Ward syndrome 136a
rotavirus vaccine 203q, 226a

roundworm 168q, 180a
Roux-en-Y gastric bypass 100q, 144a, 145a
RSV (respiratory syncytial virus) 83q, 122a, 168q, 179a
rT$_3$ (reverse triiodothyronine) 112q, 161a
RV (residual volume) 87q, 128a
rubella 170q, 184a
    MMR vaccine 203q, 226a, 291a

S
S1 lesions 303a
sacral plexus 142a
sacral spinal nerves 17q, 54a
SAH see subarachnoid haemorrhage
salbutamol 153a, 192q, 193q, 207–8a, 211a
    side effects 192q, 207a, 208a
saline 201q, 222a, 223a
saliva production 99q, 143a
salmeterol 208a
Salmonella enterica 172q, 173q, 189a
Salmonella typhimurium 172q, 186a
saltatory conduction 277q, 300a
saphenous nerve 294a
sarcomere 82q, 122a
sarcoplasmic reticulum 81q, 119a
SBAQs see single best answer questions
SCA (superior cerebellar artery) 65a, 66a
scalp layers 21q, 59a
scalp ringworm 185a
scaphoid 3q, 37a
scapula 1q, 35a
Schwann cells 81q, 120a, 248q, 259a, 300a
sciatic nerve injury 270q, 295a
SCID (severe combined immunodeficiency) 88q, 130a
scurvy 130a
secretin 97q, 101a, 140a, 141a, 146a
secretory diarrhoea 101q, 145a, 146a, 244q, 253a
seizures
    focal 280q, 302a
    psychogenic polydipsia 108q, 154a
    generalized 29q, 69–70a
Seldinger technique 48a
selection bias 231q, 236a, 237a
self-hanging 23q, 62a
semimembranosus muscles 7q, 41–2a
semitendinosus muscles 7q, 41–2a
sensitivity of a diagnostic test 229q, 233a, 290a
sepsis
    bilateral adrenal haemorrhage secondary to 114q, 163a
    high-risk criteria 266q, 267a, 292a, 293a
    microbiology 180a
    neonatal 165q, 174–5a
    neutropenic 173q, 190a
serological testing 241q, 249a
serosa (adventitia) 97q, 141a, 142a
serotonin 80q, 102q, 112q, 118a, 148a, 160a
serratus anterior 4q
serum

albumin 103q, 149a
    cortisol 111q, 159a
    C-peptide 111q, 113q, 158a, 159a, 162a
    glucagon 111q, 159a
    triglyceride 111q, 158a
severe combined immunodeficiency (SCID) 88q, 130a
Sheehan syndrome 163a
Shigella dysenteriae 172q, 186a
shingles 10q, 45a
short gut syndrome 98q, 142a
short QT syndrome 137a
short saphenous vein 9q, 45a
shoulder
    anatomy 1q, 35a
    rotator cuff 4q, 38a
    subcoracoid dislocation 1q, 4q
SIADH (syndrome of inappropriate antidiuretic hormone) 150a
sickle cell anaemia 87q, 128a
sick sinus syndrome 137a
sigmoid colon 19q, 57a
signal-transduction pathways 80q, 118a
single best answer questions (SBAQs) xvii
    mock exam paper 261–88q, 289–306a
single-blinded control trials 232q, 239a
sinoatrial nodal artery 10q
sinoatrial node 96q, 139a
sinusitis, acute 21q, 59a
sinus rhythms 90q, 132a
skeletal muscle 79q, 80q, 81q, 116a, 118a, 119a
slapped cheek disease (erythema infectiosum) 170q, 183a
SLE (systemic lupus erythematosus) 153a, 243q, 251–2a
slipped disc 271q, 281q, 296a, 303a
SMA (superior mesenteric artery) 17q, 53a, 275q, 299a
small bowel obstruction 230q, 234–5a
small intestine 19q, 56a
small saphenous vein 8q, 42a, 43a
smoking 222a, 265q, 292a
sodium bicarbonate 193q, 211a
sodium channels
    blockade 267q, 293a
    mutation 93q, 136a
    voltage-dependent 79q, 116a
    voltage-gated 79q, 84q, 94q, 116a, 117a, 123a, 138a
sodium chloride 82q, 121a, 193q, 210a
sodium/chloride symporter 103q, 149a
sodium citrate bottles 117a
sodium ion permeability, rhabdomyolysis 262q, 290a
sodium ion reabsorption 105q, 151a
sodium/potassium/ATPase pump 79q, 103q, 116a, 117a, 120a, 149a
    overdrive suppression 94q, 137a
sodium/potassium/chloride co-transporter 103q, 149a, 274q, 298a
sodium/potassium pump 196q, 216a
sodium valproate 197q, 217a
somatostatin analogues 111q, 159a

specificity of a diagnostic test 229q, 233a, 290a
sphenopalatine artery 20q, 58a
spinal cord
    C6/7 burst fracture dislocation 4q, 38a
    central cord syndrome 25q, 65a
    complete spinal cord injury 29q, 70a
    lumbar puncture see lumbar puncture
spinal nerve roots 1q, 35a
spinal shock 29q, 70a
spironolactone 157a, 196q, 198q, 216a, 219a
splenic flexure 53a
splenic vein 16q, 51a, 53a
splenomegaly 179a
splenorenal pouch/recess 17q, 54a
Staphylococcus aureus 172a, 173a
    antibiotics 220a
    cavitating pneumonia 165q, 175a
    cellulitis 166q, 176a
    endocarditis in intravenous drug users 167q, 178a, 179a
    methicillin-resistant (MRSA) 255a
statins 199q, 221a
steatorrhoea 254a
ST-elevation myocardial infarction (STEMI) 92–3q, 136a,
    269q, 295a
sternoclavicular joint 1q, 35a
sternocleidomastoid muscle injury 279q, 301a
sternum 10q, 45a
steroids 112q, 115q, 159–60a, 163–4a, 192q, 209a(t)
stratified columnar epithelial cells 89q, 131a
stratified squamous epithelial cells 89q, 131a
Streptococcus pneumoniae 165q, 168q, 175a, 179a,
    245q, 255a
Streptococcus pyogenes 166q, 172a, 176a
Streptococcus viridans 167q, 179a
streptokinase 257a
streptomycin 182a
stress response 270q, 295a
striated muscle 82q, 122a
stroke
    cerebellar 25q, 65–6a
    internal capsule 25q, 65a
    lacular 66a
    thalamus 25q, 26q, 65a, 66a
    thrombolysis 196q, 216a
subarachnoid haemorrhage (SAH) 27q, 68a, 229q, 233–4a
    diagnosis 229q(t)
subarachnoid space 69a
subcortical structures 27q, 67a
subdural space 69a
subhepatic space, right 17q, 54a
submucosa 97q, 98q, 141a, 141a
submucosal plexus 98q, 142a
subphrenic space, right 17q, 54a
subscapularis 4q, 38a
substance P 81q, 120a
substantia nigra 68a
sucrose 100q, 145a

Sudek's point 53a
sulfonylureas 198q, 218a
superficial epigastric artery 17q, 53a
superficial temporal artery 21q, 59a
superior cerebellar artery (SCA) 65a, 66a
superior gastric artery 17q, 52a, 53a
superior genicular nerve 8q, 43a
superior labial artery 20q, 58a
superior mesenteric artery (SMA) 17q, 53a, 275q, 299a
superior mesenteric vein 17q, 53a
superior oblique 72a
superior radioulnar joint 3q, 38a
superior rectal artery 53a
superior rectus 30q, 72a
supinator reflex 4q, 38a
supraorbital artery 21q, 59a
supraspinatous 4q, 38a
supraventricular tachycardia 95q, 138a
sural nerve 9q, 45a
surfactant 89q, 130a, 283q, 304a
swallowing 100q, 144a, 283q, 304a
sympathetic tone 111q, 159a
synaptic transmission 83q, 122–3a
syndesmotic sprain 44a
syndrome of inappropriate antidiuretic hormone
    (SIADH) 150a
syphilis 176a, 181a, 187a
systemic lupus erythematosus (SLE) 153a, 243q, 251–2a

T
T₃ (triiodothyronine) 160a, 161a
T₄ (thyroxine) 161a
T4 vertebral body, fracture 276q, 300a
tachy-brady syndrome (sick sinus syndrome) 137a
tachycardia
    blood flow 92q, 135a
    cardiac output 91q, 135a
    coronary artery perfusion 134a
    overdrive suppression 280q, 302a
tachycardia-induced cardiomyopathy 114q, 163a
tachypnoea 89q, 131a
taeniae coli 142a
Taenia saginata 168q, 180a
Taenia solium 168q, 180a
tanning process 155a
tapeworm 180a
tarsal tunnel syndrome 44a
tazocin (piperacillin with tazobactam) 173q, 166q, 177a, 190a
TB (tuberculosis) 169q, 181–2a, 262q, 289a
Td/IPV (tetanus, diphtheria, and polio) vaccine 203q, 226a
temporal arteritis 71a
temporal lobe 26q, 66a, 277q, 280q, 300a, 302a
tendon reflex arcs 4q, 38a
tension headache 71a
tensor fasciae latae 6q, 40a
teres major 4q, 38a, 39a
teres minor 4q, 38a

terlipressin 90*q*, 103*q*, 132*a*
testis 18*q*, 55*a*
tetanus 200*q*, 222*a*
  microbiology 179*a*
  treatment 170*q*, 182*a*
  vaccine 170*q*, 182*a*, 200*q*, 203*q*, 222*a*, 226*a*
tetanus, diphtheria, and polio (Td/IPV) vaccine 203*q*, 226*a*
tetany 81*q*, 119*a*
tetracyclines 188*a*, 206*a*
tetralogy of Fallot 133*a*
thalamus 25*q*, 26*q*, 65*a*, 66*a*
thalassaemia, alpha 246*q*, 256*a*
thenar 36*a*
thiazide diuretics 196*q*, 216*a*
third ventricle 69*a*
thirst 104*q*, 150*a*
thoracic trauma in children 278*q*, 301*a*
thoracoepigastric artery 17*q*, 53*a*
thoracotomy 280*q*, 303*a*
threadworm 180*a*
thrombin 80*q*, 118*a*
thrombolysis 196*q*, 216*a*
thromboxane A2 80*q*, 118*a*
thumb 2*q*
thyroid drugs 198*q*, 218–19*a*
thyroid gland 25*q*, 64*a*
thyroid peroxidase 112*q*, 160*a*, 161*a*
thyroid-stimulating hormone (TSH/thyrotropin) 113*q*, 161*a*
thyrotoxic crisis secondary to pituitary ischaemic
     necrosis 114*q*, 163*a*
thyrotropin 113*q*, 161*a*
thyroxine (T$_4$) 161*a*
tibial nerve 6*q*, 41*a*
tidal volume 89*q*, 131*a*
tinea capitis 171*q*, 185*a*
tinea corporis 171*q*, 185*a*
tinea pedis 171*q*, 185*a*, 306*a*
tissue factor pathway 79*q*, 117*a*
TN (trigeminal neuralgia) 31*q*, 73*a*
tobacco use 222*a*, 265*q*, 292*a*
tongue
  biting, during seizure 29*q*, 69*a*, 70*a*
  cancer 21*q*, 59–60*a*
  photograph 32*q*(*f*)
tonsillar artery 24*q*, 64*a*
tonsillectomy, bleeding after 24*q*, 64*a*
tonsillitis 288*q*, 306*a*
tonsillopharyngitis 245*q*, 254–5*a*
torsades de pointes 137*a*, 299*a*
total body water 80*q*, 117*a*
toxoplasmosis 181*a*
Toxoplasmosis gondii 169*q*, 181*a*
tracheobronchial capillaries, bleeding from 277*q*, 300*a*
tramadol 193*q*, 211*a*(*t*)
tranexamic acid 268*q*, 294*a*
transcobalamin-1 (R-binder protein) 100*q*, 144*a*
transferrin 99*q*, 143*a*

transverse colon 17*q*, 53*a*
transverse tibiofibular ligament 9*q*, 44*a*
trapezium 3*q*, 38*a*
trauma triad of death 84*q*, 123*a*
trehalose 100*q*, 145*a*
Trendelenburg position 23*q*, 62*a*
Trendelenburg test 6*q*, 40*a*
Treponema pallidum 166*q*, 172*q*, 176*a*, 187*a*
triad of death, trauma 84*q*, 123*a*
triceps 4*q*, 38*a*
Trichomonas vaginalis 166*q*, 176*a*
trichomoniasis 176*a*
trifascicular block 286*q*, 305*a*
trigeminal nerve 33*q*, 76*a*
trigeminal neuralgia (TN) 31*q*, 73*a*
triglycerides 102*q*, 147*a*
triiodothyronine (T$_3$) 160*a*, 161*a*
trimethoprim 166*q*, 176*a*, 191*q*, 206*a*, 273*q*, 297*a*
triquetrum 3*q*, 37*a*
trochlear nerve 33*q*, 76*a*
troponin phosphorylation 83*q*, 122*a*
trypsin 102*q*, 147*a*
TSH (thyroid-stimulating hormone/thyrotropin) 113*q*, 161*a*
T tubules 82*q*, 122*a*
tuberculosis (TB) 169*q*, 181–2*a*, 262*q*, 289*a*
tularemia 187*a*
T wave 91*q*, 134*a*
tyrosine 115*q*, 164*a*

U
UGI (upper gastrointestinal bleeding) 246*q*, 256*a*
ulcer, peptic 272*q*, 296*a*
ulnar artery 2*q*, 4*q*, 36*a*, 37*a*, 38*a*
  block 261*q*, 289*a*
ulnar nerve 264*q*, 291*a*
ulnar styloid process 37*a*
uncinate process 16*q*, 51*a*
upper gastrointestinal bleeding (UGI) 246*q*, 256*a*
upper oesophageal sphincter 100*q*, 144*a*
upper respiratory tract infection 106*q*, 153*a*
urea 108*q*, 154*a*
urethra 18*q*, 54*a*
urinary sphincter, external 106*q*, 152*a*
urinary tract infection (UTI) 82*q*, 166*q*, 176*a*
urine
  inability to pass 18*q*, 54–5*a*
  incontinence 29*q*, 70*a*
  osmolality 108*q*, 155*a*
  production 108*q*, 154–5*a*
uterine arteries 20*q*, 57*a*
uterine veins 57*a*
UTI (urinary tract infection) 82*q*, 166*q*, 176*a*

V
vagal manoeuvres 284*q*, 305*a*
vagus nerve 31*q*, 74*a*, 283*q*, 303*a*, 304*a*
valgus stress test 43*a*

vancomycin 173q, 198q, 218a
varicella zoster virus 183a, 303a
vasa recta 106q, 153a
vascular headache 29q, 71a
vasoactive medication 195q, 213–14a
    comparison 213a(t), 214a(t)
vasoconstriction 80q, 118a
vasopressin 26q, 66a, 195q, 214a
vasopressors 213a(t)
vasovagal syncope 95q, 138–9a
vastus intermedius 42a
vastus lateralis 42a
vastus medialis 42a
Vaughan Williams classification of drugs 191q, 207a(t)
ventilation 84q, 125a
ventilation/perfusion (V/Q) mismatch 84q, 124a, 125a
    hypoxaemia 88q, 129a, 130a, 273q, 298a
ventricles 28q, 68a, 69a
ventricular arrhythmias 299a
ventricular fibrillation (VF) 204q, 227a, 299a
ventricular pressure 91q, 134a
ventricular septal defect 295a
ventricular tachycardia 267q, 293a
ventricular volume 91q, 134a
verapamil 194q, 212a
vesicoureteric junction 18q, 55a
Virchow's triad 80q, 118a
visceral pleura 13q, 49a
visual disturbance 30q, 33q, 72a, 75–6a
    homonymous hemianopia 273q, 297a
        optic nerve lesion 284q, 305a
        right homonymous macular defect 272q, 297a
vitamin B12 (cobalamin) 100q, 144–5a, 266q, 293a, 304a
vitamin C (ascorbic acid) 99q, 143a
    deficiency 88q, 130a
vitamin D3 112q, 160a
vitamin D deficiency 160a
vitamin K 295a
vocal cords 22q, 60a
voltage-dependent sodium channels 79q, 116a
voltage-gated potassium channels 79q, 94q, 117a, 137a
voltage-gated sodium channels 79q, 84q, 94q, 116a, 117a, 123a, 138a

volvulus of large bowel 98q, 141a
vomiting
    alcohol intoxication 265q, 292a
    neurotransmitters 102q, 148a
von Willebrand's disease 287q, 306a
V/Q mismatch see ventilation/perfusion (V/Q) mismatch

W
Wallenberg syndrome 66a
warfarin 201q, 223a, 247q, 257a, 270q, 295a
Waterhouse–Friderichsen syndrome 163a
Weber's test 31q, 73a
Weil's disease 173q, 188a
Wellen's syndrome 306a
West Nile virus 177a
wheeze 84q, 124a
white coat hypertension 95q, 138a
whooping cough (pertussis) 172q, 179a, 186a
    vaccine 203q, 226a
Wolff–Parkinson–White syndrome 133a, 136a, 140a
wound infection, risk factors 268q, 294a
wrist
    anatomy 3q, 37a
    'dinner fork' deformity 109q
    fall injury 2q, 3a
    motorbike accident 3q

X
xerostomia 99q, 143a
xiphoid process/xiphisternum 10q, 45a

Y
yellow fever 173q, 188a

Z
Z line 82q, 122a
Ziehl–Neelsen stain 169q, 181a
zinc 113q, 162a
Zollinger–Ellison syndrome 115q, 164a
zona fasciculata 109q, 156a
zona glomerulosa 109q, 156a
zona reticularis 109q, 156a
zygomatico-orbital artery 21q, 59a